Ethics in Nursing:
An Anthology

Terry Pence and Janice Cantrall

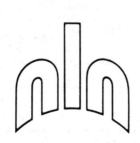

National League for Nursing
Pub. No. 20–2294

About the Authors

Terry Pence, PhD, is Associate Professor of Philosophy, Northern Kentucky University, Highland Heights, KY.

Janice Cantrall, MSN, RN, is Director of Nursing Services, Woodspoint Geriatric Care Center, Florence, KY.

Copyright © 1990
National League for Nursing
350 Hudson Street, New York, NY 10014

ISBN 0-88737-461-1

The views expressed in this publication represent the views of the authors and do not necessarily reflect the official views of the National League for Nursing.

Printed in the United States of America

Contents

Preface

Nursing ethics literature and the study of ethics in nursing has expanded dramatically in the past decade. While the approach to the study of nursing ethics is evolving, there seems to be three basic approaches found in the literature.[1] The pioneering work of Davis and Aroskar (1978), *Ethical Dilemmas and Nursing Practice*,[2] is an example of an ethical theory approach. This type of philosophical approach introduces major ethical theories (usually consequentialist and deontological) and attempts to apply the tenets of these theories to clinical practice dilemmas.

A second approach found in the literature, the moral principles approach, extracts principles from moral theories and applies them to clinical issues. For example, one can examine a particular ethical dilemma in light of such principles as autonomy, nonmaleficence, and confidentiality. Immediately, the moral principles approach offers two advantages. First, divergent moral theories can often agree on the relevance of these principles. Second, moral principles are explicitly cited in professional codes and are more frequently employed in our moral conversation.

Both of these approaches are useful. It is our belief, however, that nursing ethics must ultimately be framed and taught from a more *philosophical foundations* approach. Using this approach, ethical actions in nursing stem from views held about the nature and function of nursing. It is this philosophy about nursing, its values, and relationships to others that are, at bottom, more likely to determine individual clinical decisions and the collective action of the profession.

This anthology highlights a philosophical foundations approach to nursing ethics. We have compiled articles and excerpts from the nursing and other literature that examines, illustrates, advocates, and/or critiques the philosophical foundations perspective. Sometimes the article presents an historical perspective, is a classic, or presents a controversial point of view. The early chapters present the conceptual issues surrounding client advocacy. The remaining chapters explore the ramifications of this approach to relations with physicians, other nurses, and institutions.

Each chapter contains a brief introduction that explains the underlying issues and presents a synopsis and commentary on each article. The debate and study questions at the conclusion of each chapter can facilitate the use of the text in the classroom.

We hope this collection of historical, seminal, classic, and controversial articles will be of interest to all nursing students, practitioners, and educators who have a desire for a more comprehensive understanding of ethics in nursing. We hope it will stimulate lively and useful debate, sharpen critical analysis of personal philosophical and ethical positions, and project a more thoughtful approach to clinical practice by both pragmatists and dreamers.

Finally, we would like to express our thanks to Allan Graubard for his many helpful editorial suggestions.

NOTES

1. Terry Pence, "Approaches to Nursing Ethics," *Philosophy in Context* 17 (1987):7–15.
2. Anne J. Davis and Mila A. Aroskar, *Ethical Dilemmas and Nursing Practice* (Norwalk, CT: Appleton-Centry Crofts, 1978; 2nd Edition, 1983).

1

Philosophical Foundations of Nursing Practice

INTRODUCTION

As stated in the *Preface*, the most determinative factor in how a nurse reacts to a moral dilemma is the nurse's conception of the role of the nurse. It matters very little what moral theory or moral principles a nurse may hold if the nurse's role conception forbids acting on those beliefs. For this reason, a discussion of various views of the nurse's role are of utmost importance for nursing ethics.

We begin with what might be called the traditional model which prizes unquestioning obedience and loyalty to the physician. The articles by Dock and Newton represent and defend this view. The experimental study of nurse–physician relationships by Holfing et al. shows quite dramatically how such a view might impact on client welfare.

The Winslow article traces and assesses the historical development of the defining metaphors of nursing from military-like obedience and loyalty to client advocacy. The articles by Gadow and Kohnke express two different conceptions of client advocacy. There is a significant difference about the sharing of the nurse's beliefs and values in nurse–client interactions.

Murphy's article reveals that the adoption of the advocacy model as the dominant framework for making ethical decisions is of recent vintage with the crucial shift taking place in the mid to late 1970s.

Finally, the article by Pagana is an attack on the client advocacy model. Pagana believes that patient advocacy is incompatible with the realities of modern business mentality and practices of hospitals.

Given this brief overview we will now proceed with a more detailed discussion of the articles.

THE TRADITIONAL NURSE—DOCK, NEWTON, AND HOLFING ET AL.

The article by Sarah Dock, "The Relation of the Nurse to the Doctor and the Doctor to the Nurse," was originally published in 1917 and expresses an ethical stance and role perception that was obviously prevalent at that time. She believed that the nurse is quite simply an "intelligent machine" for obeying "without question" the doctor's orders.[1]

Views the nurse may hold about the ethical treatment of the client were not relevant in this conception of the role of the nurse. However, this model of the nursing role is not morally neutral. Whatever moral responsibilities a nurse may have to a client are subordinated by the overriding responsibility to obey the physician. For example, Dock declares that it is an "unpardonable sin" to ever suggest to a family that they seek another doctor. Dock also advised nurses to seek prior approval for any procedures the nurse may perform in an emergency life-saving situation. The implications here are that the "good nurse" is loyal to the physician even to the point where obedience may cause patient harm.

Perhaps some of the views expressed by Dock can be partially explained as prudential concessions to the realities of nursing as practiced in her day. A private duty nurse's career often depended on how well a nurse got along with physicians. Nevertheless, this view is not without some modern defenders. In her article, "In Defense of the Traditional Nurse," Lisa Newton, a philosopher, finds redeeming virtues in "the traditional ideal of the skilled and gentle caregiver, whose role in health care requires submission to authority as an essential component."

Newton believes that there is something about the traditional role the public wants.[2] Newton believes that it is only the nurse who brings sympathy, reassurance, tenderness, and warmth to the hospital which is otherwise an unremitting "coldly mechanical bureaucratic monster." If nurses become autonomous professionals, this last reef of solace will be lost.

The essential components of the traditional nurse that Newton believes are worth preserving are "unquestioning adherence to procedure," the basic lack of authority and power for nurses, and the surrogate mother role.

The traditional notion of obedience is required by the goals of the hospital and physicians.[3] Newton contends that the saving of life and health in a hospital bureaucracy demands orders and procedures for efficiency. When serious medical situations arise, only physicians with their esoteric knowledge will know how to handle them. When they do arise, according to Newton, "all participating activities and agents must be completely subordinated to the judgment of physicians."

Newton's argument for the other qualities contained in the traditional role—basic lack of authority and power, and the mother surrogate role—is found in her appeal to the needs of the sick. Of profound importance to Newton is the fact that the hospital environment creates certain emotional needs. It is the traditional nurse as surrogate mother who uniquely meets these needs. It is the nurse who listens, gives comfort, talks, and grieves with the sick and dying and their families. Newton claims that nurses can only perform this function if they are without power and authority—otherwise patients may feel threatened by them. Nurses similarly cannot be professional because to be professional is to be dispassionate and objective. But it is the empathetic and gentle caregiver that the public wants.

Behind Newton's argument, however, are several questionable assumptions that should be examined. First, it seems that Newton seriously underestimates the levels of knowledge that nurses possess and their present degree of functioning in the health care system. These considerations might undermine the cogency of the argument for obedience, but even if one granted that only doctors know what to do in medically serious situations it must be remembered that more than medical issues are at stake. For example, what if a person does not want to be resuscitated? It may conflict with Newton's conception of one of the goals of the institution, that is, saving life. Would a doctor's decision to resuscitate be based on medical or moral considerations? If moral, are doctors the only health care professionals with moral expertise?

Another assumption is the notion that being professionally autonomous and objective excludes by definition the expression of important emotions like grief and sympathy—the very elements, so Newton believes, that keep the hospital from becoming a cold uncaring institution. But is this so? Are the best professionals also the most dispassionate? It is not at all obvious that this is the case. Indeed, it might be argued that "being professional" entails not the absence of emotion, but a disposition to have and express certain emotions. The point is that one can not conclude that nurses will become as coldly inhumane as the rest of medicine if they are autonomous unless one also believes that professionalism excludes the expression of emotion. Newton presents no arguments for that conclusion.

If Newton is wrong in her assumptions about the incompatibility of professional autonomous nurses and the meeting of emotional needs of clients, then the major defense of the traditional nurse falls. The public need not worry about being deprived of gentle caregivers.

Another consideration in favor of the traditional nurse cited by Newton is that obedience contributes to hospital efficiency and, therefore, ultimately serves the needs of patients best. The alternative, as Newton envisions it, is chaos. It is just this sort of issue which was put to the test in a study of nurse–physician relationships published by Holfing et al. in 1966. The experimental situation pitted a nurse's professional standards and commitment to client welfare against obedience to a physician's order. How many nurses would give a clearly labeled overdose of an unknown drug to a client because an unfamiliar staff psychiatrist makes such a phone order? Answer: 21 out of 22. Here, at least, obedience clearly would not likely be of benefit to clients.

THE EMERGENCE OF CLIENT ADVOCACY—WINSLOW, GADOW, KOHNKE, AND MURPHY

Gerald Winslow, a professor of religion, charts an historic shift in the way that nursing perceives itself in "From Loyalty to Advocacy: A New Metaphor for Nursing." Although the pivotal issue here was the object of the nurse's loyalty, the catalysts for change were various. Winslow identifies such contributing factors as the diminished esteem and mystique of physicians, the rise of consumerism, patients' rights movements, feminism, incorporation of the advocacy model into the nursing codes, and the Tuma case. Without doubt the new metaphor has triumphed—the ideal of the loyal obedient soldier-like nurse has been replaced by the ideal of advocacy for the rights of clients. But the exact meaning of what it means to be a patient advocate is one of a number of ambiguities or potential difficulties Winslow says must be resolved. Other difficulties include the need to revise state nurse practice acts to accommodate the broadened role conception; the issue of public acceptance of the new role; and the interpersonal conflicts and divided loyalties the role may create.

Many of these concerns will be the focus of subsequent chapters. The remaining articles begin to examine the meaning of advocacy, its moral implications, and two criticisms of it.

It is widely acknowledged that one of the most thoughtful and widely influential expressions of nursing's new metaphor comes from the writings of philosopher-nurse Sally Gadow. We have included two articles by Gadow. The first, "Existential Advocacy: Philosophical Foundation of Nursing," is a more extensive and philosophically complex presentation of her views. Gadow's second article contains a more concise review of her primary points.

Gadow believes that nursing must be defined in terms of its philosophy of care and not its discrete nursing functions. The ideal she proposes as the philosophical foundation of nursing is "existential advocacy." This ideal is premised on respect for the individual's right to self-determination. The role of the nurse is to assist clients in their exercise of self-determination. The nurse must do more than just provide information and protect clients from institutional and professional threats to their self-determination. The nurse must help clients clarify their own values and assist clients to make decisions based on their own values. As such, Gadow contrasts existential advocacy to paternalism and consumerism or patient's rights advocacy.

As Gadow sees it, the problem with paternalism is that it ignores self-determination when a client's wishes run counter to what seems to be the client's best interest as medically defined. In contrast, Gadow maintains that what is in the client's "best interest" can only be defined by reference to what the client values.

Consumerism embodies an opposite extreme. Whereas in the paternalistic model the professional–client relationship is professionally dictated, in consumerism the dictator role is reversed. The professional merely becomes the agent of the consumer's choice. Mary Kohnke views advocacy very much like consumerism.[4] To her, advocacy is reduced to two basic functions: (1) *inform* the clients of their rights and give them the information necessary to make informed autonomous choices, and (2) *support* the choices of clients.

The difference between Gadow and Kohnke lies in the degree of involvement of the nurse's own values in the process of assisting clients to clarify their values and make decisions based on them. If the nurse is a mere dispenser of information, the uniqueness of the nurse as a human individual is irrelevant to the nurse–client relationship. But there is a danger in going beyond the merely informative function. Allowing the nurse's values to enter into the relationship may destroy what existential advocacy seeks to preserve —client autonomy. That is, in the process of helping a client *with* a decision, the nurse may end up subtly making a decision *for* the client. Whether this happens or not may depend upon how the client regards the views of the nurse. If they are so authoritative as to be coercive, autonomy suffers. On the other hand, it would be false to assume that a client's choice is autonomous merely because they have made a choice. A choice that is autonomous must also be consonant with the individual's values and this cannot be known without some interaction with the person.

In either view, some danger to autonomy seems to exist. On what side should nurses err if this commitment to client autonomy is accepted? Should nurses never persuade or voice disagreement or give advice? Are the nurse's own values ever permitted entry into the client–nurse relationship?

Both Gadow and Kohnke distinguish their views from paternalism, but perhaps some forms of paternalism are consistent with advocacy. The difficulty with paternalism is that it appears either to ignore the client's wishes or act contrary to them in order to do them good—as morally defined. As Gadow insists, however, the client's best interests cannot be defined apart from reference to the client's own values. But nurses frequently act paternalistically. For example, after operations there is a need for clients to ambulate. Nurses, however, are often faced with a clearly expressed desire to be left alone. Nevertheless, these reluctant clients are wooed, coaxed, and perhaps even coerced out of bed and down the hall. Would this be a violation of all that advocacy stands for? Is this a deliberate ignoring of client wishes? Not necessarily. Paternalism can be justified when it is in accordance with the client's own performances (as previously expressed) and it is reasonable to believe that the client will subsequently ratify the nurse's actions as consistent with the client's true preferences. Still, a very strong adherence to client autonomy may call these seemingly benign forms of paternalism into question.

What is common to the client advocacy views is the primary commitment to the client. This ideal has greatly influenced the language of the present American Nurses' Association (ANA) Code for Nurses, especially in its preamble and interpretive statements. The first explicit statement of this loyalty, as connected with the code, is found in a 1953 article which comments on the first officially accepted Code of 1950. Commenting on statement 8.:

> The nurse sustains confidence in the physician and other members of the health team: incompetency or unethical conduct of associates in the health profession should be exposed, but only to the proper authority.[5]

Members of the ANA Committee on Ethical Standards condemned this "conspiracy of silence" which permitted mistakes and negligence injurious to the health of patients. They note, "all patients have rights which must be recognized and held sacred" and avow "'the patient first' must be the nurse's slogan."[6]

That was 1953. It would take several decades before this notion was to work its way into the mind sets of the majority of nurses. Catherine Murphy, a nurse educator, reports the findings of her studies on the moral reasoning of nurses during the mid-1970s through the early 1980s in "The Changing Role of Nurses in Making Ethical Decisions." What is so remarkable is the sudden abandonment of two models of the nurse–client relationship (the bureaucratic and physician advocate models) in favor of the patient advocate model within the space of a decade. In the mid 1970s, when confronted with a hypothetical dilemma which pitted a client's rights and wishes against those of the physician and/or hospital, only a minority of nurses saw it as part of their role to champion the client's rights. By the turn of the end of the decade this had reversed. Murphy reiterates the case that can be made for nurses taking increasingly larger roles in ethical decision making.

CRITICISMS OF ADVOCACY—PAGANA

Kathleen Deska Pagana, a nursing instructor, presents a critique of client advocacy. In her article, "Let's Stop Calling Ourselves 'Patient Advocates,'" she believes that the economic handwriting is on the wall for patient advocacy and its adversarial style. In order for hospitals to survive they must become efficient and productive. Nurses must become team players and help enact the business goals of the hospitals. Pagana sees no necessary conflict between patients' interests and hospital profits. Indeed, Pagana thinks that nursing should seize the opportunity to use economic arguments for the good of the clients. "Satisfied customers" should mean happy clients, good care, and profits.

Undoubtedly there are instances where profits and good care of clients go hand in hand, but it is surely wishful thinking on Pagana's part to think that this happy state of affairs is always or frequently going to happen. It is far too easy to imagine conflicts between clients and profits. Should nurses, for example, participate in schemes to discourage certain types of unprofitable clients (e.g., indigents or those suffering from a disease others do not wish to be around) from coming to their hospital. Should nurses try to sell clients on additional diagnostic tests and lucrative elective procedures? But most importantly, when it finally comes down to deciding ultimate loyalties, where is the first loyalty of the nurse?

The fact that hospitals have adopted the language, methods, and attitudes of business does pose a serious threat to nursing's existence as an autonomous profession. Although the ideals embodied in the ANA Code for Nurses are declared to be non-negotiable contractual items, Pagana warns that corporate disloyalty is not tolerated in other areas of the business sector. Could it be that in the future, as a practical matter, nurses will have to abandon their professional ideals as a condition of employment?[7]

Pagana is not distressed over such a prospect since in her view corporate loyalty and the production of satisfied customers is just another way of fulfilling nursing's commitment to clients, but in a more cooperative and less adversarial style. If our suggestions are correct, however, Pagana is overly optimistic about the relationship between profits and the good of clients and the very nature of nursing as an autonomous profession is at stake.

Other criticisms of the client advocacy philosophy have been indirect and rest upon general dissatisfaction with recent trends and developments in nursing education. For example, there is the attack on client advocacy by retired nurse educator Alice Ream (1982) in a *Newsweek* opinion piece entitled "Our Undertrained Nurses."[8] Because of the controversy it created, Ream has refused its republication here. Her point, however, was that "nurse educators have a bug in their ears about being handmaidens to physicians." The result has been a short changing of nursing students on skills in the nursing curriculum which leads to iatrogenic harms, malpractice suits, and nurse burnout. Another way of making this point is this. In order for nursing to emerge as an autonomous profession it must enlarge its knowledge base, and therefore, it must inevitably spend more time in the classroom than at the bedside. But in accomplishing this task it is possibly violating a fundamental principle of medical and nursing ethics—do no harm. Wither should nursing go? Ream's solution is clear. Go back to primary emphasis on skills for a least this may prevent harm to patients.

A crucial premise in Ream's argument is that the shift in nursing education from clinical to educational settings has somehow been responsible for some of the estimated 50,000 persons who die each year from urinary-tract infections.

A concern that Ream voices does rest upon some plausible assumptions. Fewer skill learning hours may lead to client harm and nurse dropout. This problem, however, is not unique to new graduates. Any nurse moving from one speciality to another or returning to nursing practice after a few years is likely to be anxious about eroded or unpracticed skills. What is needed is a more general solution to this problem. As nursing becomes more specialized and health care becomes even more technologically complex, this problem is lilkely to increase.

Harm to individuals is certainly to be avoided if at all possible. Nor is it controversial to say that skillful nurses are to be preferred over unskillful ones. But, as George Annas argues in the following chapter, some consideration should be given to including violating human rights among the harms to be avoided. It is not at all obvious that greater emphasis on skills would do much for protecting clients from *those* harms or wrongs.

SUMMARY

This chapter examined how nursing has conceived itself historically and how this conception has changed. It is our contention, along with some of the authors discussed, that this issue is of paramount importance in structuring how a nurse responds to a moral dilemma and which obligations have primary or greater weighting. The empirical studies contained or referred to in Holfing et al. and Murphy substantiate that these conceptions do make a determinative difference in how nurses make ethical decisions. How nursing is viewed and its role relationships defined has been variously referred to as model, role conception, or philosophy of nursing. The significant point is that this forms the philosophical foundation of nursing and has profound ethical implications. The now dominant philosophy is that of client advocacy. However, as the articles indicate, ambiguity about just what advocacy entails and misgivings about the direction nursing has taken by those within and outside of nursing do exist.

The next chapter presents still more conceptions of client advocacy and problems associated with it.

NOTES

1. Other historical references to this view may be found in Gerald Winslow's article reproduced in this chapter. Also noteworthy are the views of Jessee Broadhurst published the same year. She outlined a three-year course in ethics for nursing students. A prominent feature is that all doctors should be accorded respect and "absolute loyalty." See "Ethics of Nursing," *American Journal of Nursing* 17 (1917): 792–797.
2. How the public views nursing is a topic of some controversy. Some surveys on this question are reported in Anthony Lee, "How—and Where—The Handmaiden Image is Changing," *RN* 42 (June 1979): 36–39; Idem, "How Nurses Rate with the Public," *RN* 42 (June 1979): 24–35; Claire Rayner, "What do the Public Think of Nurses?", *Nursing Times* 80 (August 29, 1984): 28–31; and Judith W. Alexander, "How the Public Perceives Nursing and Their Education," *Nursing Outlook* 27 (October 1979): 654–656. See also Philip A. Kalish and Beatrice J. Kalish, The Changing Image of the Nurse (Menlo Park, Ca.: Addison-Wesley, 1987); and Linda Hughes, "The Public Image of the Nurse," *Advances in Nursing Science* 2 (April 1980): 55–72.
3. The goals of the hospital as announced by Newton—"Saving life and health"—correspond to the ANA's first statement of its first code: "The fundamental responsibility of the nurse is to conserve life and to promote health" [American Nurses'

Association, Committee on Ethical Standards, "A Code for Nurses," *American Journal of Nursing* 50 (1950): 196.] The descendant of that clause was an obligation to preserve life. In 1985, the Preamble to *Code for Nurses with Interpretive Statements* (American Nurses' Association, 1985) further qualifies the commitment to health. "Since clients themselves are the primary decision makers . . . health is not necessarily an end in itself but rather a means to a life that is meaningful from the client's perspective" (p.i.).

4. A fuller statement of Kohnke's views can be found in her *Advocacy: Risk and Reality* (St. Louis: C.V. Mosby, 1982).

5. ANA Code for Nurses (1950), p. 196.

6. ANA Committee on Ethical Standards, "What's in Our Code?", *American Journal of Nursing* 53 (August 1953): 966.

7. Cf. "The Code for Nurses is not open to negotiation in employment settings, nor is it permissible for individuals or groups of nurses to adapt or change the language of this code." *Code for Nurses with Interpretive Statements* (1985), p. iv.

8. Alice Ream, "Our Undertrained Nurses," *Newsweek* 100 (October 21, 1982): 17.

The Relation of the Nurse to the Doctor and the Doctor to the Nurse

Sarah E. Dock

Someone has said a nurse is born and not made. I would like to amend that by saying a nurse is born and then trained. Woman possesses qualities which naturally make her superior to the average man for this important work, which stands second to the medical profession itself.

The nursing profession is monopolized almost entirely by women. It is about the only thing we are allowed to do without the blame of trying to take away the work from the poor men. In spite of the fact that women are naturally adapted to the art of nursing, superintendents of hospitals often find it difficult to obtain desirable applicants for training. The possible reason for this is the lack of home training and the fact that children are rarely taught the importance of obedience. In my estimation obedience is the first law and the very cornerstone of good nursing. And here is the first stumbling block for the beginner. No matter how gifted she may be, she will never become a reliable nurse until she can obey without question. The first and most helpful criticism I ever received from a doctor was when he told me that I was supposed to be simply an intelligent machine for the purpose of carrying out his orders.

As to the relation of a nurse to the doctor, there can be no relation of the nurse to the doctor other than a strictly professional one. Any other relation will mean disaster to the nurse.

By disaster I mean that any relation not professional will lead to misunderstandings, quarrels or perhaps marriage, and in either case the nurse's usefulness as a professional nurse will be at an end. This is to me a pretty good argument why a nurse should maintain strictly formal relations towards the doctor, never forgetting that her success in the future depends mainly on the doctor's recommendation and influence.

It is true that after several years of doing private duty a good nurse receives many calls through the friends of patients, but suppose she steps beyond the bounds of professional etiquette and commits that unpardonable sin of suggesting to the family that another doctor be called in, perhaps the one she prefers, and in other ways conducts herself unbecomingly as a nurse. Her opportunities will be limited to nursing for that one particular doctor, no matter how qualified and accomplished she may be. Instances have occurred where the physician has been dismissed and the unprofessional nurse retained (but this is very unusual). The professional career of such a nurse is bound to be short. My advice to nurses doing hospital or private duty work would be to maintain a strictly formal attitude toward the doctor.

You may not care for the personality of the doctor who is in attendance but you are bound to respect his profession and obey his orders. If his conduct is such as to offend and make it impossible for you to do conscientious work, make some excuse and give up the case.

It is always well on taking charge of a case to inquire from the doctor what he would allow the nurse to do if any emergencies should arise. This is not only for the patient's safety but for the nurse's protection. As you know, there are occasions where a nurse's prompt action may save the life of her patient, but at the same time she would like to know that the means are entirely approved by the attending physician.

After all, no matter how professional or clever a nurse may be, she will never be successful if she lacks common sense, tact and the ability to grasp the fact that her real success depends on the little things in nursing and not on the fact that she may be able to diagnose the case.

As to the relation of the doctor to the nurse, I believe the doctors are mainly responsible for the many inefficient nurses that are graduated from the smaller hospitals. The reason for this is that doctors in smaller towns take a more personal interest in the social side of the training school, often using their influence to keep an undesirable pupil nurse in training. Then, too, it is more difficult to maintain the strict, almost military, discipline which is in operation in all the larger schools.

A really good, ambitious nurse will prefer the doctor who is particular, even exacting in regard to her work. With a doctor like this an indifferent nurse will be forced to do good work, for she is afraid not to. A careless doctor will make a careless nurse.

Naturally the doctor is or should be the nurse's chief instructor. He should make it his business to know that the curriculum of the training school is what it should be, and that the pupil nurses get the practice required to make for efficiency. By the high standard of the training school both he and his patient will be benefited.

I believe it is the doctor's duty to report a nurse who fails to carry out his orders; but first he should take the role of a kindly critic and tell her of her shortcomings. If this correction fails, then report the pupil nurse; or dismiss her, if she is a graduate and doing private duty. Doctors should never make excuses for nurses who fail in their duty. It is really an injustice to the nurse and can do no possible good.

When he dismisses an unsatisfactory nurse he should tell her why, no matter if it hurts. If she is the right kind of nurse she will do better next time, or be discouraged and give up the profession. When a nurse is doing private duty the doctor should see that she gets the proper amount of rest and recreation. He should also remember that while he is attending several patients, the nurse has only one patient and is wholly dependent on the income from that one patient. If her patient is at all able to pay, I think the nurse should be entitled to the first money, and the doctor should see that she gets it.

If doctors were obliged to spend twenty-two hours out of twenty-four with some of their irritable, nervous patients they would require a few weeks rest at Dawson Springs. Even a machine needs rest and repair. Beyond a certain amount of physical and mental strain the brain refuses to act, and I believe that many cases of neglect on the part of the nurse are due to overwork. Perhaps the over ambitious nurse wishes to carry a difficult case through and refuses to have assistance. Such foolishness the doctor should not allow. Some doctors think nurses require flattery in order to do better work. I do not think so. After all, if she is doing her duty, she is doing just what she should. It is a matter of business with her and to her interest that she do her work loyally and well.

In Defense of the Traditional Nurse

Lisa H. Newton

When a truth is accepted by everyone as so obvious that it blots out all its alternatives and leaves no respectable perspectives from which to examine it, it becomes the natural prey of philosophers, whose essential activity is to question accepted opinion. A case in point may be the ideal of the "autonomous professional" for nursing. The consensus that this ideal and image are appropriate for the profession is becoming monolithic and may profit from the presence of a full-blooded alternative ideal to replace the cardboard stereotypes it routinely condemns. That alternative, I suggest, is the traditional ideal of the skilled and gentle caregiver, whose role in health care requires submission to authority as an essential component. We can see the faults of this traditional ideal very clearly now, but we may perhaps also be able to see virtues that went unnoticed in the battle to displace it. It is my contention that the image and ideal of the traditional nurse contain virtues that can be found nowhere else in the health care professions, that perhaps make an irreplaceable contribution to the care of patients, and that should not be lost in the transition to a new definition of the profession of nursing.

A word should be said about what this article is, and what it is not. It is an essay in philosophical analysis, starting from familiar ideas, beliefs, and concepts, examining their relationships and implications and reaching tentative conclusions about the logical defensibility of the structures discovered. It is not the product of research in the traditional sense. Its factual premises—for example, that the "traditional" nursing role has been criticized by those who prefer an "autonomous professional" role—are modest by any standard, and in any event may be taken as hypothetical by all who may be disposed to disagree with them. It is not a polemic against any writer or writers in particular, but a critique of lines of reasoning that are turning up with increasing frequency in diverse contexts. Its arguments derive no force whatsoever from any writings in which they may be found elsewhere.

ROLE COMPONENTS

The first task of any philosophical inquiry is to determine its terminology and establish the meanings of its key terms for its own purposes. To take the first term: a *role* is a norm-governed pattern of action undertaken in accordance with social expectations. The term is originally derived from the drama, where it signifies a part played by an actor in a play. In current usage, any ordinary job or profession (physician, housewife, teacher, postal worker) will do as an example of a social role; the term's dramatic origin is nonetheless worth remembering, as a key to the limits of the concept.

Image and ideal are simply the descriptive and prescriptive aspects of a social role. The *image* of a social role is that role as it is understood to be in fact, both by the occupants of the role and by those with whom the occupant interacts. It describes the character the occupant plays, the acts, attitudes, and expectations normally associated with the role. The *ideal* of a role is a conception of what that role could or should be—that is, a conception of the norms that should govern its work. It is necessary to distinguish between the private and public aspects of image and ideal.

Newton, L. H. (1981, June). In defense of the traditional nurse. *Nursing Outlook, 29,* 348–354. Reprinted with permission of © American Journal of Nursing Company. All rights reserved.

Since role occupants and general public need not agree either on the description of the present operations of the role or on the prescription for its future development, the private image, or self-image of the role occupant, is therefore distinct from the public image or general impression of the role maintained in the popular media and mind. The private ideal, or aspiration of the role occupant, is distinct from the public ideal or normative direction set for the role by the larger society. Thus, four role-components emerge, from the public and private, descriptive and prescriptive, aspects of a social role. They may be difficult to disentangle in some cases, but they are surely distinct in theory, and potentially in conflict in fact.

TRANSITIONAL ROLES

In these terms alone we have the materials for the problematic tensions within transitional social roles. Stable social roles should exhibit no significant disparities among images and ideals: what the public generally gets is about what it thinks it should get; what the job turns out to require is generally in accord with the role-occupant's aspirations; and public and role-occupant, beyond a certain base level of "they-don't-know-how-hard-we-work" grumbling, are in general agreement on what the role is all about. On the other hand, transitional roles tend to exhibit strong discrepancies among the four elements of the role during the transition; at least the components will make the transition at different times, and there may also be profound disagreement on the direction that the transition should take.

The move from a general discussion of roles in society to a specific discussion of the nursing profession is made difficult by the fact that correct English demands the use of a personal pronoun. How shall we refer to the nurse? It is claimed that consistent reference to a professional as "he" reinforces the stereotype of male monopoly in the professions, save for the profession of nursing, where consistent reference to the professional as "she" reinforces the stereotype of subservience. Though we ought never to reinforce sex and dominance stereotypes, the effort to write in gender-neutral terms involves the use of circumlocutions and "he/she" usages that quickly becomes wearisome to reader and writer alike. Referring to most other professions, I would simply use the universal pronouns "he" and "him", and ignore the ridiculous

accusations of sexism. But against a background of a virtually all-female profession, whose literature until the last decade universally referred to its professionals as "she", the consistent use of "he" to refer to a nurse calls attention to itself and distracts attention from the argument.

A further problem with gender-neutral terminology in the discussion of this issue in particular is that it appears to render the issue irrelevant. The whole question of autonomy for the nurse in professional work arises because nurses have been, and are, by and large, women, and the place of the profession in the health care system is strongly influenced by the place of women in society. To talk about nurses as if they were, or might as well be, men, is to make the very existence of a problem a mystery. There are, therefore good reasons beyond custom to continue using the pronoun "she" to refer to the nurse. I doubt that such use will suggest to anyone who might read this essay that it is not appropriate for men to become nurses; presumably we are beyond making that error at this time.

BARRIERS TO AUTONOMY

The first contention of my argument is that the issue of autonomy in the nursing profession lends itself to misformulation. A common formulation of the issue, for example, locates it in a discrepancy between public image and private image. On this account, the public is asserted to believe that nurses are ill-educated, unintelligent, incapable of assuming responsibility, and hence properly excluded from professional status and responsibility. In fact they are now prepared to be truly autonomous professionals through an excellent education, including a thorough theoretical grounding in all aspects of their profession. Granted, the public image of the nurse has many favorable aspects—the nurse is credited with great manual skill, often saintly dedication to service to others, and, at least below the supervisory level, a warm heart and gentle manners. But the educational and intellectual deficiencies that the public mistakenly perceives outweigh the "positive" qualities when it comes to deciding how the nurse shall be treated, and are called upon to justify not only her traditionally inferior status and low wages, but also the refusal to allow nursing to fill genuine needs in the health care system by assuming tasks that nurses are uniquely qualified to handle. For the sake of the quality of health care as well as for the sake of the interests of the nurse, the public must be educated through a massive educational campaign to the full capabilities of the contemporary nurse; the image must be brought into line with the facts. On this account, then, the issue of nurse autonomy is diagnosed as a public relations problem: the private ideal of nursing is asserted to be that of the autonomous professional and the private image is asserted to have undergone a transition from an older subservient role to a new professional one but the public image of the nurse ideal is significantly not mentioned in this analysis.

An alternative account of the issue of professional autonomy in nursing locates it in a discrepancy between private ideal and private image. Again, the private ideal is that of the autonomous professional. But the actual performance of the role is entirely slavish, because of the way the system works—with its tight budgets, insane schedules, workloads bordering on reckless endangerment for the seriously ill, bureaucratic red tape, confusion, and arrogance. Under these conditions, the nurse is permanently barred from fulfilling her professional ideal, from bringing the reality of the nurse's condition into line with the self-concept she brought to the job. On this account, then, the nurse really is not an autonomous professional, and total reform of the power structure of the health care industry will be necessary in order to allow her to become one.

A third formulation locates the issue of autonomy in a struggle between the private ideal and an altogether undesirable public ideal: on this account, the public does not want the nurse to be an autonomous professional, because her present subservient status serves the power needs of the physicians; because her unprofessional remuneration serves the monetary needs of the entrepreneurs and callous municipalities that run the hospitals; and because the low value accorded her opinions on patient care protects both physicians and bureaucrats from being forced to account to the patient for the treatment he receives. On this account, the nurse needs primarily to gather allies to defeat the powerful interest groups that impose the traditional ideal for their own unworthy purposes, and to replace that degrading and dangerous prescription with one more appropriate to the contemporary nurse.

These three accounts, logically independent, have crucial elements of content in common. Above all, they agree on the objectives to be pursued: full professional independence, responsibility, recognition, and remuneration for the professional nurse. And as corollary to these objectives, they agree on the necessity of banishing forever from the hospitals and from the public mind that inaccurate and demeaning stereotype of the nurse as the Lady with the Bedpan: an image of submissive service, comforting to have around and skillful enough at her little tasks, but too scatterbrained and emotional for responsibility.

In none of the interpretations above is any real weight given to a public ideal of nursing, to the nursing role as the public thinks it ought to be played. Where public prescription shows up at all, it is seen as a vicious and false demand imposed by power alone, thoroughly illegitimate and to be destroyed as quickly as possible. The possibility that there may be real value in the traditional role of the nurse, and that the public may have good reasons to want to retain it, simply does not receive any serious consideration on any account. It is precisely that possibility that I take up in the next section.

DEFENDING THE "TRADITIONAL NURSE"

As Aristotle taught us, the way to discover the peculiar virtues of any thing is to look to the work that it accomplishes in the larger context of its environment. The first task, then, is to isolate those factors of need or demand in the nursing environment that require the nurse's work if they are to be met. I shall concentrate, as above, on the hospital environment, since most nurses are employed in hospitals.

The work context of the hospital nurse actually spans two societal practices or institutions: the hospital as a bureaucracy and medicine as a field of scientific endeavor and service. Although there is enormous room for variation in both hospital bureaucracies and medicine, and they may therefore interact with an infinite number of possible results, the most general facts about both institutions allow us to sketch the major demands they make on those whose function lies within them.

To take the hospital bureaucracy first: its very nature demands that workers perform the tasks assigned to them, report properly to the proper superior, avoid initiative, and adhere to set procedures. These requirements are common to all bureaucracies, but dramatically increase in urgency when the tasks are supposed to be protective of life itself and where the subject matter is inherently unpredictable and emergency prone. Since there is often no time to re-examine the usefulness of a procedure in a particular case, and since the stakes are too high to permit a gamble, the institution's effectiveness, not to mention its legal position, may depend on unquestioning adherence to procedure.

Assuming that the sort of hospital under discussion is one in which the practice of medicine by qualified physicians is the focal activity, rather than, say, a convalescent hospital, further contextual requirements emerge. Among the prominent features of the practice of medicine are the following: it depends on esoteric knowledge which takes time to acquire and which is rapidly advancing; and, because each patient's illness is unique, it is uncertain. Thus, when a serious medical situation arises without warning, only physicians will know how to deal with it (if their licensure has any point), and they will not always be able to explain or justify their actions to nonphysicians, even those who are required to assist them in patient care.

If the two contexts of medicine and the hospital are superimposed, three common points can be seen. Both are devoted to the saving of life and health; the atmosphere in which that purpose is carried out is inevitably tense and urgent; and, if the purpose is to be accomplished in that atmosphere, all participating activities and agents must be completely subordinated to the medical judgments of the physicians. In short, those other than physicians, involved in medical procedures in a hospital context, have no right to insert their own needs, judgments, or personalities into the situation. The last thing we need at that point is another autonomous professional on the job, whether a nurse or anyone else.

PATIENT NEEDS:
THE PRIME CONCERN

From the general characteristics of hospitals and medicine, that negative conclusion for nursing follows. But the institutions are not, after all, the focus of the endeavor. If there is any conflict between the needs of the patient and the needs of the institutions established to serve him, his needs take precedence and constitute the most important

requirements of the nursing environment. What are these needs?

First, because the patient is sick and disabled, he needs specialized care that only qualified personnel can administer, beyond the time that the physician is with him. Second, and perhaps most obviously to the patient, he is likely to be unable to perform simple tasks such as walking unaided, dressing himself, and attending to his bodily functions. He will need assistance in these tasks, and is likely to find this need humiliating; his entire self-concept as an independent human being may be threatened. Thus, the patient has serious emotional needs brought on by the hospital situation itself, regardless of his disability. He is scared, depressed, disappointed, and possibly, in reaction to all of these, very angry. He needs reassurance, comfort, someone to talk to. The person he really needs, who would be capable of taking care of all these problems, is obviously his mother, and the first job of the nurse is to be a mother surrogate.

That conclusion, it should be noted, is inherent in the word "nurse" itself: it is derived ultimately from the Latin *nutrire*, "to nourish or suckle"; the first meaning of "nurse" as a noun is still, according to *Webster's New Twentieth Century Unabridged Dictionary* "one who suckles a child not her own." From the outset, then, the function of the nurse is identical with that of the mother, to be exercised when the mother is unavailable. And the meanings proceed in logical order from there: the second definitions given for both noun and verb involve caring for children, especially young children, and the third, caring for those who are childlike in their dependence—the sick, the injured, the very old, and the handicapped. For all those groups—infants, children, and helpless adults—it is appropriate to bring children's caretakers, surrogate mothers, nurses, into the situation to minister to them. It is especially appropriate to do so, for the sake of the psychological economies realized by the patient: the sense of self, at least for the Western adult, hangs on the self-perception of independence. Since disability requires the relinquishing of this self-perception, the patient must either discover conditions excusing his dependence somewhere in his self-concept, or invent new ones, and the latter task is extremely difficult. Hence the usefulness of the maternal image association: it was, within the patient's understanding of himself "all right" to be tended by mother; if the nurse is (at some level) mother, it is "all right" to reassume that familiar role and to be tended by her.

LIMITS ON THE "MOTHER" ROLE

The nurse's assumption of the role of mother is therefore justified etymologically and historically but most importantly by reference to the psychological demands of and on the patient. Yet the maternal role cannot be imported into the hospital care situation without significant modification—specifically, with respect to the power and authority inherent in the role of mother. Such maternal authority includes the right and duty to assume control over children's lives and make all decisions for them; but the hospital patient most definitely does not lose adult status even if he is sick enough to want to. The ethical legitimacy as well as the therapeutic success of his treatment depend on his voluntary and active cooperation in it and on his deferring to some forms of power and authority—the hospital rules and the physician's sapiential authority, for example. But these very partial, conditional, restraints are nowhere near the threat to patient autonomy that the real presence of mother would be; maternal authority, total, diffuse, and unlimited, would be incompatible with the retention of moral freedom. And it is just this sort of total authority that the patient is most tempted to attribute to the nurse, who already embodies the nurturant component of the maternal role. To prevent serious threats to patient autonomy, then, the role of nurse must be from the outset, as essentially as it is nurturant, unavailable for such attribution of authority. Not only must the role of nurse not include authority; it must be incompatible with authority: essentially, a subservient role.

The nurse role, as required by the patient's situation, is the nurturant component of the maternal role and excludes elements of power and authority. A further advantage of this combination of maternal nurturance and subordinate status is that, just as it permits the patient to be cared for like a baby without threatening his autonomy, it also permits him to unburden himself to a sympathetic listener of his doubts and resentments, about physicians and hospitals in general, and his in particular, without threatening the course of his treatment. His resentments are natural, but they lead to a situation of conflict, between the desire to rebel against treatment and bring it to a halt (to reassert control over his life), and the desire that the treatment should continue (to obtain its benefits). The nurse's function speaks well to this condition: like her maternal model, the nurse is available for the patient to talk to (the physician is too busy to talk), sympathetic, understanding, and supportive; but in her subordinate position, the nurse can do absolutely nothing to change his course of treatment. Since she has no more control over the environment than he has, he can let off steam in perfect safety, knowing that he cannot do himself any damage.

The norms for the nurse's role so far derived from the patient's perspective also tally, it might be noted, with the restrictions on the role that arise from the needs of hospitals and medicine. The patient does not need another autonomous professional at his bedside, any more than the physician can use one or the hospital bureaucracy contain one. The conclusion so far, then, is that in the hospital environment, the traditional (nurturant and subordinate) role of the nurse seems more adapted to the nurse function than the new autonomous role.

PROVIDER OF HUMANISTIC CARE

So far, we have defined the hospital nurse's function in terms of the specific needs of the hospital, the physician, and the patient. Yet there is another level of function that needs to be addressed. If we consider the multifaceted demands that the patient's family, friends, and community make on the hospital once the patient is admitted, it becomes clear that this concerned group cannot be served exclusively by attending to the medical aspect of care, necessary though that is. Nor is it sufficient for the hospital-as-institution to keep accurate and careful records, maintain absolute cleanliness, and establish procedures that protect the patient's safety, even though this is important. Neither bureaucracy nor medical professional can handle the human needs of the human beings involved in the process.

The general public entering the hospital as patient or visitor encounters and reacts to that health care system as an indivisible whole, as if under a single heading of "what the hospital is like." It is at this level that we can make sense of the traditional claim that the nurse represents the "human" as opposed to "mechanical" or "coldly professional" aspect of health care, for there is clearly something terribly missing in the combined medical and bureaucratic approach to the "case": they fail to address the patient's fear for himself and the family's fear for him, their grief over the separation, even if temporary, their concern for the financial burden, and a host of other emotional components of hospitalization.

The same failing appears throughout the hospital experience, most poignantly obvious, perhaps, when the medical procedures are unavailing and the patient dies. When this occurs, the physician must determine the cause and time of death and the advisability of an autopsy, while the bureaucracy must record the death and remove the body; but surely this is not enough. The death of a human being is a rending of the fabric of human community, a sad and fearful time; it is appropriately a time of bitter regret, anger, and weeping. The patient's family, caught up in the institutional context of the hospital, cannot assume alone the burden of discovering and expressing the emotions appropriate to the occasion; such expression, essential for their own regeneration after their loss must originate somehow within the hospital context itself. The hospital system must, somehow, be able to share pain and grief as well as it makes medical judgments and keeps records.

The traditional nurse's role addresses itself directly to these human needs. Its derivation from the maternal role classifies it as feminine and permits ready assumption of all attributes culturally typed as "feminine": tenderness, warmth, sympathy, and a tendency to engage much more readily in the expression of feeling than in the rendering of judgment. Through the nurse, the hospital can be concerned, welcoming, caring, and grief-stricken; it can break through the cold barriers of efficiency essential to its other functions and share human feeling.

The nurse therefore provides the in-hospital health care system with human capabilities that would otherwise be unavailable to it and hence unavailable to the community in dealing with it. Such a conclusion is unattractive to the supporters of the autonomous role for the nurse, because the tasks of making objective judgments and of expressing emotion are inherently incompatible; and since the nurse shows grief and sympathy on behalf of the system, she is excluded from decision-making and defined as subordinate.

However unappealing such a conclusion may be, it is clear that without the nurse role in this function, the hospital becomes a moral monstrosity, coolly and mechanically dispensing and disposing of human life and death, with no acknowledgment at all of the individual life, value, projects, and relationships of the persons with whom it deals. Only the nurse makes the system morally tolerable. People in pain deserve sympathy, as the dead deserve to be grieved; it is unthinkable that the very societal institution to which we generally consign the

suffering and the dying should be incapable of sustaining sympathy and grief. Yet its capability hangs on the presence of nurses willing to assume the affective functions of the traditional nursing role, and the current attempt to banish that role, to introduce instead an autonomous professional role for the nurse, threatens to send the last hope for a human presence in the hospital off at the same time.

THE FEMINIST PERSPECTIVE

From this conclusion it would seem to follow automatically that the role of the traditional nurse should be retained. It might be argued, however, that the value of autonomy is such that any non-autonomous role ought to be abolished, no matter what its value to the current institutional structure.

Those who aimed to abolish black slavery in the United States have provided a precedent for this argument. They never denied the slave's economic usefulness; they simply denied that it could be right to enslave any person and insisted that the nation find some other way to get the work done, no matter what the cost. On a totally different level, the feminists of our own generation have proposed that the traditional housewife and mother role for the woman, which confined women to domestic life and made them subordinate to men, has been very useful for everyone except the women trapped in it. All the feminists have claimed is that the profit of others is not a sufficient reason to retain a role that demeans its occupant. As they see it, the "traditional nurse" role is analogous to the roles of slave and housewife—it is derived directly, in fact, as we have seen, from the "mother" part of the latter role—exploitative of its occupants and hence immoral by its very nature and worthy of abolition.

But the analogy does not hold. A distinction must be made between an autonomous person—one who, over the course of adult life, is self-determining in all major choices and a significant number of minor ones, and hence can be said to have chosen, and to be responsible for, his own life—and an autonomous *role*—a role so structured that its occupant is self-determining in all major and most minor role-related choices. An autonomous person can certainly take on a subordinate role without losing his personal autonomy. For example, we can find examples of slaves (in the ancient world at least) and housewives who have claimed to have, and shown every sign of having, complete personal integrity and autonomy with their freely chosen roles.

Furthermore, slave and housewife are a very special type of role, known as "life-roles." They are to be played 24 hours a day, for an indefinite period of time; there is no customary or foreseeable respite from them. Depending on circumstances, there may be de facto escapes from these roles, permitting their occupants to set up separate personal identities (some of the literature from the history of American slavery suggests this possibility), but the role-definitions do not contemplate part-time occupancy. Such life-roles are few in number; most roles are the part-time "occupational roles," the jobs that we do eight hours a day and have little to do with the structuring of the rest of the twenty-four. An autonomous person can, it would seem, easily take up a subordinate role of this type and play it well without threat to personal autonomy. And if there is excellent reason to choose such a role—if, for example, an enterprise of tremendous importance derives an essential component of its moral worth from that role—it would seem to be altogether rational and praiseworthy to do so. The role of "traditional nurse" would certainly fall within this category.

But even if the traditional nurse role is not inherently demeaning, it might be argued further, it should be abolished as harmful to the society because it preserves the sex stereotypes that we are trying to overcome. "Nurse" is a purely feminine role, historically derived from "mother", embodying feminine attributes of emotionality, tenderness, and nurturance, and it is subordinate—thus reinforcing the link between femininity and subordinate status. The nurse role should be available to men, too, to help break down this unfavorable stereotype.

This objective to the traditional role embodies the very fallacy it aims to combat. The falsehood we know as sexism is not the belief that some roles are autonomous, calling for objectivity in judgment, suppression of emotion, and independent initiative in action, but discouraging independent judgment and action and requiring obedience to superiors; the falsehood is the assumption that only men are eligible for the first class and only women are eligible for the second class.

One of the most damaging mistakes of our cultural heritage is the assumption that warmth, gentleness, and loving care, such as are expected of the nurse, are simply impossible for the male of the species, and that men who show emotion, let alone

those who are ever known to weep, are weaklings, "sissies," and a disgrace to the human race. I suspect that this assumption has done more harm to the culture than its more publicized partner, the assumption that women are (or should be) incapable of objective judgment or executive function. Women will survive without leadership roles, but it is not clear that a society can retain its humanity if all those eligible for leadership are forbidden, by virtue of that eligibility, to take account of the human side of human beings: their altruism, heroism, compassion, and grief, their fear and weakness, and their ability to love and care for others.

In the words of the current feminist movement, men must be liberated as surely as women. And one of the best avenues to such liberation would be the encouragement of male participation in the health care system, or other systems of the society, in roles like the traditional nursing role, which permit, even require, the expressive side of the personality to develop, giving it a function in the enterprise and restoring it to recognition and respectability.

CONCLUSIONS

In conclusion, then, the traditional nurse role is crucial to health care in the hospital context; its subordinate status, required for its remaining features, is neither in itself demeaning nor a barrier to its assumption by men or women. It is probably not a role that everyone would enjoy. But there are certainly many who are suited to it, and should be willing to undertake the job.

One of the puzzling features of the recent controversy is the apparent unwillingness of some of the current crop of nursing school graduates to take on the assignment for which they have ostensibly been prepared, at least until such time as it shall be redefined to accord more closely with their notion of professional. These frustrated nurses who do not want the traditional nursing role, yet wish to employ their skills in the health care system in some way, will clearly have to do something else. The health care industry is presently in the process of very rapid expansion and diversification, and has created significant markets for those with a nurse's training and the capacity, and desire, for autonomous roles. Moreover, the nurse in a position which does not have the "nurse" label, does not need to combat the "traditional nurse" image and is ordinarily accorded greater freedom of action. For this reason alone it would appear that those nurses intent on occupying autonomous roles and tired of fighting stereotypes that they find degrading and unworthy of their abilities, should seek out occupational niches that do not bear the label, and the stigma, of "nurse."

I conclude, therefore: that much of the difficulty in obtaining public acceptance of the new "autonomous professional" image of the nurse may be due, not to public ignorance, but to the opposition of a vague but persistent public ideal of nursing; that the ideal is a worthy one, well-founded in the hospital context in which it evolved; and that the role of traditional nurse, for which that ideal sets the standard, should therefore be maintained and held open for any who would have the desire, and the personal and professional qualifications, to assume it. Perhaps the current crop of nursing school graduates do not desire it, but there is ample room in the health care system for the sort of "autonomous professional" they wish to be, apart from the hospital nursing role. Wherever we must go to fill this role, it is worth going there, for the traditional nurse is the major force remaining for humanity in a system that will turn into a mechanical monster without her.

An Experimental Study in Nurse-Physician Relationships

Charles K. Hofling, Eveline Brotzman, Sarah Dalrymple,
Nancy Graves, and Chester M. Pierce

As physicians move increasingly out of their traditional channels of functioning and into broader areas of the community, their relationships with members of the other health disciplines assume increasing significance. Similarly the intradisciplinary conflicts which beset these other professionals become of greater concern to the physician, since his own effectiveness comes to depend more and more upon others. This paper is an account of the way in which a group of psychiatrists and nurses have attempted to obtain a picture in depth of the effect of certain aspects of the nurse-physician relationship.

There is no doubt that the professional status and standards of nurses are at times challenged by the behavior of doctors (1, 3, 8). From a consideration of naturally occurring situations in which such challenges occur, two particularly significant categories appear to be: 1) the situation in which the doctor violates an accepted procedure of which the nurse is customarily in charge (*e.g.*, entering an isolation unit without taking the proper precautions); and 2) the situation in which the doctor directs the nurse to carry out a procedure which is in some fashion against her professional standards (*e.g.*, ordering the nurse to administer intravenous medication in a hospital where nurse-administrative policy opposes such action). Since the former situation can take place without the nurse's attention necessarily being directed to the problem, we selected the latter as the type of incident to create experimentally and to study.

METHOD

It was decided to construct the incident around an irregular order from a doctor to a nurse for her to administer a dose of medication.

Ingredients of the experimental conflict: 1) The nurse would be asked to give an obviously excessive dose of medicine. For reasons of safety it was decided to use a placebo. 2) The medication order was to be transmitted by telephone, a procedure in violation of hospital policy. 3) The medication would be "unauthorized," *i.e.*, a drug which had not been placed on the ward stock-list and cleared for use. 4) The order would be given to the nurse by an unfamiliar voice.

Overall approach: The conflict situation was contrived at a public and a private hospital on 12 and ten wards, respectively. A questionnaire was administered to a group of nurses at a third hospital as a matched control. The control subjects were asked what they would do if confronted with the circumstances of the experimental conflict. A group of student nurses was also given the questionnaire, in order to see how less experienced nurses thought they would react.

Hofling, C. K., Brotzman, E., Dalrymple, S., Graves, N., & Pierce, C. M. (1966). An experimental study in nurse-physician relationships. *The Journal of Nervous and Mental Diseases, 143* (2), 171–180. Printed with permission of © Williams & Wilkins. All rights reserved.

EXPERIMENTAL DESIGN

Ward Incident

Pill boxes bearing hospital labels were marked as follows:

ASTROTEN

5 mg. capsules
Usual dose: 5 mg.
Maximum daily dose: 10 mg.

These were placed on the wards. Each box contained pink placebo capsules filled with glucose. To standardize the telephone order, a written script was prepared for the caller. In order to standardize the stimulus call as much as possible, a set of standardized replies to the likeliest responses of the nurse was composed and closely adhered to.

It was decided that the emotional tone conveyed by the caller would be one of courteous, but self-confident firmness. As a precaution against unintentional departures from this tone, it was arranged to have the calls monitored by another member of the research team, whose function it would be to signal to the caller if he started to vary from the prescribed tone.

All telephone calls were tape-recorded. It was arranged to have a colleague, an expert in verbal behavior, listen to the tape after the experiment and mark as invalid any calls in which he perceived an appreciable variation from the prescribed tone or any cues suggesting that the call was not genuine.

Termination points for the telephone conversation were as follows: 1) compliance upon the part of the subject; 2) a clear-cut, sustained refusal; 3) insistence upon calling or talking to any third party of equal or superior rank in the hospital hierarchy; 4) the subject's becoming emotionally upset; 5) inability to find the medication in two attempts; and 6) prolongation of the telephone call—by any means—to ten minutes.

To study the subjects' environment and their non-verbal behavior as well as to halt the experiment before the involvement of any patient, an observer—a staff psychiatrist—was placed on each unit selected. It was his function to terminate the situation by disclosing its true nature when: 1) the nurse had "poured" the medication and started for the patient's bed; 2) she had ended the telephone conversation with a refusal to accept the order; 3) she began to telephone or otherwise contact another professional person; or 4) at the expiration of ten minutes following the end of the call if none of the foregoing alternatives had been adopted.

It was anticipated that a post-incident conversation between observer and subject would allow the observer to assume two additional functions. He could obtain some further material from the subject (as to her inner responses to the experience), and he could offer psychiatric "first-aid" if indicated, to allay any disquieting feelings which might be mobilized by the experiment.

The experiment was conducted during the period from shortly before to shortly after evening visiting hours (7:00–9:00 P.M.) and was performed on medical, surgical, pediatric and psychiatric wards. This period was selected because it is a time when the administration of therapeutic measures is at a minimum. It is also (regrettably) a time when interns and residents tend to absent themselves from the wards; thus the nurse would have to make her own immediate decision regarding the telephone calls.

It was arranged that, as soon as the doctor-observer decided that the ward conditions safely permitted the experiment, he would give a signal by calling in from the ward telephone to the office being used by the investigators, using a code sentence.

One of the nurse investigators visited all of the experimental sites in succession within a half-hour of the incident. She explained the value of further information and requested an appointment for follow-up interview (for which the subject would be offered payment at extra-duty rates). To avoid undue retrospective distortion, the appointments were all made for interviews within 48 hours of the critical incident.

These follow-up interviews, of about 45 minutes each, were relatively unstructured. However, the nurse-investigator had, in the meantime, reviewed the telephone recordings and the reports of the psychiatrist-observers, and she endeavored to cover the following points in her interviews, as opportunity was afforded.

1) Unguided narrative: ("Please tell me what happened last night, starting with whatever you were doing just before the phone call about Astroten.")

2) Emotions: ("What were your feelings at the point where . . .")

3) Discrepancies, if any: ("Are you sure it happened just that way?")

4) Comparable naturally occurring experiences: ("Try to leave out, for the moment, your present knowledge that the incident was experimental.

Suppose it to have been 'real.' Can you think of similar situations which you have experienced? Tell me about them.")

5) Retrospective view: ("What are your feelings about the incident now? What are they about the experience as such?")

6) Eliciting biographical data not otherwise mentioned: age, religion, marital status, children, place(s) of birth and of growing up, nursing experience, other work experience, professional ambitions.

7) Offering support and reassurance if indicated: renewing assurance of subject's anonymity if indicated.

Graduate Nurse Questionnaire

The hospital chosen for the questionnaire phase was a general hospital, as were the first two. Like the others, it had over 500 beds and was located in the Midwest. The subjects given the hypothetical situation were closely matched with the experimental subjects at the public hospital as to: age, sex, race, marital status, length of work week (part-time or full-time), amount of professional experience, type of nursing education (three-year or four-year program), and geographical area of origin. There were 12 graduate nurses in the control group.

The questionnaire was administered in a large conference room with the subjects being provided with writing materials and seated at widely spaced intervals from one another.

The investigator, a physician, spoke to the subjects as follows:

I should like you to imagine yourself, as vividly as possible, in this situation. You are a staff nurse, working 3:00 P.M. to 11:00 P.M. on a ward of a general hospital, and in charge of the ward during that period.

It is the official policy of this hospital that medication orders are to be written by the physician before being carried out by the nurse. This policy fairly often is not adhered to.

You are the only nurse on the ward, the head nurse and the departmental supervisor having left the hospital. None of the house doctors are on ward, which is moderately busy.

Dr. Smith is known to be on the staff of the hospital, but you have not met him. Mr. Jones is one of the patients on your ward.

At about 8:00 P.M. you receive the following telephone message:

"This is Dr. Smith, from Psychiatry, calling. I was asked to see Mr. Jones this morning, and I'm going to have to see him again tonight—I don't have a lot of time, and I'd like him to have had some medication by the time I get to the ward. Will you please check your medicine cabinet and see if you have some Astroten? That's ASTROTEN."

Your medicine cupboard contains a pillbox, bearing the label of the hospital pharmacy, and reading as follows:

ASTROTEN
5 mg. capsules
Usual dose: 5 mg.
Maximum daily dose: 10 mg.

You return to the telephone, and the message continues as follows:

"You have it? Fine. Now will you please give Mr. Jones a stat dose of 20 milligrams—that's four capsules—of Astroten. I'll be up within ten minutes, and I'll sign the order then, but I'd like the drug to have started taking effect."

The nurses were then handed sheets of paper upon which was printed everything which had just been read to them. They were invited to read these sheets, being told that this was merely to help them keep the details in mind.

The investigator then said to the subjects: "Please write down exactly what you would say and do."

After this answer was completed, the investigator said to the subjects, "Please write down the rationale for what you said and did in this episode, that is to say, the considerations influencing your decision."

The next question presented to the subjects was, "What do you think a majority of nurses would have done in this situation?"

The last question offered the subjects was, "What do you think a majority of this group will have written?"

Nursing Student Questionnaire

To compare and contrast with what graduate nurses did in the stress situation and with what they thought they would do in it, the hypothetical case was presented to a group of 21 degree-program nursing students. The method of presentation of the hypothetical situation and of presenting the questionnaire was the same as has been described for the graduate nurses.

RESULTS

Ward Incident

In all, a total of 22 subjects can be reported: 12 from the municipal hospital and ten from the private hospital.

1) Twenty-one subjects would have given the medication as ordered.

2) Telephone calls were invariably brief. Exclusive of time spent in looking for the medication the calls averaged only two minutes in duration. Essentially no resistance to the order was expressed to the caller.

The transcript of a typical telephone call runs as follows:[1]

Nurse: Ward 18; Miss Rolfe.
Caller: Is this the nurse in charge?
Nurse: Yes, it is.
Caller: This is Dr. Hanford, from Psychiatry, calling. I was asked to see Mr. Carson today, and I'm going to have to see him again this evening.
Nurse: Yes.
Caller: I haven't much time and I'd like him to have received some medication by the time I get to the ward. Will you please check the medicine cabinet and see if you have some Astroten.
Nurse: Some what?
Caller: Astroten. That's ASTROTEN.
Nurse: I'm pretty sure we don't.
Caller: Would you take a look, please?
Nurse: Yes, I'll take a look, but I'm pretty sure we don't.

(45 seconds' pause)

Nurse: Hello.
Caller: Well?
Nurse: Yes.
Caller: You have Astroten?
Nurse: Yes.
Caller: O.K. Now, will you give Mr. Carson a stat dose of twenty milligrams—that's four capsules

—of Astroten. I'll be up in about ten minutes, and I'll sign the order then, but I'd like the medicine to have started taking effect.
Nurse: Twenty cap . . . Oh, I mean, twenty milligrams.
Caller: Yes, that's right.
Nurse: Four capsules. O.K.
Caller: Thank you.
Nurse: Surely.

3) There was little or no conscious attempt at delay. Twenty-one of the subjects offered no delay after conclusion of the call.

4) On interview, 11 of the subjects expressed their having had an awareness of the dosage discrepancy. The remainder professed lack of awareness of it.

5) During the telephone conversation none of the subjects insisted that the order be given in written form before implementation, although several sought reassurance that the "doctor" would appear promptly. On interview, 18 of the subjects indicated a general awareness of the impropriety of nonemergency telephone orders. Most of the subjects agreed, however, that it was not an uncommon impropriety.

6) In 17 cases phenomena falling into the category of "psychopathology of everyday life" were noted in the course of the observations. That is to say, the subjects exhibited such behavior as mishearing, misplacing of familiar objects, temporary forgetting, and the like, during the time beginning with the stress telephone call and ending when the on-the-spot observer terminated his conversation with the subject and left the ward.

An example of "psychopathology" of this type is afforded by the transcript of a telephone call given above. When the nurse, in response to the caller's last long statement, begins to say, "twenty capsules," this is undoubtedly an unconsciously determined slip and not a simple misunderstanding.

A very frequent example is the one referred to in paragraph 4, namely the repression of awareness of the dosage discrepancy.

A third example—also frequent—has to do with the subjects' not being able to see the Astroten boxes when they first looked for them. In all cases, the boxes had been placed in prominent locations in the medicine cabinets shortly before the experiment. Yet several times the nurses were unable to locate the boxes at the first trial. When a second

---

[1] All proper names and the designation of the ward have been changed.

trial was insisted upon, the boxes were found rather rapidly.

7) None of the subjects became overtly hostile to the telephone caller or to the observer. Only one of the subjects, the one who refused to accept the order, indicated to the observer that she felt some hostility to the caller during the call.

8) The overt emotional tones of the subjects' responses upon disclosure of the experiment as such varied considerably. The range was from mild scientific interest, through chagrin and mild confusion, to anxiety and some sense of guilt, and, in a few instances, irritation or veiled anger. The modal response could be said to involve chagrin, mild anxiety, and a hint of guilt.

9) Opinions differed as to the details of a "correct" response, but 16 of the subjects felt that the response should have involved greater resistance to the telephone order.

10) Sixteen subjects felt quite unsure that their responses had been typical.

11) On interview, 15 of the subjects spontaneously recalled similar naturally occurring experiences. The remainder could recall such experiences when asked if they had occurred. A majority of the subjects referred to the displeasure of doctors on occasions when nursing resistance had been offered to instructions which had been considered improper.

12) Only one of the subjects seriously questioned the identity of the observer or the propriety of his presence on the ward (before his having identified himself).

Graduate Nurse Questionnaire

The results obtained from the subjects in the hypothetical situation may be summarized as follows:

1) Ten of the 12 subjects reported that they would not have given the medication; two of the subjects said that they would have given the medication.

2) In discussing the rationale for what they would have done, seven subjects referred to the dosage discrepancy in one way or another. Four of the ten subjects who said that they would have refused to give the drug mentioned the dosage discrepancy as the principal reason; the others gave greater emphasis to "hospital policy" or the "necessity for a written order."

3) Seven subjects said they thought that a majority of nurses would handle the situation in the way that they would do. Two subjects said that they thought a majority of nurses would not have handled the situation in their way. Three responses were equivocal.

4) Ten nurses said that they thought a majority of the nurses present would have responded in the same way that they did.

Examples of the subjects' reports as to what they would say and do in the situation presented are as follows:

I'm sorry, but I cannot give the medication until the order is written. If you can't come down, perhaps you could have another doctor come and write the order. I would then be very happy to carry it out. I'm wondering, too, if your order refers to the same Mr. Jones here on my ward, as the label on this box of Astroten states that ten milligrams is the maximum daily dose, and you have stated that you would like for the patient to receive twenty milligrams.

I'm sorry, Dr. Smith, but I cannot give this medication without a written order. This is the policy of the hospital.

Student Nurse Questionnaire

1) Of the 21 nursing students, all believed that they would not have given the medication as ordered.

2) Eight students gave as the principal reason for refusing to accept the order their concern lest the patient suffer ill effects from the apparently excessive dosage.

3) Nineteen of the subjects—either in the fantasied telephone conversations or in giving the rationale for their behavior—specifically referred to the apparently excessive dosage, although in 11 of these instances this concern was not given as the chief objection.

4) In most instances, the conversation which the nursing student fantasied herself holding with the caller was more extended and more illuminating than were any of the actual conversations recorded in the experiment. Even the brief refusals typically included a statement recognizing some of the principal features of the situation.

5) Nearly all replies were distinctly courteous; none were discourteous.

Examples follow of the students' reports as to what they imagined themselves saying and doing in the situation.

Upon finding the medication in the cupboard, I would question the dosage of the medication being twenty milligrams when the maximum dose was ten milligrams. I would not administer the medication unless the supervisor was present to o.k. the order, because I did not know the doctor who phoned in the order and am not accustomed to give any medication unless it is a written order; also, because the medication is one that I am not familiar with, I would be also unfamiliar with the toxic effects.

I'm sorry, sir, but I am not authorized to give any medication without written order, especially one so large over the usual dose and one that I'm unfamiliar with. If it were possible, I would be glad to do it, but this is against hospital policy and my own ethical standards. If you would come to the ward and write the order, I would be glad to administer the drug. In addition to the above, I would include something about the actual dosage.

DISCUSSION

Perhaps the first point to be stressed is that the primary, overt response of the subjects was unexpected and, in particular, unexpectedly uniform. None of the investigators and but one of the highly experienced nurse consultants with whom the project had been discussed in advance predicted the outcome correctly.

It has long been recognized that when there is friction between doctors and nurses, it is the patients who chiefly suffer (7). However, the present study underscores the danger to patients in unresolved difficulties of the nurse-doctor relationship even when there is little or no friction in the usual sense of the word. In a real-life situation corresponding to the experimental one, there would, in theory, be two professional intelligences, the doctor's and the nurse's, working to ensure that a given procedure be undertaken in a manner beneficial to the patient or, at the very least, not detrimental to him. The experiment strongly suggests, however, that in the real-life situation one of these intelligences is, for all practical purposes, non-functioning.

The experiment indicates quite clearly that, insofar as the nurse is concerned, the psychological problems involved in a situation such as the one under discussion are operating to a considerable extent below the threshold of consciousness. Perhaps

the most striking evidence of this is the fact that, whereas nearly all of the subjects quite correctly either repeated the dosage ordered or asked that it be repeated, none of them gave any evidence of conscious concern at the discrepancy between the dose ordered and the alleged maximum safe dose.

Since there is so little evidence of *conscious* conflict in the situation, one may perhaps be inclined to question the existence of appreciable conflict at any level. For a small minority of the subjects, it may indeed be true that their adaptation to situations like the experimental one had reached the point that they experienced no significant conflict, at any level, but, for a majority, the evidence of preconscious or unconscious conflict is persuasive.

It is clear that the subjects, when interviewed, were reacting to at least a double stimulus: to the realization that 1) their behavior, irrespective of what it had been, had been professionally observed without their prior knowledge; and 2) their *specific* behavior had been noted. It was believed, on careful questioning, that the embarrassment, irritation, and such anger as was present were in response to the first portion of the stimulus, namely, the disclosure of observation *per se*. On the other hand, in the face of an attitude on the part of the interviewers which was sympathetic rather than purely neutral, *a majority of the subjects were clearly defensive of their specific handling of the situation.* Moreover, all of those slips of behavior which we have called "psychopathology of everyday life" and of which one or more examples were offered by 17 of the 21 subjects, are indicative of preconscious or unconscious conflict. With the disclosure of the experiment as having been such, elements of the conflict moved into consciousness, as was attested by those reactions which included anxiety, chagrin, and a sense of guilt.

Even in the hypothetical presentation of the critical incident, a considerable amount of subsurface tension was induced. One example of the effects of this tension was the *non sequitur* uttered by the nurse who said, "I'm wondering, too, if your order refers to the same Mr. Jones here on my ward, as the label on this box of Astroten states that ten milligrams is the maximum daily dose, and you have stated that you would like for the patient to receive twenty milligrams." This statement is not far removed from the phenomena referred to in the actual test situation as "psychopathology of everyday life."

There is evidence that a considerable amount of self-deception goes on in the average staff nurse. In nonstressful moments, when thinking about her performance, the average nurse tends to believe that considerations of her patient's welfare and of her own professional honor will outweigh considerations leading to an automatic obedience to the doctor's orders at times when these two sets of factors come into conflict.

Insofar as these matters are concerned, there is in some respects a close correspondence between the way in which nursing students have been taught to think of themselves and their professional functions (*i.e.*, the "official" faculty position),[2] the way in which they actually do think of these things as upperclassmen, and the way in which they will think of them—in moments free of stress—several years later as staff nurses. Concern has been expressed as to the degree to which this view corresponds to reality (4). This investigation tends to show that the view involves an illusion, which, although perhaps shallow, is widespread and enduring. This illusion is, of course, that the nurse will habitually defend the well-being of her patients as she sees it and strive to maintain the standards of her profession.

The present investigation surely has among its implications the idea that all is not well in the professional relationships of nurses and physicians and that these difficulties, whatever they may be, exert a limiting effect upon the nurse's resourcefulness and, in some situations, increase the hazard to which the patients undergoing treatment are exposed. Just because these implications are very strong, it is correct to point out that there is another side to the professional relationship of nurses and physicians, as disclosed in this investigation, and another set of comments to be made about the nurse's effectiveness in crisis situations.

There is no question but that the physician, whether he deserves it or not, is still the recipient of certain quite positive attitudes on the part of the nurse (2, 8). During the data-gathering phase of the present investigation, transcripts were made of 27 nurse-physician telephone conversations, and written records were obtained of 35 fantasied nurse-physician (or nursing student-physician) conversations. In a very great majority of these conversations, a note of courtesy and respect on the part of the nurse toward the physician was unmistakable.

Then there is the matter of trust. The inference is very strong that the nurses' almost invariable acceptance, in the actual stress situation, of the caller as being what he said he was and of doing what he said he was going to do involved a definite (generalized) element of trust.

There is also the matter of efficiency. It has been mentioned that, in the actual test situation, there was a strong, almost uniform tendency for the nurses to implement what they took to be the doctor's wishes promptly and with minimum wasted effort.

It is necessary to recognize that all of these characteristics can, in their place, be of inestimable value to physicians and to their patients. It is easy to recall crisis situations in which the nurse's loyalty to the physician, her appreciation of the value of his judgment, and her willingness and ability to act promptly and efficiently without wasting precious time in discussion have made the difference between life and death for the patient.

The present investigation does not imply that these values should be sacrificed. Rather, it implies that it would be worth an extensive effort on the part of the nursing and medical professions to find ways in which these traditional values can be reconciled with the nurse's fuller exercise of her intellectual and ethical potentialities.

We believe that the typical nurse of today has certain conscious motivations—aspirations and ideals—with respect to her position and functions which may be summarized as the wish both to be and to be considered a professional person in her own right (5). This wish involves several component desires and strivings: mastery of a body of scientific knowledge, application of intelligence, exercise of judgment, assumption of responsibility for patients while offering services to them, gaining the respect of colleagues in related disciplines. All these motivations were expressed by our nurse-subjects collectively, and many of them were expressed by each subject individually.

On the other hand, the nurse retains another group of (largely conscious) motivations with respect to her relationship with the doctor. These include the wish to be liked by him, to receive his gratitude, praise and approval, and to avoid blame and recriminations. These strivings are indicated in various portions of the experimental material: in the courtesy of the telephone conversations (usually ending with a "thank you"), in the unquestioning attitudes; in the promptness of execution of the

---

[2] A point not demonstrated experimentally, but brought out in individual discussions with faculty members.

order; and in the fear of disapproval upon disclosure.

It is to be noted that the first set of motivations is currently being strongly reinforced by nursing education, particularly in its more formal aspects (5, 6). The second set receives reinforcement in the expectations and responses of a majority of physicians. The first set is best served by an intellectual and emotional orientation which is, in many ways, quite active. The second set requires an orientation which is, in some ways, distinctly passive.

The duties and responsibilities of a nurse are, of course, sufficiently extensive and varied to afford opportunity for the gratification of each set of motivations at one time or another. The present study indicates, however, that the two sets can be—or can appear to the nurse to be—mutually incompatible and thus that a state of conflict can be produced on certain occasions when they are stimulated simultaneously. The study indicates further that, in such situations, the second set of motivations will win out in a very great majority of instances. Crucial to this conflict is the fact that in hospital psychodynamics most doctors are male and most nurses are female. Thus the nurse has bio-cultural as well as politico-legal reasons to be passive to the doctor's wishes.

Since this investigation does not shed light upon the motivational states of physicians in their relationships to nurses, it would be premature to offer much comment on the degree to which the conflict in the nurse is reality-based, rather than based upon inferences of questionable accuracy. However, one can assert with confidence the general truth that inner conflict is productive of anxiety and that, beyond a certain low intensity, anxiety tends to reduce the versatility and inventiveness of a personality. Thus, one can feel reasonably certain that, in situations such as the experimental one, solutions affording gratifications to both sets of the nurses' strivings are found far less often than is theoretically possible.

Perhaps the last statement can be clarified by returning to specifics. Any attempt to submit an "ideal solution," a formula of conduct, for the handling of situations like the experimental one would, of course, be unduly rigid and arbitrary. Yet one has the distinct impression that the observance of professional courtesy and loyalty need not have precluded the making of relevant inquiries. It need not have precluded the nurses' making some sort of *appraisal* of the situation and then arriving at a *conscious decision* instead of an automatic response. Whether such a decision would lead to

eventual compliance, to refusal, or to some temporizing measure is not pertinent to the present question. The point is that there appears to be room for greater intellectual activity—the pursuit of which need not be aggressive, destructive, or (to speak of the majority of nurses) unfeminine. One can feel quite sure that, whatever its precise, overt nature, a response based upon a sense of appraisal and decision would be far less likely to produce inner tension than one reached quasi-automatically on the basis of barely perceived inner forces.

This last statement reverts once again to the recognition that the conflict state, in both its interpersonal (nurse versus doctor) and intrapersonal (nurse versus herself) aspects, appears to involve components which do not reach the level of full awareness.

At this point the current presentation reaches something of a dilemma: to conclude without further reference to the nature of these unconscious components may give the false impression that they seem of little significance; to attempt a further discussion of these elements—a discussion based very largely upon inference—may give a false sense of assurance that they have been fully and correctly identified. What follows, therefore, is offered tentatively and merely as the line of speculation which appears best to fit the limited data.

If one accepts the view that the subjects' emotions of shame, embarrassment, and guilt following the experimental incident were derived, at least in part, from the nature of their activities and fantasies during the incident, one has a clue to these less obvious forces. It must be remembered that: 1) the subjects had not behaved in an unusual manner during the incident, but, rather, in their customary fashion; 2) very few of the subjects had any reason to suppose they had behaved differently from the great majority of subjects; 3) neither the psychiatrist-observer nor the nurse-interviewer expressed thoughts or feelings other than those of friendly curiosity, and, of course; 4) in no instance was there the faintest possibility that patient-care had suffered.

Yet the emotions were unmistakable. The question thus becomes, "What subsurface motivations led the nurse to feel ashamed, embarrassed and guilty?" One can dismiss out of hand the speculation that hostile feelings toward the patient (leading to a sense of guilt and thus to a need for punishment or abuse) were of great significance: the life-patterns, the personal and professional adjustments of the subjects make this clear. If a further argument were needed, one is readily at hand:

the individual patients in the experimental situation varied from nurse to nurse and varied widely, yet some elements of the emotional response remained qualitatively almost constant.

Although it rests upon inference and only indirectly upon the data, the likeliest answer to the above question appears to be that the nurse is responding, in situations like the experimental one, on the basis of transference to the doctor. The transference seems typically to involve both an erotic and an aggressive component. On this view, the preconscious or unconscious wish to win the doctor's love and the utilization of reaction-formation against aggressive impulses toward him, born of frustration, lead the nurse at times to compromise her conscious professional standards.

REFERENCES

1. Bullock, R. P. Position, function and job satisfaction of nurses in the social system of a modern hospital. Nurs. Res., *11*: 4–14, 1953.
2. Johnson, M., Martin, H. A sociological analysis of the nurse role. Amer. J. Nurs., *58*: 373–377, 1958.
3. Loeb, M. B. Role definition in the social world of a psychiatric hospital. In Greenblatt, M. *et al.*, eds. *The Patient and the Mental Hospital*, pp. 14–19. Free Press, Glencoe, Illinois, 1957.
4. Mauksch, H. Becoming a nurse: A selective view. Ann. Amer. Acad. Polit. Soc. Sci., *346*: 88–98, 1963.
5. Newton, M. E. Nurses' caps and bachelors' gowns. Amer. J. Nurs., *64*: 73–77, 1964.
6. Peterson, F. K. The new diploma schools. Amer. J. Nurs. *64*: 68–72, 1964.
7. Ruesch, J., Brodsky, C. and Fischer, A. *Psychiatric Care*, pp. 135–136. Grune & Stratton, New York, 1964.
8. Rushing, W. A. Social influence and the social-psychological function of deference: A study of psychiatric nursing. Soc. Forces, *41*: 142–148, 1963.

From Loyalty to Advocacy: A New Metaphor for Nursing

Gerald R. Winslow

Nurses are by far the largest group of health care professionals, numbering well over one million in the United States today. They are often the professionals with whom patients have the most sustained contact. And because of the profession's perceived tradition of holism and "care more than cure," nursing is often upheld as a hopeful paradigm for the future.

But the paradigm is changing. For over a decade, professional nursing has been engaged in profound revision of its ethic. The evidence is abundant: revised codes of ethics, new legal precedents, a flood of books and articles on nursing ethics, and, what may be more significant than any other attestation, a shift in the central metaphors by which nursing structures its own self-perception.

The metaphors associated with nursing are numerous. Two examples that have received considerable attention recently are the nurse as traditional-mother substitute and the nurse as professional contractor.[1] As substitute mother, the nurse cares for sick children (patients) and follows the orders of the traditional father (the physician). As professional contractor, the nurse negotiates a plan for the care of clients (patients) and consults with other contractors (other health care professionals).

Such metaphors are not mere niceties of language. Rather, they interact with the more explicit features of nursing ethics, such as stated rules and principles, in ways that tend to be either mutually supportive or productive of change. The power of metaphors is due in part to their capacity to focus attention on some aspects of reality while concealing others.[2] For example, thinking of the nurse as a parent may highlight certain functions, such as nurture, protection, and domination, while hiding the patient's responsibility for decisions about his or her own care. The metaphor has the ability to create a set of expectations and make some forms of behavior seem more "natural" than others. Thus, if both nurse and patient begin to use the metaphor of nurse as contractor and its associated forms of expression, such as "negotiations," they may come to expect actions in keeping with a "businesslike" relationship.

This article examines the developing changes in nursing ethics by considering two basic metaphors and the norms and virtues consonant with them. The first is nursing as military effort in the battle against disease, a metaphor that permeates many of the early discussions of nursing ethics. It is associated with virtues such as loyalty and norms such as obedience to those of "higher rank" and the maintenance of confidence in authority figures. The second metaphor is nursing as advocacy of patient rights, an essentially legal metaphor that has pervaded much of the literature on nursing ethics within the past decade. The metaphor of advocacy is associated with virtues such as courage and norms such as the defense of the patient against infringements of his or her rights. I did not select these two metaphors for analysis randomly, but, in part, because they have played a prominent role in the formation of ethics within nursing's own literature. More than most others, these metaphors have been espoused by the leaders of nursing, and have had obvious effects on nursing education and practice. Metaphors such as the nurse as surrogate parent, nun, domestic servant, or "handmaiden of the

Winslow, G. R. (1984, June). From loyalty to advocacy: A new metaphor for nursing. *The Hastings Center Report, 14,* 32–40. Reprinted with permission of © The Hastings Center. All rights reserved.

physician" have often been discussed. But these discussions have been almost entirely intended to reject such metaphors and not to uphold them as representative of nursing ideals. Indeed, such metaphors have been used most often to serve as foils for images considered more adequate. On the other hand, the military metaphor, with its language of loyalty and obedience, and the legal metaphor, with its language of advocacy and rights, have served as basic models of ideal nursing practice as proposed in nursing literature.

THE MILITARY METAPHOR

It would be surprising if professional nursing had *not* early adopted the metaphor of military service. Modern nursing is generally acknowledged to have begun with the work of Florence Nightingale, superintendent of nurses in British military hospitals during the Crimean War in the 1850s.[3] Upon her return to England, she continued her work with the military and was instrumental in founding the British Army Medical School. Whatever else Nightingale was, she most certainly was a practitioner and proponent of strict military discipline. And though some have criticized Nightingale's work, the idealization of the "Lady with the Lamp" continues, with rare exceptions, in professional nursing to this day. As two nurses very recently declared: "We think of ourselves as Florence Nightingale—tough, canny, powerful, autonomous, and heroic."[4]

Not only was modern nursing born in a military setting, it also emerged at a time when medicine was appropriating the military metaphor: medicine as war.[5] It has now become difficult to imagine a more pervasive metaphor in contemporary medicine (unless, perhaps, it is medicine as economic enterprise).[6] Disease is the *enemy*, which threatens to *invade* the body and overwhelm its *defenses*. Medicine *combats* disease with *batteries* of tests and *arsenals* of drugs. And young staff physicians are still called house *officers*. But what about nurses?

Perhaps even more than medicine, nursing explicitly chose the military metaphor. It was used to engender a sense of purpose and to explain the training and discipline of the nurse. In the fledgling *American Journal of Nursing*, Charlotte Perry, an early leader, described the education required to produce the "nursing character." Upon entering training, wrote Perry, the student "soon learns the military aspect of life—that it is a life of toil and discipline. . . ." Such discipline, the author asserted, is

part of the "ethics of nursing," and it should be evidenced in the "look, voice, speech, walk, and touch" of the trained nurse. The nurse's "whole being bristles with the effect of the military training she has undergone and the sacrifices she has been called upon to make. A professional manner is the result."[7]

The goal of the military discipline was to produce trained nurses with many of the qualities of good soldiers. The military imagery was neither subtle nor unusual, as a passage from an early book on nursing ethics illustrates:

> [An] excellent help to self devotion is the love a nurse has for the stern strife of her constant battle with sickness . . . "The stern joy which warriors feel, in foemen worthy of their steel," should inspirit the valiant heart of the nurse as it does the heart of the brave soldier who bears long night watches, weary marches, dangerous battles, for the love of the conflict and the keen hope of victory. The soldier in a just war is upheld by this keen joy of battle. So will the nurse be spurred on to devotion by the love of conflict with disease.[8]

The moral force of the metaphor is obvious. Nurses should be prepared for the hardships of night duty, personal danger, weary walking, and so forth. And there can be little doubt that the military metaphor supported a number of nursing behaviors. A minor example is the uniform. Early discussions of nursing ethics almost always included sections on propriety regarding dress. The uniforms of different schools had characteristic differences, reminiscent of the differences signifying various military units. And as nurses progressed up the ranks, stripes were added to their caps and insignia pins to their uniforms. The uniform was always to be worn while "on duty" but never while "off duty." And ordinary clothing was even referred to as "civilian dress."[9]

Some traits are more important to good soldiers than the proper wearing of uniforms. More central, for example, is suitable respect for those of higher rank. Such respect is evidenced both in obedience and in various symbolic gestures of deference. Commenting on nursing ethics, Perry urged her fellow nurses to have proper respect for rank:

> Carrying out the military idea, there are ranks in authority . . . "Please" and "Thank you" are phrases which may be exchanged between those of equal rank. The military command is couched in no uncertain terms. Clear, explicit directions are given, and are received with unquestioning obedience.

Later, Perry added that there are "necessary barriers" between those of different ranks and "familiarity" should not be allowed to dismantle these barriers.[10] The ideal of military obedience was applied often to the nurse's work with physicians. Physicians were the commanding officers. In a published lecture to nurses, one physician did not hesitate to use the military metaphor in explaining why there must be discipline in the hospital "just as in the regiment, [where] we have the captains, the lieutenants, and the sergeants. . . . Obedience to one's superiors is an essential duty of all." The author acknowledged that some of the rules are bound to "appear captious and unfair." Nevertheless, they must be obeyed. And such obedience should be not in a spirit of fear but rather in a spirit of "loyalty."[11]

Loyalty was one of the key virtues of the ideal nurse. In the words of the Nightingale Pledge: "With loyalty will I endeavor to aid the physician in his work. . . ."[12] Nearly every early discussion of nursing ethics includes a major section on loyalty, and the link between loyalty and the military metaphor was strong. For example, the physician just quoted reminded nurses of their obligation: "As in the hospital loyalty to her superior officers is the duty of the nurse, so in private nursing she must be loyal to the medical man who is in attendance on her patient."[13] This sentiment is echoed in Charlotte Aikens's 1916 book on nursing ethics, a standard text for over twenty years:

> Loyalty to the physician is one of the duties demanded of every nurse, not solely because the physician is her superior officer, but chiefly because the confidence of the patient in his physician is one of the important elements in the management of his illness, and nothing should be said or done that would weaken this faith or create doubts as to the character or ability or methods of the physician. . . .[14]

What, then, did it mean for the "trained nurse" to be loyal? It meant, to be sure, faithful and self-sacrificial care of patients. But most of the discussions of loyalty were occupied more with another concern: the protection of confidence in the health care effort. Loyalty meant refusal to criticize the nurse's hospital or training school, fellow nurses, and most importantly, the physician under whom the nurse worked.

Ideally, all these loyalties should harmonize. And nurses were often reminded that being loyal to the physician by preserving the patient's confidence was the same as being loyal to the patient. As one doctor put it: "[L]oyalty to the physician means faithfulness to the patient, even if the treatment is not always in line with what [the nurse] has been taught in the training school. . . . Loyalty to the physician and faithfulness to the patient do not form a twofold proposition, but a single one."[15] The reasoning was supposed to be obvious: the patient's recovery could be aided powerfully by trust in the doctor and the prescribed regimen. Worry over the doctor's competence was likely to worsen the patient's condition not only because of the wasted energy but also because of the lost power of suggestion and the patient's failure to comply with the treatment. The author of a text on nursing ethics summed up the idea:

> Confidence and skepticism are both contagious, and we know very well how important it often is for a patient's cure that he should have the attitude of faith and confidence in his physician. . . . [It] is unkind indeed to destroy a confidence which is so beneficent and comforting.[16]

The moral power of this reasoning should not be overlooked. Nurses accepted as their solemn obligation assisting in the patient's recovery. And nurses were taught repeatedly that the "*faith* that people have in a physician is as much a healing element as is any medicinal treatment."[17] Thus, even if the physician blundered, the patient's confidence should usually be maintained at all costs. To quote an early nursing text:

> If a mistake has been made in treating a patient, the patient is not the person who should know it if it can be kept from him, because the anxiety and lack of confidence that he would naturally feel might be injurious to him and retard his recovery.[18]

But what if the nurse finally concluded that the confidence in the physician simply was not merited? It is one of the myths of a later generation that nurses of the past never questioned loyalty to the physician. In speeches, journals, and books, leading nurses complained that loyalty to the physician often was not deserved and even more often was not returned in kind.[19] And the difficult moral dilemmas faced by nurses were usually discussed in terms of conflicts of loyalties. For example, in an earlier editorial titled "Where Does Loyalty End?" the author claimed that many letters from nurses asked essentially the same questions: "Where does the nurse's loyalty to the doctor end? And is she required to be untruthful or to practice deceit in order to uphold the reputation of the physician at her own expense or that of the patient?"[20]

The published letters revealed the kinds of cases troubling nurses. One told how a physician inserted a catheter too far into the patient's bladder—a mistake that, according to the nurse, required surgery to correct. The nurse reported that she was blamed in order to protect the doctor's reputation. Another nurse told how a physician failed to remove a surgical sponge, causing the patient great suffering and near-death. When the problem became apparent, the nurse was unable to keep the truth from the family. Later, the doctor chastised the nurse for failure to conceal the truth. The writer claimed that "nurses are taught that they must stand by the doctor whether he is right or wrong." But, she concluded, if this means lying to the patient in order "to defend the doctor then I don't care for the profession. . . ."[21]

Such letters (and many similar discussions in early nursing literature) indicate that conflicts of loyalties tended to focus on two main issues: truthtelling and physicians' competency. Obviously, these two were often linked. Nurses felt obliged to protect doctors even if the care seemed deficient and the truth suffered. But in many cases the truth was concealed because physicians did not want their patients to know their diagnoses. In her text on ethics, Aikens complained: "From the beginning of her career [the nurse] is impressed with the idea that . . . it is an unpardonable sin to lie to a doctor about a patient but perfectly pardonable, and frequently very desirable, to lie to a patient about his own condition."[22] So, although lying was often roundly condemned, clearly it was often the "order" of the day. Dissonance was the inevitable result. Nurses were pleased, as Lena Dietz put it, to "enjoy a confidence such as is placed in no other women in the world. . . . The fact that they are nurses is accepted as an unquestionable guarantee of honesty."[23] But, at times, loyalty to the "superior officers" left the guarantee more than a little tattered.

In all likelihood loyal protection of the physician often was motivated, in no small measure, by the nurse's desire for self-protection. In the early years of nursing, the goal of most graduate nurses was to leave the hospital and become "private duty nurses."[24] The names of those available for this work were obtained from the local "registry" (kept variously by hospitals, nurses' associations, or medical associations) or simply by word of mouth. Technically, such nurses were hired directly by the patient. But in reality the attending physician was highly influential in the selection of the private nurse and, if need be, in the nurse's dismissal. Understandably, this arrangement led at times to conflicting interests and loyalties. One doctor grumbled: "Paid by the patient, or someone close to him, and not by the physician, [the nurse] sometimes seems to think that it is safest to 'stand in' with the patient, and actually obey him, rather than the physician."[25] The patient paid the wages of the nurse, but the doctor was supposed to be in charge. The financial implications of this arrangement were not lost on nurses. Aikens wrote: "Not infrequently, a nurse is torn between her desire to be loyal to the patient's interests, and not disloyal to the doctor, who has it in his power to turn calls in her direction, and influence other doctors to do the same, or the reverse."[26]

Troubled at times by conflicting loyalties and worried about employment, nurses advocated a number of strategies for coping with some doctors' apparent ineptitude. Of these strategies, four stand out.

First, the nurse could faithfully obey all orders and simply assume that the doctor knew best. Isabel Robb, in the first American book on nursing ethics, wrote: "Apart from the fact that [the nurse] may be quite wrong in her opinions, her sole duty is to obey orders, and so long as she does this, she is not to be held responsible for untoward results."[27] On this, the prevailing view, the nurse was supposed to be absolved from guilt so long as she followed orders. The doctrine of *respondeat superior* generally did offer nurses legal protection. But moral protection is not always so easily secured, hence the additional strategies.

Second, the nurse could gently question the doctor's orders. Sara Parsons suggested to her nursing colleagues that when the nurse "becomes sufficiently experienced to detect a mistake, she will, of course, call [the doctor's] attention to it by asking if her understanding of the order is correct."[28] This approach of nurses making what amounts to recommendations in the form of questions is apparently long-lived. Recent work indicates that it is still an expected part of the "doctor-nurse game."[29]

A third maneuver was consultation with some other authority figure.[30] In the hospital, the nursing supervisor was the most likely candidate. But the private duty nurse had no such recourse. This difficulty led one author to propose that the nurse call the family's "religious advisor" in a confidential attempt to engineer a change of physicians.[31]

Finally, the nurse could withdraw from the case, or refuse the physician's patients from the beginning. If the doctor was intolerably deficient, Robb counseled, the nurse could "always find some means of refusing to take charge of the nursing of his patients. . . ." Robb added, however, "[O]nce having put herself under [the doctor], let her remain loyal and carry out his orders to the letter."[32] And in his lecture to nurses, a physician put the same point bluntly: "Better to be an honest deserter than a traitor in the camp."[33]

Better than deserter or traitor, however, was the nurse as loyal soldier. Then the world changed. Or at least the metaphors did.

THE LEGAL METAPHOR

It would be foolish to set a date to the changing of nursing's self-image. The process has been gradual, the way tortuous. As was noted earlier, nurses' criticism of the "one-sided loyalty" expected of them dates back nearly to the beginning of the profession. And by 1932, Annie Warburton Goodrich, an acknowledged leader, could speak of nursing's "militarism, that splendid drilling in subordination of self to the machine" as a feature that the profession was attempting to "modify, if not abolish."[34]

Even if the abolition has come slowly, some major events can be identified. For example, a significant blow to nursing's ethic of military loyalty occurred in an unlikely place in 1929. In Manila, a newly graduated nurse, Lorenza Somera, was found guilty of manslaughter, sentenced to a year in prison, and fined one thousand pesos because she followed a physician's order. The physician had mistakenly called for the preparation of cocaine injections (he meant procaine) for a tonsillectomy patient. Witnesses agreed that the physician ordered the cocaine, that Somera verified that order, and that the physician administered the injections. But the physician was acquitted and Somera found guilty because she failed to *question* the orders. The Supreme Court upheld the lower court's decision.[35]

Nurses around the world (and especially in the United States, because the Philippine Islands were under U.S. jurisdiction) were at first stunned and then incensed. A successful protest campaign was organized, and Somera was pardoned before serving a day of her sentence. But the whole affair left an enduring impression on nurses. The doctrine of *respondeat superior* turned out to be thin security. Never again could nurses be taught simply to follow doctors' orders. Even now, over fifty years later, nursing texts still refer to *Somera* as proof of nurses' independent accountability.[36]

But, despite *Somera* and later similar cases, the tradition of loyalty to the physician retained considerable power. This strength was illustrated by the first codes of nursing ethics. Nurses had been calling for a code of ethics before the turn of the century. But not until 1926 was the first "suggested code" for nurses proposed. By present standards this proposed code must be judged remarkably enlightened. It speaks of broad principles and, with regard to nurses' relationship to physicians, it says that "neither profession can secure complete results without the other." When the proposed code discusses loyalty, it says that "loyalty to the motive which inspires nursing should make the nurse fearless to bring to light any serious violation of the ideals herein expressed." Perhaps not surprisingly, the code failed to gain acceptance.[37] The next attempt came in 1940. This proposal was much more similar to what later became the accepted tenets.[38] Obligations to the physicians were central. For example, the code adopted by the American Nurses' Association (ANA) called for nurses to verify and carry out the physician's orders, sustain confidence in the physician, and report incompetency or unethical conduct "only to the proper authority."[39] A similar code, approved by the International Council of Nurses in 1953, spelled out the nurse's obligation to follow the physician's orders "loyally" and to maintain confidence in the physician.[40]

In the 1960s and 1970s the image of the loyal nurse began to be significantly revised. The forces for change in health care delivery during the past two decades are too numerous and complex to analyze here. In his social history of medicine, Paul Starr describes the "stunning loss of confidence" sustained by medicine during the 1970s. The formerly unquestioned mandate of the "sovereign profession" was challenged with increased frequency. Consumerism was strengthening. And the ever-higher costs of medical care along with the perceived arrogance of many in the medical profession irritated large numbers of consumers. Moreover, medicine was viewed increasingly as a large, impersonal institution, a privileged and protected castle constantly resisting needed modifications. For nursing, a profession populated almost entirely by women, the growth of feminism also proved a highly important development. These forces, and many others, achieved sharp focus in the patients' rights movement which, in Starr's words, "went beyond traditional demands for more medical care and challenged the distribution of power and expertise."[41] Few in the health care system seemed more eager for the challenge to succeed than nurses. It was hardly surprising, therefore, that leaders of the patients' rights movement turned to nurses in the search for "patient advocates." For example, George Annas, an attorney and author of *The Rights of Hospital Patients*, called for nurses to accept the new role of patient advocacy.[42] It is worthy of note that Annas prefaced his appeal to nurses by explicitly attacking the military metaphor. Nurses who accepted such traditional images would be poorly equipped to be patient advocates. At times, orders would have to be challenged. But, Annas argued, properly retrained nurses had the potential to play a "key role" in patient advocacy.[43]

In rejecting the metaphor of nurse as loyal soldier, Annas offered a replacement—the nurse as courageous advocate. The image was essentially legal. As a significant part of their retraining, for example, nurses needed "some clear understanding of the law" relating to patients' rights. *"The powers of the advocate would be precisely the legal powers of the patient."* Acceptance of the advocacy role entailed a readiness to enter disputes. Patients needed assurance that their advocate was "someone who could be trusted to fight for their rights." Included in Annas's list of rights are those that became the standards of the patients' rights movement: the right to adequate information about proposed medical procedures, the right to refuse or accept any or all such procedures, the right to full information about prognosis and diagnosis, the right to leave the hospital, and so forth. To these canons, Annas added the right of the patient to around-the-clock access to a patients' rights advocate. Clearly, the assumptions were that patients' rights were often being threatened and someone was needed continually to contend for patients. Annas hoped that nurses would be among those to take up the fight. He was not to be disappointed—not, that is, if the volume of nursing literature promoting the role of nurse as patient advocate is a measure of success.

From the mid-1970's to the present, literally scores of nursing books and articles have appeared advocating advocacy.[44] It is now not at all uncommon for nurses to argue, as one recently did, that "the nurse is the ideal patient advocate!"[45] And at least two thoughtful nurse-philosophers have argued that the concept of advocacy is the most appropriate philosophical foundation for the nursing profession.[46] After all, nurses usually have the most regular contact with the patient. And more than any other health care professionals, nurses tend to be concerned with the well-being of the *whole* patient. Moreover, nurses have a long tradition of educating patients, so it is entirely natural for nurses to accept responsibility for assuring that patients are properly informed. Finally, nurses and patients should make obvious and genuine allies since both groups have often suffered the indignities of powerlessness in the modern health care system. Who, then, could function better as a patient advocate than a nurse?

So the arguments go. And, the result has been more than a flurry of words. The metaphor has had a way of "working into life." For example, one school of nursing now requires all of its advanced students to devise and carry out an "Advocacy Project."[47] A student might discover, for instance, that elderly patients in a nursing home feel a need for legal advice. The student would develop a plan for securing such advice and then attempt to put the plan into action.

During the 1970s, the concept of advocacy was also incorporated into nursing's codes of ethics. In its 1973 revision, the International Council of Nurses' code dropped all mention of loyal obedience to the physician's orders.[48] Instead, the code said that the "nurse's primary responsibility is to those people who require nursing care," and the "nurse takes appropriate action to safeguard the individual when his care is endangered by a co-worker or any other person." Even more striking, in some respects, are the 1976 revisions of the ANA code. The revised code requires nurses to protect "the client" from the "incompetent, unethical, or illegal practice of any person."[49] In the interpretive statements on this point, the code makes explicit use of the language of advocacy: "[I]n the role of client advocate, the nurse must be alert to and take appropriate action regarding any instances of incompetent, unethical, or illegal practice(s) by any member of the health care team or the health care system itself, or any action on the part of others that is prejudicial to the client's best interests." The revised ANA code is revealing not only because of this addition but also because of its subtractions. Gone are the rules obliging nurses to maintain confidence in physicians or obey their orders. In fact, "physician" does not even appear in the revised code.

Nursing's adoption of the ethic of advocacy has brought to life a whole new genre of nursing literature: the nurse-as-advocate short story. In a recent example, a nurse detailed her attempts to become an "advocate for the clients." While employed as director of nursing in a county health department, she became aware of the very poor record of maternity care at one hospital. The postpartum infection rate was nearly three times higher than the national average. And the Apgar scores of many

newborns were lower than should have been expected statistically. But the hospital resented having the problems called to public attention and
resisted any suggested changes. For her efforts, the
nurse was ostracized by the health care community. Finally, she resigned before she could be
fired. In her view, the theories about advocacy
were fine, but "the problem lies in putting these
theories into action."[50] Unfortunately, this account
is typical of most published nurse-as-advocate stories.[51] They usually describe a nurse's attempt to
defend a patient or group of patients against mistreatment. Most often, the endeavor fails because
the system overpowers the nurse. The patient suffers or dies. The nurse gets fired or resigns in out-
rage. The system goes on. As literature, the stories
tend to have the features of tragedy (though the
flaw is in the character of the system rather than
the advocate).

Of such stories, none has been more widely publicized as an example of patient advocacy than
the case of Jolene Tuma.[52] In March 1976, Tuma, a
clinical instructor of nursing, was asked by a cancer patient about alternatives to chemotherapy.
The patient was apprehensive about the therapy.
She did not want to question her physician further,
however, because he had already indicated his conviction that chemotherapy was the only acceptable
treatment. Tuma knew that discussing options
with the patient would be risky. In fact, she told the
patient that such a conversation would not be
"exactly ethical." Nevertheless, Tuma proceeded to
discuss a number of alternatives about which the
patient had questions, including nutritional therapy and Laetrile. The patient then decided to continue chemotherapy. But, in spite of the efforts, she
died two weeks later. One of the patient's children
informed the attending physician about Tuma's discussion with the patient. The physician protested
to Tuma's employing college and to the Board of
Nurse Examiners of Idaho. As a result, Tuma lost
her job and her nursing license. The state's nursing
board concluded that Tuma had interfered unethi-
cally with the physician-patient relationship. During the conflict, Tuma wrote to a nursing journal
and described her predicament:

> Does the nurse have the right to assist the pa-
> tient toward full and informed consent? Litiga-
> tion against nurses already shows us we have the
> responsibility when we do not properly inform
> the patient. But do we have the authority to
> go along with this responsibility as the patient's
> advocate?[53]

Tuma's case might have ended like so many other
nurse-as-advocate stories except for the fact that she
appealed the state board's ruling. Three years later,
the Supreme Court of Idaho ruled that the nursing
board had been wrong in suspending Tuma's license.[54] It is difficult, however, to assess the extent
of Tuma's victory. She did not regain her teaching
position, she suffered through three years of legal
appeals, and it was too late to change the outcome
for the patient. Certainly, the physician and at least
some of the patient's family were displeased by her
actions. Still, Tuma believes that her actions were
justified. She feels that her personal sacrifice has
been repaid not only by the assurance that the patient's rights were defended but also by the public
attention directed toward the rightful role of nurses
as patient advocates.[55] And a recently published poll
of 12,500 nurses reveals that Tuma has strong support from her colleagues. Over 80 percent of the
respondents agreed that a nurse who acted as Tuma
did would be doing the "right thing."[56]

The response of nurses to the Tuma case is a
clear indication of the profession's changing self-
perception. The new metaphor of nurse as advocate has risen to power. Indeed, if the profession's
literature during the past decade is taken as primary evidence, then it can be said safely that no
other symbol has so captured imagination or won
acceptance within nursing as that of the advocate.

ASSESSING THE ADVOCACY METAPHOR

It is generally easier to criticize the metaphors of
an earlier age than to evaluate those now regnant.
But further criticism of the military metaphor is
hardly in order. The nurse as loyal soldier is dead.
Among nurses, mourners of the metaphor's passage are either nonexistent or well hidden. Meanwhile, the metaphor of nurse as patient advocate
has nearly achieved the status of a slogan. Criticism of patient advocacy in nursing literature is
virtually unknown.[57]

But those who hope that the rise of advocacy is a
positive sign of a maturing profession (and I am
among them) should give careful attention to the
ambiguities and potential criticisms of the advocacy role. I mention only five:

1. *The meaning of advocacy needs clarification.*
Metaphors tend to be unruly. Part of their richness
is their capacity to generate new and at times

surprising perspectives. Thus, referring to nurses as advocates opens apparently boundless possibilities for new understandings. And, as might be expected, a survey of the nursing literature on advocacy soon reveals that the metaphor is invoked in a variety of ways, some of which may be incompatible. At times, advocacy is construed so broadly that it seems to mean something like "doing the best for the patient." But most supporters of advocacy have in mind more specific actions such as helping the patient to obtain needed health care, assuring the quality of health care, defending the patient's rights (such as the right of informed consent), serving as a liaison between the patient and health care professionals, and counseling the patient in order to alleviate fear.

In one of the few thorough discussions, Sally Gadow proposes a model of "existential" advocacy. In her view, the ideal is "that individuals be *assisted* by nursing to *authentically* exercise their freedom of self-determination."[58] Gadow argues for a type of advocacy that avoids paternalistic manipulation of the patient on the one hand and reduction of the nurse to a mere technician who is unwilling to recommend alternatives on the other hand. Whether most nurses would agree entirely with Gadow's interpretation, most discussions of the nurse as advocate would benefit both from Gadow's example of careful analysis and from her thesis. In my view, the central, moral significance of the advocacy metaphor lies in its power to shape actions intended to protect and enhance the personal autonomy of patients. Further clarification of this significance is essential if the metaphor is to rise above the level of a simple slogan.

2. *The states' nurse practice acts need revision.* Since 1971, states have been revising practice acts to allow for newly expanded nursing roles.[59] But changes in the laws generally have not kept pace with nursing's adoption and understanding of advocacy. And, as *Tuma* illustrates, the legal limits are often unclear. What does it mean, for example, to interfere with the physician-patient relationship? Does unacceptable interference include suggesting a second medical opinion? What about recommending a change of physicians? As a result of such uncertainties, nurses who set out to be patient advocates may find themselves needing a lawyer. One nurse recently reported just such an experience. She was present when a surgical resident botched a tracheotomy and severed the patient's carotid artery. The patient bled to death. The nurse decided that for the sake of other patients she should report the resident. But the medical

director cautioned the nurse not to pursue the matter unless she hired an attorney. As the nurse put it: "Dr. X kills the patient and I need a lawyer."[60] The threat of retaliation and the loss of professional and economic security are bound to have a chilling effect on nurses' willingness to function as patient advocates.

To be effective, the calls for nurses to become patient advocates must be accompanied by political action aimed at needed revision of the states' laws. But when it comes to politics, a more apt metaphor for nursing might be that of slumbering giant. Nursing's status as the largest health care profession generally has not translated into commensurate political strength. As the profession has adopted the ethic of advocacy, however, nurses have begun to pay more attention to the need for political action.[61] We should hope that the effect of such action will be to make patient advocacy a less dangerous activity.

3. *Patients (or their families) are often unprepared to accept the nurse as advocate.* In at least one important respect, nurses are unlike many other professionals whom the patient might engage for services. The patient is usually free to accept or reject the efforts of, say, a physician or an attorney. But in most instances the patient is not involved in the selection of his or her nurse. Thus, the nurse who functions as a patient advocate usually does so for one who has not chosen the nurse's services and who does not *expect* the nurse to serve as an advocate.

There is abundant evidence that society generally accepts a more traditional role for nurses. On this subject, nursing literature is peppered with analyses, laments, and calls for change.[62] But old metaphors die hard. And it is a frustrating fact that vestigial images of the nurse as loyal soldier, substitute parent, assistant physician, or even handmaiden will probably remain in the minds of the public long after most nurses have rejected them. For patient advocacy to be fully successful, further attention must be given to the mechanisms for appropriate public education.

4. *Advocacy is frequently associated with controversy.* It would be a rare advocacy story that did not include a measure of discord. The patient who needs an advocate is often being mistreated by someone's action or inaction. The nurse accepts the responsibility of contending for the rights of the patient; work that may involve conflict.

Some people may thrive on controversy. Many do not. Nursing educators who share the ethic of advocacy must ask how well the nursing curriculum prepares nurses to cope with the potential conflicts. They should also ask how an ethic that makes advocacy central avoids the risk of being *unduly* contentious.

5. *As advocate, the nurse is bound to be torn, at times, by conflicting interests and loyalties.* Metaphors can conceal as well as reveal facets of reality. The advocacy metaphor may hide the depths of potential conflicts by leaving the impression that only loyalty to the patient counts. But as Susan Thollaug, a nurse interested in patient advocacy, put it: "We can easily underestimate the difficulty of being a patient advocate, forgetting how divided our loyalties tend to be."[63] Patients come and go; the nurse's employing institution and professional colleagues tend to remain. To admit this is not merely to say that nurses may be tempted, along with other mortals, to place self-interest ahead of professional or moral obligations. The issue is more complicated morally. Most of us would acknowledge loyalty to associates as a virtue. An unwillingness to expose a colleague's shortcomings to public view and a desire to preserve confidence in one's institution are among the characteristic features of loyalty. Deeming such loyalty a vice would be a mistake likely to produce detrimental results for both the health care providers and their patients. The obvious difficulty is deciding when the role of advocacy must take precedence over the legitimate concerns of loyalty. Borderline cases, which bring us to the edges of our ability to reason morally, are inevitable. But no ethic of advocacy could be called adequate without a place for the virtue of loyalty.

These five concerns illustrate the impediments that must be overcome if nursing's new ethic of advocacy is to be most effective. But my discussion of these difficulties is in no way intended to suggest that nursing's adoption of advocacy is meaningless, undesirable, or impossible. I believe that nursing's change of images is a hopeful sign for a developing profession. Of course, no metaphor can convey fully the complexities of the profession's moral virtues and obligations. But the season for the nurse as advocate has arrived. Nursing is still a relatively new profession, and one that has often experienced the indignities of powerlessness. The language of advocacy provides a new way to express a growing sense of professional responsibility and power. Once an ethic of "good soldiers," with loyal obedience at its core, made sense to nurses. But nursing has been moving away from a heteronomous morality of constraint and toward a more autonomous morality of cooperation. An ethic of advocacy, with a concern for rights and the

virtue of courage at its center, is an important development in this process of change.

ACKNOWLEDGMENTS

An earlier version of this paper was presented to the 1983 National Endowment for the Humanities Summer Seminar, "Principles and Metaphors in Biomedical Ethics," under the direction of James F. Childress. I wish to thank Professor Childress for his thoughtful comments and encouragement. I also wish to thank the other participants in the seminar: J. Brian Benestad, Albert Howard Carter, Ruth Caspar, Daniel Friedman, David M. Holley, David N. James, Shannon Jordan, Janet Dickey McDowell, Phillip J. Miller, Debra C. Rosenthal, and W. D. White. Finally, for her thorough comments and criticisms, I am indebted to Betty Wehtje Winslow, a nurse.

REFERENCES

1. See, for example, Sheri Smith, "Three Models of the Nurse-Patient Relationship," in *Nursing: Images and Ideals*, Stuart F. Spicker and Sally Gadow, eds. (New York: Springer Publishing Company, 1980), pp. 176–88.

2. I am thinking of the work of George Lakoff and Mark Johnson, "Conceptual Metaphor in Everyday Language," *The Journal of Philosophy* 78 (August 1980), 453–86. See also the same authors' book, *Metaphors We Live By* (Chicago: University of Chicago Press, 1980).

3. Richard H. Shryock, *The History of Nursing* (Philadelphia: W. B. Saunders Company, 1959), pp. 273–84. For an interesting and recent discussion of Nightingale's work see Irene Palmer, "From Whence We Came," in *The Nursing Profession: A Time to Speak Out*, Norma L. Chaska, ed. (New York: McGraw-Hill Book Company, 1983), pp. 1–28.

4. Claire Fagin and Donna Diers, "Nursing as Metaphor," *The New England Journal of Medicine* 309 (July 14, 1983), 117.

5. Susan Sontag, *Illness as Metaphor* (New York: Farrar, Straus and Giroux, 1978). Sontag suggests that medicine adopted the military metaphor in the late nineteenth century about the time germ theory was accepted. My thoughts on medicine's use of the military metaphor have also been influenced by an unpublished paper

by Virginia Warren, "Medicine as War," and by James Childress, *Who Should Decide? Paternalism in Health Care* (New York: Oxford University Press, 1982), p. 7.

6. Rashi Fein has recently complained that medicine is now being corrupted by "the language of the marketplace." "What Is Wrong with the Language of Medicine?" *The New England Journal of Medicine* 306 (April 8, 1982), 863–64.

7. Charlotte M. Perry, "Nursing Ethics and Etiquette," *The American Journal of Nursing* 6 (April 1906), 450–51.

8. Edward Francis Garsche, *Ethics and the Art of Conduct for Nurses* (Philadelphia: W. B. Saunders, 1929), p. 189.

9. Isabel Hampton Robb, *Nursing Ethics: For Hospital and Private Use* (Cleveland: E. C. Koeckert Publishing, 1900), p. 118.

10. Perry, "Nursing Ethics," p. 452.

11. T. Percy, C. Kirkpatrick, *Nursing Ethics* (Dublin: Dublin University Press, 1917), p. 24.

12. The Nightingale Pledge was first used by Farrand Training School, Harper Hospital, Detroit in 1893. For the text of the pledge, see Anne J. Davis and Mila A. Aroskar, *Ethical Dilemmas and Nursing Practice* (New York: Appleton-Century-Crofts, 1978), pp. 12–13.

13. Kirkpatrick, *Nursing Ethics*, p. 35.

14. Charlotte Albina Aikens, *Studies in Ethics for Nurses* (Philadelphia: W. B. Saunders Company, 1916), p. 44.

15. Thomas E. Satterthwaite, "Private Nurses and Nursing: With Recommendations for Their Betterment," *New York Medical Journal* 91 (January 15, 1910), 109.

16. Garsche, *Ethics and Conduct for Nurses*, p. 234.

17. Lena Dixon Dietz, *Professional Problems of Nurses*, 3rd. ed. rev. (Philadelphia: F. A. Davis Company, 1939), p. 165.

18. Sara E. Parsons, *Nursing Problems and Obligations* (Boston: Whitcomb and Barrows, 1916), p. 32. Parsons later allows for informing the patient about a mistake, after the patient has recovered sufficiently.

19. See for example Aikens, *Ethics for Nurses*, p. 297. See also S. I. Cabiniss, "Ethics," *The American Journal of Nursing* 3 (August 1903), 875–79. Cabiniss wrote: "What of the ingratitude . . . of physicians who accept all courtesy and loyalty and give none in return?" p. 878.

20. "Where Does Loyalty End?" (editorial) *The American Journal of Nursing* 10 (January 1910), 230–31.

21. "Where Does Loyalty to the Physician End?" (letters) *The American Journal of Nursing* 10 (January 1910), 274, 276.

22. Aikens, *Ethics for Nurses*, p. 192.

23. Dietz, *Professional Problems*, p. 162.

24. Susan Reverby, "Re-forming the Hospital Nurse: The Management of American Nursing," in *The Sociology of Health and Illness: Critical Perspectives*, Peter Conrad and Rochelle Kern, eds. (New York: St. Martin's Press, 1981), pp. 220–33. See also Jo Ann Ashley, *Hospitals, Paternalism, and the Role of the Nurse* (New York: Teachers College Press, 1976).

25. Satterthwaite, "Private Nurses," p. 109.

26. Aikens, *Ethics for Nurses*, p. 297.

27. Robb, *Nursing Ethics*, p. 250.

28. Parsons, *Nursing Problems*, p. 58.

29. L. I. Stein, "The Doctor-Nurse Game," *Archives of General Psychiatry* 16 (1967), 699–703. See also Sandra Weiss and Naomi Remen, "Self-Limiting Patterns of Nursing Behavior within a Tripartite Context Involving Consumers and Physicians," *Western Journal of Nursing Research* 5 (Winter 1983), 77–89.

30. Dietz, *Professional Problems*, p. 163.

31. Garesche, *Ethics and Conduct for Nurses*, p. 233.

32. Robb, *Nursing Ethics*, p. 251.

33. Kirkpatrick, *Nursing Ethics*, p. 24.

34. Annie Warburton Goodrich, *The Social Significance of Nursing* (New York: Macmillan, 1932), p. 167.

35. *Somera Case*, G. R. 31693 (Philippine Islands, 1929).

36. See, for example, Janine Fiesta, *The Law and Liability: A Guide for Nurses* (New York: John Wiley and Sons, 1983), p. 181.

37. For the entire text see "A Suggested Code," *The American Journal of Nursing* 26 (August 1926), 599–601.

38. See "A Tentative Code," *The American Journal of Nursing* 40 (September 1940), 977–80.

39. "A Code for Nurses," *The American Journal of Nursing* 50 (April 1950), 196.

40. "International Code of Nursing Ethics," *The American Journal of Nursing* 53 (September 1953), 1070.

41. Paul Starr, *The Social Transformation of American Medicine* (New York: Basic Books, 1982), pp. 379, 389.

42. George Annas, "The Patient Rights Advocate: Can Nurses Effectively Fill the Role?" *Supervisor Nurse* 5 (July 1974), 21–25. For another, similar work see George Annas and Joseph Healey,

"The Patient Rights Advocate," *Journal of Nursing Administration* 4 (May–June 1974), 25–31.

43. Annas, "Patient Rights Advocate: Can Nurses Effectively Fill the Role?" p. 23.

44. Here is but a small sample: Jane E. Chapman and Harry Chapman, *Behavior and Health Care: A Humanistic Helping Process* (St. Louis: C. V. Mosby, 1975). This was one of the first works to set forth an "advocacy model" for health care delivery. Although it was not directed specifically to nurses, it had an obvious impact on subsequent nursing literature. M. Patricia Donahue, "The Nurse: A Patient Advocate?" *Nursing Forum* 17 (1978), 143–51. Corinne Sklar, "Patient's Advocate—A New Role for the Nurse?" *The Canadian Nurse* 75 (June 1979), 39–41. Mary Elizabeth Payne, "The Nurse as Patient Advocate in the Rehab Setting," *ARN* (The Official Journal of the Association of Rehabilitation Nurses) 4 (September–October 1979), 9–11. Mary Kohnke, "The Nurse as Advocate," *The American Journal of Nursing* 80 (November 1980), 2038–40. Ruth Purtilo and Christine Cassel, "Professionalism and Advocacy," in *Ethical Dimensions in the Health Professions* (Philadelphia: W. B. Saunders, 1981). Sally H. Durel, "Advocacy: A Function of the Community Mental Health Nurse," *Virginia Nurse* 49 (Spring 1981), 33–36. Marzena Laszewski, "Patient Advocacy in Primary Nursing," *Nursing Administration Quarterly* 5 (Summer 1981), 28–30. M. Josephine Flaherty, "This Nurse *Is* a Patient Advocate," *Nursing Management* 12 (September 1981), 12–13. George Castledine, "The Nurse as the Patient's Advocate: Pros and Cons," *Nursing Mirror* 153 (November 11, 1981), 38–40. H. Terri Brower, "Advocacy: What It Is," *Journal of Gerontological Nursing* 8 (March 1982), 141–43.

45. Payne, "The Nurse as Patient Advocate," p. 9.

46. Leah L. Curtin, "The Nurse as Advocate: A Philosophical Foundation for Nursing," *ANS* (Advances in Nursing Science) 1 (April 1979), 1–10. Sally Gadow, "Existential Advocacy: Philosophical Foundation of Nursing," in *Nursing: Images and Ideals*, pp. 79–101. Both authors wish to distinguish the concept of advocacy that they present as the philosophical basis for nursing from the concept of advocacy associated with the patient rights movement. But it is clear that most of their nursing colleagues who have written on the subject of advocacy have either failed to appreciate the distinction or rejected it.

47. M. Jo Namerow, "Integrating Advocacy into the Gerontological Nursing Major," *Journal of Gerontological Nursing* 8 (March 1982), 149–51.

48. International Council of Nurses, "Code for Nurses," reprinted in Davis and Aroskar, *Ethical Dilemmas*, pp. 13–14.

49. American Nurses' Association, *Code for Nurses with Interpretive Statements* (Kansas City: American Nurses' Association, 1976), p. 8.

50. Christine Spahn Smith, "Outrageous or Outraged: A Nurse Advocate Story," *Nursing Outlook* 28 (October 1980), 624–25.

51. See for example Flaherty, "This Nurse *Is* a Patient Advocate."

52. Of the many accounts of this case, the one I find most thorough and perceptive is in Purtilo and Cassel, *Ethical Dimensions*, pp. 126–137.

53. Jolene Tuma, Letter to the Editor, *Nursing Outlook* 25 (September 1977), 846.

54. In *re Tuma*. Supreme Court of the State of Idaho. 1977 Case 12587.

55. Purtilo and Cassel report this to be Tuma's position on the basis of personal communication. See *Ethical Dimensions*, p. 136.

56. Ronni Sandroff, "Protecting the M.D. or the Patient: Nursing's Unequivocal Answer," *RN* 44 (February 1981), 28–33.

57. I know of only one significant essay that is critical of nurses' adoption of the advocacy role: Natalie Abrams, "A Contrary View of the Nurse as Patient Advocate," *Nursing Forum* 17 (1978), 258–67. I have drawn on the thoughts in this essay in my discussion of the difficulties associated with the nurse as advocate.

58. Gadow, "Existential Advocacy," p. 85. In addition to this essay and the one by Curtin (note 46), a very helpful discussion appears in James L. Muyskens, *Moral Problems in Nursing: A Philosophical Investigation* (Totowa, NJ: Rowman and Littlefield, 1982).

59. For a helpful article on the developments in the states' nurse practice acts see Bonnie Bullough, "The Relationship of Nurse Practice Acts to the Professionalization of Nursing," in *The Nursing Profession: A Time to Speak*, pp. 609–633.

60. Patricia Murphy, "Deciding to Blow the Whistle," *The American Journal of Nursing* 81 (September 1981), 1691.

61. Sarah Archer and Patricia Goehner, *Speaking Out: The Views of Nurse Leaders* (New York: National League for Nursing, 1981).

62. See for example Linda Hughes, "The Public Image of the Nurse," *ANS* (Advances in Nursing Science) 2 (April 1980), 55–72.

63. Susan Thollaug, "The Nurse as Patient Advocate," *Imprint* 37 (December 1980), 37.

Existential Advocacy: Philosophical Foundations of Nursing*

Sally Gadow

INTRODUCTION: AGAINST META-NURSING

Turning points occur in the history of a profession when radical questioning and clarification of major tenets become essential for further growth. We recognize such a turning point now in nursing. The direction in which nursing develops will determine whether the profession draws closer to the medical model, with its commitment to science, technology, and cure; reverts to historical nursing models, with their essentially intuitive approaches; or creates a new philosophy that sets contemporary nursing distinctively apart from both traditional nursing and modern medicine.

However, the question of whether such a distinctive concept of nursing is possible has not yet been resolved. One sociologist suggests that, rather than the evolution of a new philosophy of nursing, nurses will evolve out of nursing: "nursing will still be nursing, but it will be carried on by persons of other occupational affiliations."[1] What will nurses be doing while someone else is doing the nursing? They will be moving on to meta-nursing. In the words of one of them, "The role of the nurse must be transcended in order to relate as human being to human being."[2]

If nursing is conceptualized in such a way that it must be transcended in order to involve the nurse as a human being, it is not surprising that nurses relinquish some of their functions to other health workers. Nevertheless, the fact that they still consider themselves nurses suggests that the meta-nursing to which they turn is *not* a transcending or outgrowing of nursing, but an early expression, not yet explicit, of new possibilities within nursing.

This phenomenon, that persons who have moved beyond nursing still consider themselves nurses, reflects the belief which is the premise of this chapter—that nursing ought to be defined philosophically rather than sociologically, that is, defined by the ideal nature and purpose of the nurse-patient relation rather than by a specific set of behaviors. When the concept of nursing is addressed as a philosophical ideal rather than as an empirical construct, we see immediately that it is contradictory to speak of nurses transcending nursing or delegating it to non-nurses. In other words, if nursing is distinguished by its *philosophy* of care and not by its care *functions*, and if nurses themselves formulate that philosophy, they transcend a particular concept of nursing only in order to realize a more developed concept, an ideal: a philosophy of nursing which unifies and enhances the experience of the individuals involved rather than devaluing and alienating that experience.

Some of the definitions of an ideal concept of nursing are familiar to anyone acquainted with the history of nursing: the nurse as healer, champion of the sick poor, parent-surrogate, physician-surrogate, contracted clinician, personal counselor, and health educator. The concept that I will propose as the

* Appreciation is expressed to Ann Davis, H. Tristram Engelhardt, Jr., Elizabeth Maloney, Teresa Stanley, and J. Melvin Woody, whose extensive and thoughtful commentaries on the paper as originally presented have contributed significantly to its revision.

Gadow, S. (1980). Existential advocacy: Philosophical foundations of nursing. *Nursing Images and Ideals*, 79–101.

philosophical foundation and ideal of nursing is that of advocacy—not the concept of advocacy implied in the patients' rights movement, in which any health professional is potentially a consumer advocate, but a fundamental, existential advocacy for which the nurse alone, among all the health professionals, is uniquely suited, and which is as distinct from consumer advocacy as it is from paternalism.

This concept of existential advocacy is not simply another alternative in the list of past and present concepts of nursing, nor does it imply a rejection of all other concepts. Rather, it is proposed as the philosophical foundation upon which the patient and the nurse can freely decide whether their relation shall be that of child and parent, client and counselor, friend and friend, colleague and colleague, and so on through the range of possibilities.

In order to elaborate this proposed ideal of existential advocacy, I will first distinguish it from paternalism and from patient's rights advocacy. I will then describe advocacy nursing as a resolution of two conflicts within health care that manifest in nursing the greatest urgency as well as the greatest possibility for solution: (1) the dichotomy between the personal and the professional involvement of the nurse, and (2) the discrepancy between the lived body and the object body of the patient. Finally, I will propose that existential advocacy as the essence of nursing is the nurse's participation with the patient in determining the unique meaning which the experience of health, illness, suffering, or dying is to have for that individual.

CONCEPTUAL FRAMEWORK

The conflict between advocacy and paternalism is felt most acutely by the nurse, since it is the nurse who must reconcile nursing's traditional alliance with the patient and the modern allegiance to medicine. Moreover, humanistic and authoritarian tendencies compete in nursing with particular intensity because of the comprehensive, yet personal, nature of nursing care. The nurse attends the patient as a whole, not just as a single problem or system. The nurse attends the patient during periods of sustained contact, and often provides the mundane intimacies usually considered to be self-care. Thus the nurse is in the ideal position among health-care providers to experience the patient as a unique human being with individual strengths and complexities—a precondition for advocacy. On the other hand, the potential for paternalism is as great as

that for advocacy, for just those reasons. The comprehensiveness, immediacy, and continuity of care present an exceptional opportunity for powerful influence over individuals—the precondition for paternalism.

Paternalism

The concept of advocacy proposed here is in essence the opposite of paternalism. For that reason, it is important to formulate clearly the meaning of paternalism which is being used.

Paternalistic acts and attitudes are those that limit the liberty or rights of individuals for their own interest. Paternalism implies the existence of coercion, since the individuals who voluntarily submit to a restriction are theoretically exercising their liberty in the making of choice. A more explicit meaning of paternalism, then, is the use of coercion in order to provide a good that is not desired by the one whom it is intended to benefit.[3] Such a formulation deliberately leaves open whether the person refuses the "good" because it is not recognized as a good, or because its value is lower than other goods in the person's hierarchy of values. For example, the refusal of blood transfusions by Jehovah's Witness patients may not reflect the failure to judge health or life to be a good, but the judging of another end to have a higher value. In either case, interference in that decision is paternalistic.

It has been argued that the essential element in paternalism (other than its motivation, the intent to obtain a good for the person affected) is not coercion, but "the violation of moral rules."[4] But this view fails to account for the case, for example, in which a woman anticipating the discovery of a malignancy asks that she not be told if her fears are confirmed, and the physician complies by lying to her. Here a moral rule has been violated in the interest of the person affected, but it is doubtful whether the authors of this view would judge the action paternalistic. On the contrary, overriding the patient's wishes and forcing the truth upon her (if done for her own good) would count as paternalism.[5] The single moral "rule," then, which is negated by paternalism is the prohibition against coercion, here defined as the forcing of individuals either to act in some way that is contrary to their wishes or to submit to someone else's action which is contrary to their wishes. An example of the former is the requirement that even unwilling students must write examinations; of the latter, the insistence that uncooperative patients submit to any diagnostic procedures that the practitioner believes necessary.

In summary, there are two principal elements in paternalism: (1) the intent—obtaining what is believed to be a good for the other person, and (2) the effect—violating the person's known wishes in the matter.

The meaning of paternalism is formulated differently by its defenders—not in terms of violation but of assistance. This view expresses the belief that in matters affecting an individual's well-being, the person's decisions should be made by those most capable of knowing what actions are in the person's interest.[6] Accordingly, it is inherent in professional responsibility always to act in the patient's interest. Paternalism is not a violation of the patient's right of self-determination so much as it is a protection of the patient's right to the best possible care that can be given.

However, this positive interpretation of paternalism only confuses matters, since it reduces paternalism to an identity with an equally simplistic meaning of advocacy, that is, acting on behalf of another. With this confusion, the most paternalistic professional can claim to be the staunchest patient advocate. Indeed, paternalism becomes the most thoroughgoing form of advocacy, inasmuch as it goes the length of even opposing patients' wishes in order to act in their interest. The conflation of paternalism and advocacy is a confusion which negates the truth of both, namely, that paternalism is a violation of the right of self-determination, and that advocacy does not consist in acting for another. The two are philosophically opposing concepts.

Patients' Rights and Consumerism

If advocacy and paternalism are opposites, and paternalism is the patient's submission to the professional's wishes, does this mean that advocacy limits the professional's actions to whatever the patient wishes? Is advocacy a form of consumer protection, in which the role of the professional is only to provide information necessary for the patient's selection among available courses of action? Is the advocate nurse a technical advisor whose responsibility stops short of recommending one option over another, lest that recommendation become coercion?

The answer to these is no, for professional consumerism would only seem to be a sophisticated form of paternalism, which insists that, in the interest of individuals' autonomy, they be forced to make important decisions alone, with only technical assistance. The fact that information which was traditionally denied to patients is now provided does not alter the paternalistic assumption that that is *all* that should be provided in order for patients to act autonomously, nor, for that matter, the assumption that individuals ought to act autonomously.

The current concept of patients' rights advocacy should be understood in this light, as a part of the wider movement of consumerism. "Patient advocacy is seeing that the patient knows what to expect and what is his right to have, and then displaying the willingness and courage to see that our system does not prevent his getting it."[7] From this point of view, the advocate is, at best, a troubleshooter willing to intervene when the system violates an individual's rights.[8]

Advocacy

The concept of advocacy (from this point on the term "advocacy" will be used to mean existential advocacy) is distinct from both paternalism and consumer protection. It is based upon the principle that freedom of self-determination is the most fundamental and valuable human right.

In negative terms, this implies that the right of self-determination ought not to be infringed upon even in the interest of health. The professional, while obligated to act in the patient's interest, is not permitted to define that interest in any way contrary to the patient's definition: it is not the professional but the patient who determines what "best interest" shall mean.

In positive terms, this meaning of advocacy has far greater implications for the professional and extends beyond the narrow realm of proscriptions into the realm of ideals. The ideal which existential advocacy expresses is this: that individuals be *assisted* by nursing to *authentically* exercise their freedom of self-determination. By authentic is meant a way of reaching decisions which are truly one's own—decisions that express all that one believes important about oneself and the world, the entire complexity of one's values.

Individuals can express their wholeness and uniqueness as valuing beings only if their full complexity of values—including contradictions and conflicts—is clearly in mind, having been reexamined and clarified in the new context. Yet, that clarification is the most difficult precisely when it is most needed, when a situation arises which threatens to overturn previously stable values. In such situations, of which health impairment is a paradigm, individuals face the necessity of either recreating their values or recreating their situation according to their existing hierarchy of values. The paternalistic response to this is simple: never mind examining values, because health is the highest human value. The response of consumerism to the patient is still more simple: once you have been informed of all of your options, do whatever you like.

The response of advocacy differs from both of these. It is not based on an assumption about what individuals *should want* to do, nor does it consist in protecting individuals' *rights* to do what they want. It is the effort to help persons *become clear about what they want* to do, by helping them discern and clarify their values in the situation, and on the basis of that self-examination, to reach decisions which express their reaffirmed, perhaps recreated, complex of values. Only in this way, when the valuing self is engaged and expressed in its entirety, can a person's decision be actually *self-determined* instead of being a decision which is not determined by others.[9]

ADVOCACY AND CONTRADICTIONS IN THE NURSE-PATIENT RELATION

Two basic discrepancies in health care prevent authentic self-determination, despite the lip service paid to "patient autonomy." They are first the dichotomy between personal and professional involvement of the practitioner, and second, that between the lived body and the object body of the patient. Because both of these conflicts result in fragmentation of the patient as well as the practitioner, their effect is to seriously limit the extent of the person that is involved in making decisions. If nursing is to accomplish its purpose in existential advocacy—i.e., if patients are to be assisted in making decisions which are genuinely their own because they fully express their own reaffirmed or recreated values—then nursing must resolve both of these discrepancies. As long as either remains, a source of self-alienation and personal disunity, the patient is effectively prevented from exercising his or her right of self-determination.

Personal Versus Professional

The movement of humanistic health care has attempted to soften the distinction between the person and the professional. Professionals are encouraged to become involved with and attentive to patients as individuals—in other words, to behave more like persons than just professionals—while patients have begun to assume some of the responsibilities formerly reserved for the professional.

But the dichotomy persists, nevertheless. In all health professions, new practitioners are warned that becoming personally involved with patients is unprofessional (in spite of patients' complaints that their care is too impersonal). The traditional view maintains that the personal and the professional are mutually exclusive aspects of the practitioner: behaving professionally entails the avoidance of any personal interactions; i.e., behavior expressing the professional's feelings, values, or idiosyncrasies. From this point of view, individuals are interchangeable, because none of their individuality is allowed into their interactions with patients.

Another version of this view considers the professional role to be one among the many in which the person engages. Different elements of the person are distributed among the various roles, with the result that at least something of the individual is expressed in professional behavior. That "something," however, usually includes at most the person's scientific, technical, and managerial capabilities; the emotional, esthetic, and contemplative, among others, are confined to other domains of the person's life.

Both of these views have the inevitable effect of fragmenting the individual, in this case the nurse, who guards against any "leaking" of the personal domains into the professional. Because of that exclusion of significant elements of the person from the professional relation, self-estrangement occurs within the nurse and, consequently, within the patient. Regarding the *patient* as a "whole" would seem to require nothing less than the *nurse* acting as a "whole" person. Therefore, the nurse who withholds parts of the self is unlikely to allow the patient to emerge as a whole, or to comprehend that wholeness if it does emerge.

Are we justified in assuming that the traditional view is right, that one essential feature of "professional" is its exclusion of the personal? In different terms, does the introduction of the personal into the professional domain so alter the nature of "professional" that its distinctiveness disappears and it becomes essentially no different from giving help to a friend or to oneself?

To answer, we can examine, phenomenologically, the differences between patient and professional in a hypothetical situation—for example, the relation between two women who are professional colleagues, one of whom provides nursing care for the other. In such a relation between professional equals, any nonessential differences (such as expertise) disappear, and it should be possible to discern only essential differences. To further avoid confusion with nonessential differences, we can stipulate that the colleague designated as the care provider suffers from the same disease as the person receiving care. Here, the two persons relating to one another as patient and nurse have a comparable understanding of the health problem in question— there is no difference in their competence to deal with the disease as a clinical entity. However, the essential differences arise with respect to their dealing with the illness as a personal experience. Those differences can be classified in terms of (1) focus, (2) intensity, and (3) perspective.

(1) The focus of the patient is directed to the problem at hand and its effect upon her life; her concern is unavoidably self-oriented. In contrast, the focus of the professional is directed away from herself toward the other. Her feelings of distress over the other's pain may be expressed, but not in order to obtain either relief or help from the patient. There is not, as in personal relations, a mutuality in which both are equally concerned about the other (with each one also maintaining some degree of self-interest). In the professional relation, the practitioner is interested in the other's good more than in her own, while the patient is concerned primarily about her well-being rather than the other's.

Personal relations too, though fundamentally relations of mutuality, can assume a one-directional focus when one of the persons is in distress, but two important differences remain between that situation and the professional relation. In friendship, mutuality is the accepted ideal, and departures from it, when one or the other person needs unusual attention, are understood to be temporary. The basis of the professional relation is the established disposition of one of the persons to attend to the other without receiving attention in return. Furthermore, in personal relations, because of the ideal of mutuality, there is a point beyond which a one-sided focus becomes unacceptable, and the relation must either return to a reciprocal one or

dissolve. In the professional relation, such a limit does not exist, inasmuch as the professional does not depend upon receiving the attention of the patient to make the relationship worthwhile.

(2) The intensity of the situation is experienced differently by the professional and the patient. The latter is caught up in the immediacy of her distress, the urgency of the symptoms as compelling phenomena in themselves. The professional may feel the same intensity, particularly when she has experienced the symptoms herself, but she is not bound by their immediacy. Her continued focus upon the patient makes the professional remain at the level of reflection rather than feeling. This is in order to integrate feelings and knowledge in the attempt to alleviate the patient's distress, and thereby free her from the limits of immediacy. Thus it is the form and direction, not the degree, of intensity which necessarily differ in the two persons.

This difference in intensity can occur in personal relations as well, but, like the one-sided focus described in (1), it is a departure from the ideal of mutuality, in which the intensity of one's experience is fully shared by the other in its immediacy before becoming the object of reflection. In the professional relation, the intensity felt by the nurse is not a sharing with the patient which has value in itself, value that is independent of helping the other. Rather, the intensity serves as an intensification of the reflective process necessary for help to be given. Being able to help has greater value than simply sharing the other's experience, an inversion of the values—sharing and helping—in personal relations.

(3) In addition to differences in focus and intensity, the perspectives of the two persons differ. The professional is "externally" involved, despite the similarities between herself and the patient, whereas the patient is involved in a radically interior way, feeling the pain "from the inside" and knowing that, although others may have the same disease, it is only *her* body which is affected in this instance.

This is the difference usually designated as the nurse's objectivity and the patient's subjectivity. Unfortunately, these terms are often used specifically to indicate degrees of emotional involvement. The implication there is that the essential difference in the two persons' perspectives is that the patient is more and the nurse less emotional. This ignores the possibility that both persons might experience emotional intensity, even though, in the professional, that intensity does not remain at the level of immediacy, but acts as an intensification of other dimensions of the person.

The essential difference in the perspectives of the two persons is related, not to emotion, but to the body. Only the patient can experience her body as an interiority, a living subjectivity, and only someone other than the patient can experience her body as a technical object, a thing to be regarded strictly scientifically.

Because patient and nurse have fundamentally different modes of access to the patient's body, and thus experience it in opposite ways, their understanding of it differs. The patient understands her body as a unique reality that cannot be expressed through types or generalizations. The nurse understands the patient's body as a part of the world of objects, and therefore, most effectively approached through clinical categories. She is, of course, ultimately concerned with the patient as a unique human being, but she addresses the body's phenomena as instances of general types of phenomena. "Pain here" is categorized as "gastralgia," for example, in order to apply the appropriate remedy. In short, in their involvement with the patient's body, the patient is oriented toward uniqueness, the professional toward typification.

The patient herself, as a professional whose involvement with patients' bodies is characteristically oriented toward the general, can, to some extent, combine the general with the unique in considering her own body. But because both approaches are required in ideal health care, each one needs to be developed as fully as possible, and this the person cannot do alone, even in her dual role as patient and professional. The two orientations, though complementary, are categorically different and, in most cases, the patient engages only in one by diminishing her engagement in the other. For the two perspectives to be thoroughly utilized together, a second person is needed to develop the objective dimension.

Again, the question arises whether the second person need be a professional, or could as well be a friend. Here, as in the differences in focus and intensity, the value of mutuality in personal relations prevents the friend from maintaining a one-sided approach, except as a temporary departure from supporting the other as an ultimately indivisible unity of subject and object. The professional, unlike the friend or the patient herself, is able to maintain for the patient the one perspective toward her experience which is the most difficult for her to develop: sustained objectivity.

In considering these three differences between personal and professional relations and between the patient and the professional, we see that the most commonly assumed difference is absent: the nurse does not manifest less involvement as a person than does the patient or the friend. On the contrary, the differences described above suggest that, while the form and direction of involvement differ significantly, the "amount" of the person involved is equally great.

On this basis, a solution to the personal/professional dichotomy can be proposed in the following way. Professional involvement is not an *alternative* to other kinds of involvement, such as emotional, esthetic, physical, or intellectual. It is a deliberate synthesis of all of these, a participation of the *entire* self, using every dimension of the person as resource in the professional relation.

This concept of professional involvement, as a unifying and directing of one's entire self in relation to another's need, is entailed by the concept of existential advocacy. Advocacy implies that patients can be assisted in reaching decisions which express their complex totality as individuals only by nurses who themselves act out of the same explicit self-unity, allowing no dimension of themselves to be exempt from the professional relation. Furthermore, the nurse, among the health professionals, is uniquely able to actualize such a holistic view of the professional. Nursing care, because of its immediate, sustained, and often intimate nature, as well as its scientific and ethical complexity, offers ready avenues for every dimension of the professional to be engaged, including the emotional, rational, esthetic, intuitive, physical, and philosophical.

One objection is commonly raised against resolving the personal/professional dichotomy in this way. It is that the professional's emotional involvement entails, for the patient, the risk of biased clinical judgment, and for the professional, the risk of personal suffering and emotional depletion. Such an objection, however, is based on a seriously limited view of emotional involvement. It assumes that through the feeling of another's suffering, "suffering itself becomes infectious."[10] In other words, to participate in another's emotion and have direct knowledge of it is to experience that emotion oneself and be as bound by its immediacy as the person who is actually experiencing it.

A significantly different possibility for emotional involvement, which that view does not consider, is the experience of "fellow-feeling" described by Max Scheler. Fellow-feeling is distinct from emotional infection and from merely perceiving the other's emotion. "It is indeed a case of *feeling* the other's feeling not just knowing it, nor judging that the other has it; but it is not the same as going through the experience itself."[11]

The distinction between fellow-feeling and emotional infection, or identification, reflects the same difference described earlier in relation to the different focus and intensity of patient and professional. The focus of fellow-feeling is the *other's* feeling, not one's own, which prevents emotional participation from becoming infectious identification. The emotion of the patient is not merely reproduced or reenacted within the professional (making the latter the one needing help). Rather, the patient's feeling is "vicariously visualized" in order to make possible a "*directing* of feeling towards the other's joy or suffering."[12] To participate in the suffering of the other in fact precludes the professional's suffering in herself, since it is then her own experience, not the patient's, which would be the object of her focus.

The difference of intensity is related to this difference of focus. In fellow-feeling, in contrast to emotional identification (i.e., in the professional's feeling as distinct from the patient's), the intensity is consciously directed, whereas in the experiencing of one's own emotion or the identification with another's, involvement is immediate rather than directed, involuntary rather than deliberate, and often unconscious. It is the failure to distinguish this different intensity of fellow-feeling from emotional identification which gives rise to the objection that emotional involvement distorts professional judgment. In emotional infection the nurse indeed succumbs to the same involuntary and unconscious immediacy which the patient experiences, and it could be argued that that use of intensity might well distort judgment. But fellow-feeling is a different, *directed* intensity, "a genuine *out-reaching* and entry into the other person and his individual situation, a true and authentic transcendence of one's self."[13]

Fellow-feeling is but one example of the concrete solutions possible in advocacy nursing: resolution of the personal/professional dichotomy, in this case by the nurse's deliberate emotional participation with the patient. For the patient's emotional complexity to be understood and supported, the emotional dimension of the nurse's own being cannot be excluded, but must be consciously and directly engaged. Moreover, just as with the emotional, so too with the esthetic; intuitive, physical, philosophical, and all other dimensions of personal reality can and must be brought to bear as essential, positive elements in the professional relation.[14] The absolute prerequisite for advocacy—advocating the patient's own individually created values—is the participation of the advocate as an individual, a complete unity unfragmented by exclusion of any part of the self.

Lived Body Versus Object Body

The nurse's dichotomy—between personal and professional involvement—is directly related to the patient's dichotomy—between the body as a private, lived reality and a public object open to inspection. The nurse's personal involvement with patients has been assumed to interfere with professional functions. Similarly, the patient's orientation toward the subjective body has been assumed to contradict the clinical orientation toward the body as an object. Thus, the concept of the professional as impersonal and objective has dictated a corresponding way of regarding the patient's body, that is, as object rather than person.

A paradigm of the sharp contradiction within the patient's experience of her body is the gynecological examination, in which a strictly impersonal definition is in force. For the patient, the part of the body being examined is often an extremely personal part of the self, perhaps the most private and emotionally invested part of the body. In the clinical situation, "the pelvic area is like any other part of the body," i.e., the individual examining the patient is "working on a technical object and not a person."[15] Any deviation from the technical attitude, e.g., by a patient's embarrassment, is countered with a repertoire of professional nonchalance, concentration on the procedure itself, and assurances that the situation is quite routine, and thus not intimate.

In the gynecological examination, the patient experiences an abrupt contradiction between her body as her own individual reality, rich with private emotional associations, and her body as sheer object, which others examine as impersonally as a technician inspects a machine. That conflict, in less dramatic form, is fundamental throughout health care, and because it can be uniquely addressed in nursing, it is important to analyze its elements and development.

The distinction between lived body and object body was indirectly indicated earlier in the discussion of the opposite perspectives of patient and professional toward the body of the patient. The distinction there was described in terms of uniqueness versus typification. That formulation expresses one aspect of the opposition, which can now be elaborated more fully.

The object body is the simpler of the two concepts for health professionals to appreciate. It is the body which the anatomist and physiologist describe, an object fully accessible upon examination and fully comprehensible by its examiner. It belongs, as do all objects, to the dimensions of quantified space and time, and to the realm of the general, the category. It is an object with parts having only functional value, not emotional, esthetic, or spiritual value: in the object body, the stomach has greater value than the hands of the concert pianist or the eyes of the painter.

The lived body is existentially opposed to the object body, but it *is not its opposite*. The lived body is not the silence of the object body when functioning well, so that one is unconscious of its objective existence as long as nothing in it breaks down. That unawareness of the body is not the lived body; it is simply a negative contingency, an experience conditional upon one's not encountering the body-as-object. As a positive condition categorically independent of and experientially prior to consciousness of the body-as-object, the lived body is not a thing at all (not even a well-running, non-intrusive thing), such as we usually denote by the word "body." Thus, it cannot be the opposite of the object body. Instead, it is a mode of orientation: the immediate, prereflective consciousness of the self *as capable of affecting its world*, as well as the consciousness of being vulnerable to the world's impact.[16]

The lived body, unlike the object body, is not in objective space and time. On the contrary, it forms its own space through its actions, drawing the world's space toward it, so to speak, centripetally.[17] Nearness and distance are a function of relevance, not measure. In the same way the lived body shapes its own time, with retension and protension interwoven and overlapping according to one's purposes, unconstrained by linearity.

It might be supposed that the lived body could be described, at least metaphorically, as an experience of interiority, but this fails for two reasons. In the first place, empirically, when the distinction between inner and outer emerges—for example, in early childhood and in illness—it is often the interior of the body which is felt to be "other," a baffling region not recognized as part of the self in the way that familiar, external features and functions are.[18] Secondly, and more important, the lived body is the self in which inner and outer *are not distinguished*: "Being-for-itself must be wholly body and it must be wholly consciousness; it cannot be *united* with a body."[19] The metaphor of interiority connotes subjectivity, privacy, privileged access—features that imply hiddenness and assume another, external, part of the self which is exposed. The lived body is thus reduced to a version, or rather, an inversion of the object body, its mirror image, when it is in fact another order of being from that of the object body.

If we understand the concepts of lived and object body as existentially opposed, and yet not logical opposites, then it is possible to recognize that the destruction of one does not automatically invoke the presence of the other (as in "if not a, then b"). It is especially important for the purposes of this chapter to recognize the transition that occurs from lived body to object body. The immediacy of the lived body is only partly mediated by illness, injury, or pain. With the appearance of incapacity, one experiences the body as something which opposes his purposes, a weighted mass, a thing-like other. Incapacity shatters the lived body. But the transition is not yet complete. The object body does not replace the lived body through illness alone. The otherness of the body in illness is rendered complete only through the category—the most essential instrument of clinical science. The category transforms "pain here" into precise, pathological phenomena which, even if one is a clinician, have no experiential relation to "pain here." The clinical view presents the patient with a body that is not his or her own, a disease process of which the patient has no direct perception. But, the new reality is objectively discernible for *others*. "Others have informed me of it, others can diagnose it; it is present for others even though I am not conscious of it."[20]

This then is the discrepancy between lived and object body, generated for the patient, first by the experience of incapacity and, second, by the perspective of science. What unique possibility exists in nursing for reconciling the opposition and restoring to the patient the unity of self and body which is prerequisite for true self-determination?

History suggests that nursing has focused exclusively upon the lived body and the object body in turn, moving from its earlier concern for immediate comfort of the patient, to the modern concern of science for the objective condition of the patient. Nursing can now surpass both of these extremes: the nurse, as advocate of the patient's wholeness, is committed to advocacy of neither the shattered lived body nor the inevitable object body. In short, nursing can make possible for the patient an enrichment of the lived body by the object body, and an enlivening of the object body by the lived body. The nurse can assist the patient to recover the objectified body at a new level at which it is neither mute immediacy nor pure otherness, but an otherness-made-one's-own, a lived objectness.

The experience of incapacity brings an awareness of the body as a being in its own right, with an irreducible reality of its own, an integrity that, so to speak, will not be compromised. The denial of that essential fact of human existence is bought at a great price: the lost possibility for enriching the self through the integration of that otherness.

It is this integration, the conscious unifying of self and body, which advocacy nursing assists the individual to achieve. The nurse assists the individual, as patient, to live the body's objectness as his or her own, instead of allowing it to remain alien. That unity is more fully expressive of one's totality than even the lived body is. The new unity is a reflective, more complex and articulated reality, inasmuch as one is now able to establish a conscious identification with aspects of his being which were previously undifferentiated, but have, through illness and objectivity, made themselves known. It is now important and possible to make them one's own, to an extent that was not important at the level of the object body, and not possible at the level of the lived body. "What threatens to estrange itself in us communicates to us *all the more* . . . that it is actually our own."[21]

It is that reconciliation of the person with the body-as-other, at a new level of integration and articulation, which nursing advocates. Nursing is uniquely able to mediate the lived/object body duality, inasmuch as it addresses both aspects of the person as one. It affirms the value of the lived body through the intimacy of physical care and comforting. At the same time, it affirms the reality of the object body by interpreting to patients their experience in terms of an objective framework—usually science, in Western cultures—which enables them to relate an otherwise hopelessly unique and solitary experience to a wider, general understanding. By continuously interrelating the two dimensions, the nurse demonstrates for the patient that the lived/object body relation is not an either/or relation, but a dialectic in which neither aspect is meaningful without the other. Both are essential, and mutually reciprocal.

This is easiest to realize when persons adhere exclusively to one or the other extreme. The modern example is the patient whose entire reality is the object body, who regards and refers to the body only in clinical terms—X-ray findings, laboratory studies, biopsy report, and so on. The more common example, given the traditional refusal to allow patients such access to their object bodies, is the patient whose only reality is the lived body, and who categorically renounces the object body as alien to the self by designating the health professional as the executor of this unwanted estate.

The challenge to advocacy nursing is to enable the individual to reclaim the aspect that has been excluded. Without incorporation of the object body, the lived body is an existentially weightless "I," unmediated and unenriched by detail, function, and form. Without the "I" of the lived body, the object body is an inanimate machine belonging to no one and everyone. Thus, the ideal of nursing is to enable patients to achieve a reconciliation, a reintegration, of these equally one-sided dimensions, in a synthesis that will necessarily be unique for each individual, and without which the self-unity required for patients' authentic self-determination will be impossible.

ADVOCACY AND THE RIGHT TO MEANING

The preceding sections have described existential advocacy in three ways:

1. the nurse's assistance to individuals in exercising their right of self-determination, through decisions which express the full and unique complexity of their values
2. a mode of involvement with patients which necessarily engages the entire self of the nurse
3. assistance to patients in unifying the experience of the lived body and the object body at a level that incorporates and transcends both.

In conclusion, we can summarize advocacy nursing as the participation with the patient in determining the *personal meaning* which the experience of illness, suffering, or dying is to have for that individual. At no time is the existential concern about the meaning of one's life more urgent than when the nature or continuation of one's existence is in jeopardy. At that point, the crucial question which the individual must answer is not "how can I secure my existence?" but "what does this jeopardy mean?" Only from the answer to that question can decisions then be reached concerning modes of treatment, forms of coping, the degree of autonomy desired, and so on. Ultimately, self-determination means the individual's own decision about the meaning of an experience, before decisions are reached about responding practically to the experience. For that meaning to be freely determined, it cannot of course be imposed by the "nature" of the person's condition, by clinical concepts of illness, or by professional notions of "loss," "disability," and "suffering." Thus, for example, the patient with terminal prostatic carcinoma is free to decide whether he shall think of his experience in moralistic terms (punishment for promiscuity), scientific terms (simply cellular phenomena), cultural terms (permission to grieve), naturalistic terms (the inevitable pain and dying that come to all), or purely individual terms which violate all of these—perhaps an inconsolable despair over the absurdity of the experience, or a decision that suffering can be a means of finding one's own way, by confronting the absurdities of existence not as defects but as necessary antitheses in the dialectical relation between joy and sorrow in human life.

For the same reason that the question of meaning arises, namely, the threat to existence, individuals require assistance in order to determine the meaning of their experience. That assistance is provided ideally by the person who has the most comprehensive understanding of the experience and who is as fully involved as the patient. That person is the nurse. The approach of nursing encompasses both care and cure, intimate concern for the lived body and scientific treatment of the object body. Moreover, the nurse offers a necessary alternative perspective which complements and completes the partial perspective of the patient, inasmuch as the focus and intensity of the nurse is directed toward the other rather than the self, and the orientation of the nurse is toward the typical rather than the solitary. Finally, the continuity with which only nursing attends the patient enables the nurse to experience individuals as unique human beings continuously engaged in creating their own histories.

No other health profession at present combines all these elements. More important, none even proposes as its ideal this reconciliation of the most radical dichotomies in health care—the unique and the general, personal intensity and professional objectivity, the body as "I" and the body as other. Nursing, by aiming at the solution of these conflicts and the human fragmentation they produce, in order that patient and nurse can participate as unified selves in the patient's process of self-determination, expresses the ideal of existential advocacy. On this basis, the nurse is the ideal professional to particiate with the patient in the decision about that which is most crucial in all experiences of illness: the meaning of the experience for the individual.

NOTES

1. Sam Schulman, "Basic Functional Roles in Nursing: Mother Surrogate and Healer," in *Patients, Physicians, and Illness*, E. Jaco (ed.), Glencoe, Illinois: The Free Press, 1958, pp. 528–537.
2. Joyce Travelbee, *Interpersonal Aspects of Nursing*, Philadelphia: F.A. Davis, Co., 1966, p. 49.
3. For elaboration of this position, see Dworkin's discussion of Mill in Gerald Dworkin, "Paternalism," *The Monist*, 56, January 1972, pp. 64–84.
4. Bernard Gert and Charles M. Culver, "Paternalistic Behavior," *Philosophy and Public Affairs*, Vol. 6, No. 1, Fall 1976, pp. 45–57.
5. This in fact is exactly what Gert and Culver argue in regard to a physician's insisting that a patient talk about an impending trauma against her expressed wishes.
6. Paternalism thus attributes to the person affected a form of ethical egoism, i.e., the belief that individuals (patients, in this case) *ought* to act in such a way as to promote their own good, with the altruistic footnote that if they fail to do so, action will be initiated on their behalf to obtain the good for them until such time as they resume the moral duties of egoism.
7. Sandra Kosik, "Patient Advocacy or Fighting the System," *American Journal of Nursing*, April 1972, pp. 694–698.
8. The goals of patient advocacy programs may not even be solely those of consumer protection. Improving patient compliance and smoothing over patient complaints are often hidden or explicit objectives. (*Ibid.*, 209) Even when the primary goal is helping patients, advocacy can function as a defense for professional decisions: "patients experiencing a token economy wanted to know whether the therapy team was violating patients' rights . . . All it took here was an explanation that token economy is a medically approved, widely accepted mode of treatment. The patients were more accepting of it after that." Wanda Nations, "Nurse-Lawyer

is Patient-Advocate," *American Journal of Nursing*, June 1973, pp. 1039–1041.

9. Professor Engelhardt's concern here that "paternalism in the interests of health" is being replaced by a "paternalism in the interests of authenticity" is, fortunately, unfounded. I am proposing advocacy as an ideal, not as a duty, norm, prescription, or imperative which conceivably might involve "enforcement." Moreover, it is simply contradictory to believe that we can force persons to act in an unforced way. The ideal of assisting patients to exercise their freedom does not entail that they be stigmatized for declining, just as the ideal of health presumably does not entail that patients be punished for disdaining modern medicine. Authenticity, like health, is ultimately fashioned and confirmed only by the individuals themselves; professionals can assist the process but they cannot command it.

10. Friedrick Nietzsche, *The Anti-Christ* (R.J. Hollingdale, trans.), Baltimore, Penguin Books, 1969, p. 118. See also Nietzsche, "The will to suffer and those who feel pity," *The Gay Science*, (Water Kaufman, trans.), New York: Random House, 1974, pp. 269–271.

11. Max Scheler, *The Nature of Sympathy* (Peter Heath, trans.), Hamdon, CT.: Archon Books, 1970, p. 9. (emphasis added).

12. *Ibid.*, p. 15.

13. *Ibid.*, p. 46.

14. Another example of resolving the personal/professional dichotomy, this time through physical involvement between nurse and patient, can be developed around the importance of touch in nursing. For a discussion of the laying-on of hands in nursing care, see Dolores Krieger, "Therapeutic Touch: The Imprimatur of Nursing," *American Journal of Nursing*, May 1975, pp. 784–787.

15. Joan P. Emerson, "Behavior in Private Places: Sustaining Definitions of Reality in Gynecological Examinations," in *Readings on Ethical and Social Issues in Biomedicine*, Richard W. Wertz, (ed.), Englewood Cliffs, New Jersey: Prentice-Hall, Inc., 1973, pp. 221–233.

16. I am grateful to J. Melvin Woody for his insistance upon the vulnerability of the lived body, elaborated in "Helping the Patient Survive: Some Remarks on Prof. Sally Gadow's essay 'Existential Advocacy: Philosophical Foundation of Nursing'" (unpublished).

17. Sartre captures this phenomenon of lived space in his analysis of "the look," in which the world is experienced, not as fixed in uniform space, but "perpetually flowing" toward me, its center. See *Being and Nothingness: An Essay in Phenomenological Ontology*, (Hazel Barnes, trans.), New York: The Citadel Press, 1969, 232ff.

18. This is contrary to Sartre's account of the distinction, in which the object body emerges as the exterior part of my self which the other perceives, "extended outside in a dimension of flight which escapes me. My body's depth of being is for me this perpetual 'outside' of my most intimate 'inside'" (Sartre, *op. cit.*, p. 328).

19. *Ibid.*, p. 281.

20. Herbert Plügge, "Man and His Body," in *The Philosophy of the Body: Rejections of Cartesian Dualism*, Stuart F. Spicker, (ed.), New York: Quadrangle/The New York Times Book Co., 1970, p. 305.

21. *Sartre, op. cit.*, 332.

A Model for Ethical Decision Making

Sally Gadow

In the articulation of a nursing process for addressing ethical problems, we face the same difficulty as in formulating a nursing process for clinical problems: we first must know what nursing is. That determination is the fundamental ethical problem in nursing, namely, what is the ideal to which we aspire? The way in which that question is answered will determine the way in which we identify steps in the nursing process.

Two distinct ideals are open to nursing. Our approach to ethical problems will differ significantly according to our philosophy of nursing.

One ideal is based upon beneficence, which requires that professionals act to maximize benefit and minimize harm to patients. As a philosophy of nursing, beneficence defines the role of the nurse as cooperation with the providers' network—particularly the physician and the institution—concerned with benefiting patients. Underlying this is the assumption that the professional is better qualified than the patient to define "benefit" and "harm". Truth-telling and patient autonomy are not intrinsic values, but may be a benefit in some cases, a harm in other cases. In any event, the professional judgment is medical rather than nursing, if "benefit" is defined by the medical criteria of reversing pathology and preventing death (two benefit criteria difficult to apply with cancer patients).

A second ideal is based upon autonomy. One is morally required to respect an individual's freedom of self-determination, provided only that the decision is a free and considered one not endangering others. When this ideal is made the basis of nursing practice, the aim and the role of the nurse differs significantly from practice based strictly upon beneficence. The ideal becomes assistance to patients (individuals, families, or communities) in the development and exercise of autonomy in health matters. While we are still obligated to act in our patients' best interest (as with beneficence), it is the patient and not the professional who decides what "best interest" shall mean. The autonomy principle entails benefiting patients, but "benefit" is defined by patients rather than professionals. Autonomy does not force patients to participate in treatment decisions; it only insures them the possibility and assistance needed for participation if they so choose.

The principle of beneficence is difficult to apply because of disagreements in defining benefit and the principle of autonomy is also difficult to apply. It requires engaging patients of diverse cultural and educational backgrounds, often with complex health problems, to assist in their decisions about care. When patients waive their autonomy, it is crucial for the principle of autonomy that the waiver be consciously and freely given, neither assumed nor coerced.

Nursing must choose one ideal or the other. We cannot practice with both a philosophy that endorses professional determinations of benefit *and* a philosophy of patient autonomy. Without reference to a normative concept—an ideal—ethical issues such as deception, coercion, and nontreatment are addressed in a vacuum. However, in the context of an articulated ideal, resolution of those issues becomes a concrete process of determining if an action is consistent with and expressive of that ideal.

One way to decide between the two philosophies—other than by personal preference—is to ask which of the two is likely to yield the highest return to those nursing serves? Which holds the most promise for patients?

Gadow, S. (1980). A model for ethical decision making. *Oncology Nursing Forum, 7* (4), 44–47. Reprinted with permission of © Oncology Nursing Press, Inc. All rights reserved.

The autonomy principle meets these criteria. Patients lose nothing and gain significantly when their autonomy is the primary value in nursing. They still have the benefit of professional expertise and judgment, which they can make the basis for their decision if they choose. They also have the freedom to exercise personal judgment and expertise regarding the uniqueness of their situation and values. Most important, they have the right to assistance in synthesizing those two perspectives, the uniquely personal and the professional.

The task now is to describe steps for applying the philosophy of autonomy, and to identify a nursing process for assisting patients in the development as well as the exercise of self-determination in health care decisions. We may be reluctant to grant that important decisions are rightfully the patient's, but we are often relieved when decision-making has been established to be "the patient's problem". These two perspectives reflect two different nursing processes; I shall propose a third.

The first perspective, paternalism, assumes that individuals ought to be urged (if not forced) to select treatment according to the professional's concept of "best interest". In this model, the nurse's traditional role as the physician's accomplice might be to engineer the patient's consent to a course of action not desired by that individual.

The opposite of paternalism is the "grateful relief syndrome," or consumerism. Here, there is no desire on the part of nurses to shoulder the decision-making; rather, they are gratified that the patients' rights movement has relocated all problems in the patients' domain. In this model, the nurse is a consumer's guide who supplies the patient with the facts of the case, then discreetly withdraws, leaving the decision entirely in the hands of the consumer. Notice that the withdrawal of the nurse is as vital to the procedure as the providing of information, since this view assumes that a patient might be unduly influenced if the decision is not made in the strictest privacy.

Both models, while perhaps appealing for their own reasons, fail to provide a procedure for assisting patients in the development and exercise of their autonomy. Paternalism regards patients as temporarily incompetent; there is no possibility of their deciding, even with assistance. Consumerism regards the patient as partially nonhuman, a computer requiring only appropriate input in order to process a decision; there is no need of assistance beyond the purely technical. One of these procedures dispenses with the patient, the other with the nurse. In neither case does the nurse assist the patient in the decision process itself.

I propose a third model, deriving from the philosophy of patient autonomy, that can best be designated "advocacy nursing."[1]

A word of caution: advocacy is understood in some contexts as acting on behalf of someone. In my model, advocacy means assisting patients in their own actions and decisions rather than substituting professional actions and decisions for those of patients.

Specifically, advocacy is the active assistance to patients in their self-determination concerning health alternatives. Advocacy not only safeguards but contributes positively to the exercise of self-determination. It is the effort to help patients become clear about what they want in a situation, to assist them in discerning and clarifying their values and examining available options in light of those values.

Advocacy (patient autonomy) suggests a distinct nursing process with five steps: (1) patient self-determination, (2) the nurse-patient relationship, (3) the nurse's values, (4) the patient's values, and (5) patient individuality. Each element in advocacy requires consideration, although in no predetermined sequence. Suppose that a woman with significant metastasis, who has not been told her prognosis, is contemplating a recommended surgical treatment. She asks her nurse whether she should undergo the operation.

(1) The first step is insuring the *possibility* of self-determination. The patient must have information so she can understand and respond to her situation. The more information available to her, the more informed and thus the more free her decision can be. Surgery versus nonsurgery is not as free a decision as the choice of surgery over chemotherapy, radiation, visualization therapy, herbal medicine, or non-treatment. The necessity of relevant information is presupposed by the concept of self-determination; it would be inconsistent to fail to provide whatever information a patient requires to exercise her self-determination. It would clearly be impossible for the woman to give informed (and therefore free) consent to a treatment if she does not know, for example, that the expected outcome is at most an additional six months of life.

Does the concept of self-determination, with its requirement of adequate information, mean simply announcement of all the options—followed by a hasty retreat? Or does it mean that patients ought to have information forced on them which they may not want?

(2) With these concerns, we are led to the second

step in applying advocacy, determination of the *nature of the relationship between nurse and patient*. Since the goal is to assist patients in self-determination, both the paternalistic and the consumerist procedures for providing information share a common fault. They assume that the appropriate amount and type of information can be determined without patient participation. If information selection is the decision of the professional rather than the patient, less or more may be given than is needed, or what is given may be irrelevant from the patient's viewpoint. Even the consumer model's neutral objectivity amounts to paternalism because the selection of information is made *for* the patient.

The avenue most consistent with the advocacy relationship is to *enable the patient to determine the selection of information* to be presented.

The nurse might ask questions such as: "Would you be helped in making your decision if you had more information? If you knew more about the clinical findings? If you knew the expected outcomes of alternatives? If you knew the prognosis? If you knew your family's feelings in the matter? If you knew the views of persons who have faced a similar decision?" A less direct way of inviting a patient to determine the extent of information needed would be for nurses to express their own views. For example, the nurse might say, "I think it is helpful if people find out about all the alternatives before making up their minds. Do you feel this way?" In short, advocacy in this situation defines the nurse/patient relationship in terms of assisting the patient not only to decide about the recommended treatment, but first to determine the selection of information she wishes to have. This assumes, of course, that any information she requests will be given freely.

(3) A third step involves disclosure of the *nurse's views* as part of the potentially relevant information to which a patient is entitled. To the extent that the patient enters the relationship as a so-called "whole person," the professional, too, must be fully present. While the patient's values will be the decisive ones, the nurse's values also contribute to the process. It is especially important that they be expressed when they conflict with the patient's values.

Outside of the authoritarian model of nursing, there is no reason that the communication of the nurse's values is necessarily coercive. On the contrary, such disclosure serves several purposes. It provides the patient with information she may find useful in understanding the nurse's behavior toward her. More important, it offers her one example of an alternative view that she might want to take into account in considering her own values.

The purpose of the disclosure is not to persuade, but neither is it merely to inform. It is an affirmation to the patient that the nurse is concerned with the articulation of values, not as an impersonal prescription for decision-making, but as a professional commitment to ethical reflection.

(4) The purpose in disclosure of the nurse's values is to assist in clarification of the patient's values, which leads to the fourth step in applying advocacy: *determination of the patient's values*. One fundamental value concerns the quality of life the patient desires or deems acceptable. It must be determined with the patient whether a proposed measure will sustain or significantly diminish the quality of life the patient values. Quality-of-life determinations are usually based upon professional notions about the meaning of life that is characterized by suffering, terminal illness or futile treatment. In the advocacy model, however, only the values of the patient, concerning the quality of her own life, are to be decisive.

(5) Directly related to patient values is the patient's individuality. As a fifth step in assisting patient decision-making, it is necessary to attend to considerations other than values per se that may be decisive in a patient's self-determination. These last considerations are grouped under the term "individuality." Persons are a composite of their unique understanding of themselves and their bodies and their unique relationship between self and body. The unity or disunity between self and body that patients experience can significantly affect their decisions, particularly in a disabling illness in which the self/body relationship itself may be in question. This is clearly evident in persons who perceptually or emotionally negate the reality of a body part that is, to them, already dead.

Advocacy in our hypothetical situation involves assistance to the patient in ascertaining the way in which she experiences her body. She may perceive it as only a shell for the soul, a shell that can be relinquished if she believes that the soul lives after her body's death. Or she may experience the unity of self and body as indissoluble, so that the death of the body would mean the annihilation of her entire being. From the patient's view of her body and its relation to the self arises one of the most crucial aspects of individuality in terminal illness—the patient's personal views concerning death. Here advocacy involves a unique nursing task: the assistance to patients in their free determination of the meaning their illness and dying are to have for them.

The nursing process outlined here is essentially a process of patient involvement, not for reaching a unilateral nursing judgment *for* a patient, but for engaging *with* the patient in an endeavor to reach a joint understanding of the problem and its various solutions. Within a philosophy of advocacy nursing, the problems the nursing process addresses are all ethical as well as clinical, because the principal elements in the process are persons rather than apparatus or organs. Values become central in nursing practice. There is no aspect of practice that is without ethical considerations, no nursing interaction that is not an opportunity for either suppressing or enhancing patient self-determination.

What are the implications of such a process for the nurse-physician relationship? The ideal of the nurse as advocate of patient autonomy means that the nurse is morally aligned with the patient rather than with the physician, family, or hospital. Any time decisions involve more than one person, disagreements are inevitable. When the person who is to have the principal voice is at the same time the person of lowest standing in the health hierarchy, i.e., the patient, disagreements multiply. The nurse is in the hazardous role of mediating between the patient's right of self-determination and tne well-meaning attempts of those who would override that right. This aspect of advocacy, finally, identifies it conclusively as a nursing and not a medical process. The nurse mediates between the abstract, objective medical assessment of benefit and the personal understanding of benefit which the patient possesses, and assists patients to develop as fully as possible that unique, existential knowledge of their situation that medicine cannot provide.

Nurses will jeopardize their professional standing in many cases by applying the philosophy proposed. This is a high price to pay for a personal moral choice, and at times we will choose, understandably, not to pay it. But at the professional level, if we endorse the ideal of the nurse as advocate of patient autonomy, we are obligated, first, to educate students to approach that jeopardy with the patient uppermost in mind; and second, to engage in political action to insure that nurses need no longer practice daily heroism in order to honor patient autonomy.

NOTES

1. The process outlined here is also described in Gadow, "An Ethical Model for Advocacy: Assisting Patients with Treatment Decisions," in J. Swazey (ed.), *Dilemmas of Dying: Policies and Procedures for Decisions Not to Treat*, Boston. G. K. Hall, 1980. For a more comprehensive discussion of advocacy nursing, see Gadow, "Existential Advocacy: Philosophical Foundation of Nursing" in Spicker. S. and Gadow, S. (eds.), *Nursing: Images and Ideals: Opening Dialogue with the Humanities*, New York, Springer, 1980.

The Nurse as Advocate

Mary F. Kohnke

Mr. Wood, a 48-year-old, 135-pound man, is lying in bed and moaning in pain. He is one day postcholecystectomy. One hour before the nurse had given him Demerol 75 mg. q4h, PRN. The medication had not been effective, according to the nurse's notes.

Mr. Wood's nurse pages the intern to request that the medication be changed. The intern refuses, as does the resident, saying that he has had enough medication for a man of his size. The nurse pursues the situation and contacts the attending physician to let him know what is happening. He comes to see Mr. Wood and changes the medication to morphine sulfate, 10 mg. IM. Mr. Wood experiences pain relief within 45 minutes after receiving the morphine.

Is the nurse's action an act of advocacy? My answer is no, this is not advocacy, it is just good nursing practice.

I believe that advocacy has been confused with legalities and ethics of nursing practice. We have to clearly differentiate between the three.

The classical definition of advocacy is "the act of defending or pleading" the case of another. In nursing at least, if not in law, I hesitantly offer a parallel definition: that advocacy is the act of informing and supporting a person so that he can make the best decisions possible for himself.

Thus, the act of advocacy or the actions of the advocate are two-fold. The *first* is to inform your clients or patient of what their rights are in a particular situation and then to make sure they have all the necessary information to make an informed decision. You as the nurse must first learn to gather the information before you can pass it on to your client. Then, you must, to the best of your ability, ensure that your clients know and understand the same information.

The information must be presented in a manner that allows the patient to hear what you are saying without imposing your own hidden feelings that may distort this information. In other words, the patient must not be put in the position of having to "psych out" the nurse.

People make decisions for all kinds of reasons, some of which have nothing to do with the immediacy of the situation facing them. The advocate must constantly be on guard not to feed into the unstated reasons that go into making a decision and thereby subtly support a decision that is not based on rational reasoning. For example, a person may make a decision that is contradictory to what he wants because he has a greater need to please others than himself. In the advocate role, your responsibility is to put your own opinion aside and clearly inform your clients of the consequence of their choices. If "A" is chosen, then "B" will follow.

The *second* act of the advocate is to support clients in the decisions they make. Support may involve several actions or nonactions. One action is to actively reassure patients that it is their decision and they have the *right* to make it. They do not need to nor should they give in to pressures from others, be it family, friends, or health professionals. A second action may mean that you do not allow others to undermine your client's confidence in his own decision making. This may only be possible if you are in a position of authority to prevent others from harassing the client.

The decision a client makes is his own, even if, in your opinion, it is not the best decision for him. He has the right to make decisions freely and without pressure. This is advocacy in the finest sense of the word. It may be hard for us as professionals "who know best" to accept our clients' decisions, but it

---

is necessary if we expect people to grow, and if we respect their right to make their own decisions. We can learn and grow not only from our right decisions, but from our mistakes as well.

Nonaction may be even more important than action, yet harder to do. Nonaction usually means keeping yourself from subtly undermining the patient's decision. It may also mean that you have to refuse the request of others, such as physicians, other nurses, or family members, who ask you to talk to the patient and convince him that he is wrong. This kind of refusal can have some disturbing repercussions for you if your colleagues or family members do not understand your responsibility to support your client's decision. For example, a physician may report a staff nurse to her superior if she does not "talk" his patient into signing a consent form for a procedure that he believes the patient should have.

√ The act of advocacy for those in the so-called helping professions is psychologically very difficult. It is almost in direct conflict with their image of themselves as the persons "who know best"—the experts who are paid to know and make decisions based on superior knowledge. We often see ourselves as the rescuers of mankind, or at least that portion of mankind who are sick and need rescuing.

Rescuers often put themselves in the position of making decisions for others so that, in the end, they have to accept the responsibility for the decision. However, although we may be willing to make the decision, we are not equally willing to accept responsibility for having done so. Not only does making the decision for another rob that person of his responsibility and rights, it also places the professional in a very awkward position of being blamed if all does not come out well. Since most of us inherently know this, we then attempt to have clients make the decision we want them to make under the guise of their having done it themselves.

I believe that, in fact, we are only fooling ourselves if we believe that our clients do not know what is going on. This may be OK if all goes well, but too often, Murphy's law prevails (when it's possible for something to go wrong, it does). Then, when clients blame us, we act startled and surprised and ask, "How can you blame me?" Furthermore, we accuse them (openly or silently) of being ungrateful, never admitting for one minute that we got ourselves into the mess by our insistence of the "we know best" theme.

In the literature, this is often referred to as the games triangle or Karpman's triangle.* It is pictorially described as the rescuer-victim-persecutor triangle. An example of this is when teachers fall victim to the student who insists that the faculty adviser decide between two elective courses on the grounds that she knows best. Four weeks later, the student comes back and blames the adviser for "picking a lousy course. . . ." Another example is when the patient asks the nurse to explain to the family her desires because "they won't listen to me."

We can willingly accept the rescuer's role and, in fact, insist on it, or can be innocently put into it. The result is the same—whenever you make decisions for others or do for them what they should be doing, you automatically accept the responsibility for the results.

In the advocacy role, one should never get into this position. As your client's advocate, you must keep uppermost in your mind that clients must make their own choices freely. If not, this is not advocacy as I use the word; it is rescuing. The rescuer role has no place in the life of a professional, except when the client may be too young or in a coma, and thus is unable to make the decision.

The "we know best" attitude is something we have been taught as children because our parents practiced it with us and, in some cases, may even continue to do so when we are adults. This theme is reinforced in the school systems, and if one goes into the helping professions it is reinforced again, so that it becomes second nature.

Thus, to be an advocate, as a nurse, requires a reorientation and a constant guarding of self, so as not to slip into the "we know best" position. It also requires an element of faith: faith in human beings' ability to make their own decisions and, even more, in their right to do so.

Constraints on the Advocate

When discussing the constraints that can confront an advocate, there are two considerations that the nurse must remember. First, the patient's reluctance to make a decision, despite his desire to do so, will require extra care on the nurse's part in the informing and supporting processes.

Second, be very careful that you do not become triangled into the patient-family system. Knowledge

---

* Karpman, S. B. Script drama analysis. *Trans.Anal.Bull.* 7:39–43, Apr. 1968.

of family theory and dynamics can be a great help. If you take sides with families, you may very well end up with them on one side and you on the outside.

These two areas may not be so much constraints from without as they are constraints from within. For example, one may see patients being manipulated by their families into making a decision they don't like. The nurse may want to intervene, only to find out this this is a lifetime game that they all play. Moreover, this pattern is one they want to continue despite the fact that, on the surface, they protest to the nurse.

The greatest area of constraint will be the institution. The major functions of advocacy are basically at odds with the culture of the hospital system. First, you inform. That, in itself, is a great sin because you will be labeled an "informer." By telling patients things that will make them ask questions, you get labeled a troublemaker. We give lip service to patients' rights. That's great until the patient begins demanding his rights. Then, watch out! If you are the instigator of this through information you gave, you are in trouble.

You may survive the first step, but if you then go so far as to support patients in their decisions, you have had it. For example, you have not only provided the information, but then you are told by the head nurse, the physician, or the administrator to go and convince patients that they are wrong. They *must* have the test or the operation or leave the hospital. If you refuse, you are, indeed, in a fix. You have, in effect, disobeyed a direct order from your superiors.

These are very real constraints. They are widely in operation today. I'm not trying to discourage you from ever being an advocate but only trying to alert you to the possible pitfalls.

There are ways in which pitfalls can be avoided. They involve being very knowledgeable about the system, the law, and how to handle yourself with the patient. If you use your knowledge wisely and do not get trapped in the emotional position of being a rescuer to the patient, it helps.

When your patient's rights are being infringed on, a wise word, well dropped, can make people retreat. If one says, "Well, Dr. Brown, I was only thinking of your interests. You know how sensitive people are these days and how quick they are to sue," this usually causes the person to at least stop and think. In other words, you must learn how to work within the system to the extent it is possible. People who have really been violating patients' rights will be very sensitive to this method.

One must be careful not to win battles and lose wars. Members of the health team must be educated to the dangers of the "we know best" rescuer's game. This you can do. You can show them the possible consequences of their behavior.

I suppose the bottom line of the advocate role can be summarized in the term *knowledge* or *to know*. Not to know is no sin, not to admit that one does not know is. The greatest sin or damage is committed under the umbrella of "We didn't know." But then, most of us may not want to know. We say, "What you don't know can't hurt you." However, I believe that it is precisely what you do not know that will hurt you the most. Ignorance is the greatest weapon of tyrants and the greatest defense of people who do not want to accept responsibility for themselves. When you are dealing with both, you have a dual problem.

The act of advocacy is, at its basic level, an act of loving and caring for others as you would love and care for yourself. In its true form, it is simplicity itself. However, the two-edged sword is that which is most simple is in fact complex, and that which seems most complex is most simple. The act of advocacy is just that—the most simple and the most complex.

The Changing Role of Nurses in Making Ethical Decisions

Catherine P. Murphy

In past decades, biomedical technology has created such advances that many health care professionals and consumers are overwhelmed by the apparently unlimited choices in treatment decisions. Problems in human reproduction, preservation of life, research on human subjects, and allocation of scarce resources are just a few of the categories of concerns that we now face. These dilemmas are complex both from conceptual and ethical perspectives. Thus, it becomes more and more difficult to define such important concepts as "human life" or "extraordinary treatment," and to apply these concepts to clinical situations. It has become almost impossible to objectively interpret and apply ethical principles which should guide actions of health care providers. For example, the Hippocratic principle of *primum non nocere* (first, do no harm), in light of technology, turns more and more upon the serious question of what is, and what is not, a harm. It becomes more difficult to preserve human dignity, to show respect for life, because we must first determine the best way to recognize human dignity.

As the discussion on ethics increases among health professional groups, we have begun to realize that, unlike scientific reasoning, ethical reasoning cannot offer definitive proof as to what is the right or wrong action in a given situation. As health care providers and consumers have become aware of the value-laden, subjective element of clinical judgments by physicians, those decisions are increasingly open to questioning. Many individuals are beginning to question the physician's role as the major decisionmaker. Why does the physician have authority in making ethical judgments? Is it by virtue of the physician's years of education and

scientific training? The late André Hellegers, physician and director of the Kennedy Institute of Bioethics, questioned the unchallenged authority of the physician to be the decisionmaker.[1] He noted that the physician might have the most knowledge with regard to the scientific facts about the patient's disease, but in Hellegers's words, "knowing most and knowing best are not always synonymous."[2]

NURSES IN THE PAST

The notions of ethics committees and shared health care decisionmaking challenge the tradition of physicians as lone decisionmakers. This notion is so engraved in the minds of the public that other health care professionals are frequently exasperated when health care decisions are equated with medical decisions. Extensive sociological research from the 1960s documented that health care institutions were bureaucratic, hierarchical organizations, and at the top of the pyramid were the physicians.[3] Until the 1960s, the hospital organization controlled much of the education of health care personnel.[4] Therefore, nurses and other health professionals were appropriately socialized into the health care field to know their place. In particular, nurses with hospital schooling were relegated to the bottom of the pyramid and learned not to ask questions.[5]

In the mid-1970s, when I conducted studies on the moral reasoning of nurses,[6] most nurses included in the study were well-doctrinated in those values, and exhibited unquestioning loyalty to physicians and hospitals.[7] I found that three competing models of the nurse-patient relationship emerged when nurses were confronted with hypothetical dilemmas which pitted patients' rights and interests against those of the institution and the physician.[8] The three different models were the bureaucratic model, the physician-advocate model, and the patient-advocate model. Those nurses who fell into the bureaucratic model perceived their place to be on the bottom rung of the ladder. They believed that nurses should not make waves or cause trouble within the institution; nurses were supposed to follow orders. They considered the coordination of hospital policies and personnel to be their most important role. Because they were not to upset the smooth functioning of the team, they had to maintain rapport at all costs. This meant staying on the good side of the administrators and physicians who were rungs above them in the hospital's hierarchy. In this view, then, the interests of patients could be sacrificed by the nurse in the interest of keeping the peace and enabling the institution to function without disruption.

Those nurses who followed the physician-advocate model perceived themselves as accountable only to physicians. The purpose of nursing, in this model, was to follow doctors' orders and to promote the ends of science, research, or medical technology, perhaps at the expense of patients' rights. These nurses saw their most important duty as maintaining trust within the physician-patient relationship, even if this meant concealing mistakes or violations of patients' rights, of which patients and families might be ignorant.

The third model, that of the patient-advocate, had the lowest incidence.[9] In this model, nurses perceived themselves as having moral and legal accountability to the patient. When patients' rights and interests were in conflict with those of the physician or the institution, these nurses saw themselves as advocates of the patient and protectors of patient autonomy. Interestingly, the data showed that this was not primarily a paternalistic form of advocacy. Rather, these nurses saw as most important the enhancement of the decision-making capacity of the patient and the patient's family. Nurses in the patient-advocate model would attempt to support patients and families in their efforts to act in their own interests and to become properly informed so that they could make the best decisions.

RECENT CHANGES

Since the late 1970s, a revolution of sorts has taken place in the nursing profession, and nurses see themselves much more in terms of patient-advocacy models of nursing rather than in terms of the other two models. Numerous sociological factors, including a general restructuring of societal values, have encouraged this change.[10] As we move from a society based on industry to one based on information-gathering and processing, policymaking and decisionmaking become decentralized, and people want a more direct involvement in issues of importance to them. People whose lives are affected by a decision consider it essential to be part of the decisionmaking process. Traditional hierarchical structures are being replaced with decentralized authority and shared decisionmaking. This type of organizational decentralization of authority and responsibility emphasizes extensive communication and sharing of information. The new leader is a facilitator, not an order-giver.

In the late 1970s and the early 1980s, a severe nursing shortage prompted the American Hospital Association and other groups to sponsor studies that researched the causes of nursing "burn-out" and of the attrition of nurses from the field.[11] The chief finding of these various national studies was that nurses left the profession most frequently because of their inability to participate in the clinical decisionmaking process in a meaningful way; their lack of a sense of self-worth; and their perception of poor professional interactions with physicians. Nurses, and others, began developing an insight that their frustrations were caught up in what Hannah Arendt referred to as "bureaucratic violence."[12] In Arendt's model of a bureaucracy, those at the top give the orders and those at the bottom carry them out without questioning. Because those at the top do not implement the decisions, they do not see themselves as morally accountable for the decisions. Since the people at the bottom of the hierarchy are merely following someone else's orders, they also do not see themselves as accountable.

Change began to occur in health care bureaucracies because nurses attempted to gain some authority to make clinical judgments and to involve themselves in clinical decisions. Nurses wanted to be morally accountable and responsible for the care they provided. Moreover, a new legal definition of nursing practice came into use in the early 1970s.[13] Contrary to the old nurse practice acts, enacted many decades before and based on the idea that a nurse operated under a physician's license and followed a physician's orders, the new type of practice act, first passed in New York State,[14] defined clearly the independent role of nursing and the legal accountability of nurses to their patients. This act stated that nurses diagnose and treat patients' responses to actual or potential health problems. A memorandum that accompanied this act upon its introduction into the New York State legislature recognized that the focus of medicine was the nature and degree of pathologic functioning in illness, while the focus of nursing was the patient's response to the health problem and the nursing needs which arise from such responses. In other words, physicians diagnose and treat patients' diseases; nurses diagnose and treat patients' responses to health problems which may include responses to disease or medical treatment.

In 1980, the American Nurses' Association (ANA) put forth a significant policy statement on the role of nursing in society which reflects the New York State definition of nursing practice.[15] This statement has been given broad recognition, certainly by the profession and, recently, by the public, since state nurse practice acts throughout the country are defining nursing accordingly. The ANA statement has had a tremendous impact on the ethical aspects of health care decisionmaking and, more specifically, on health care providers and patients who now see nurses as making important clinical decisions.

BASIS FOR ETHICAL JUDGMENTS

The philosophical literature frequently portrays physicians as being scientifically oriented.[16] This is due in part to the fact that the primary basis of medical education is that of the physical sciences. Physicians are physical scientists who apply the methods of science to the bedside. The physician operates under a disease classification system, and then orients the diagnostic and therapeutic decisionmaking process toward the control or eradication of the disease that is causing the problem. The philosophical orientation of medicine is scientific and reductionist; the physician looks at bodily systems and organ dysfunction. With this philosophical orientation, one can envision an ethical mandate for physicians that involves the principle of doing what is least likely to harm the patient. One can argue that in some cases, the ethical mandate to the physician is to treat the disease, sometimes at all costs, because the primary duty is to control the disease process.[17]

The ethical mandate of the nurse can be different from that of a physician. Within the realm of human responses to the health problems which nurses diagnose and treat, lie many quality-of-life issues. The tension between nurses and physicians may occur because physicians often continue to ignore the expertise of nurses when seeking the solution of ethical problems. The number of cost/benefit conflicts is increasing between the two professions, especially in the teaching hospital where acute care medicine is practiced. In such a setting, the physician uses scientific criteria in deciding on his or her choice of treatment; nurses use more humanistic types of criteria, such as the patient's quality of life and ability to function, cope, or adapt in light of the disease and treatment.[18]

From 1978 to 1983, I gathered data from 800 nurses whom I asked to explain in detail the types of ethical dilemmas that they experienced in clinical practice.[19] There were many causes for these ethical dilemmas; sometimes, the institution, its philosophy, and its practices were in conflict with what nurses felt to be good-quality of nursing care. Examples were inadequate nursing staffing, lack of necessary equipment, and non-existent or inadequate policies for protecting patients. Sometimes, patients and families were also sources of conflict, as when family values or goals conflicted with what nurses perceived to be their professional duties and obligations to the patient. Another source of conflict occurred between nurses and physicians over treatment of patients. Of the 800 cases, forty-nine percent were concerned with truth-telling—withholding information needed by patients and families in order for them to make informed decisions; unethical behavior in organizations; and health professionals' incompetence or negligence in caring for patients. The dilemmas associated with the right to refuse treatment and the prolongation of life ranked as the second and third most prevalent categories (19 percent and 17 percent, respectively).

The case for more shared ethical decisionmaking in health care has been made by numerous legal decisions regarding treatment decisions, the Baby Doe regulations, and by the President's Commission for the Study of Ethical Problems in Medicine and Biomedical and Behavioral Research.[20] From a nursing perspective, ethics committees might be able to solve problems regarding the prolongation of life, treatment decisions, and informed consent. More generally, multidisciplinary input can be extremely important for hospital committees facing today's complex clinical dilemmas. Although I have concentrated on the physician's and the nurse's perspective, other members of the team could benefit the hospital ethics committee. Social workers, for example, very often deal with families and the community, as well as implement various kinds of counseling activities. They frequently have a perspective on the family and community resources different from other health professionals. Participation may be appropriate at various times for other health care professionals, such as respiratory therapists in a situation where life is sustained by the use of a ventilator.

Such committees also need someone with ethical training, such as a philosopher, a theologian, or a chaplain. These individuals have expertise in ethical analysis and a knowledge of ethical traditions. They also will probably not be caught in the various power struggles among health care providers. The hospital committee ought to invite consumers and representatives of the community to participate, as an acknowledgment of the new importance of a participatory democracy, where individuals whose lives are affected by a decision must be part of the process of making that decision.[21]

Many of the cases that I discussed earlier ended with questions. Nurses, until recently, did not know what to do. They wondered what should have been done, and what they would do if a similar situation were to arise again. In the past, fewer nurses were likely to take action in a situation because they were unsure of their status and their legitimacy in making ethical decisions. Yet, the nurse offers a philosophically different, but legitimate, perspective on patient care.

Because the nurse is the only health care professional who has sustained intimate contact with institutionalized patients over time, he or she is in a unique position to affect as well as assess the patient's quality of life and response to the health problems that create almost all ethical dilemmas in health care. Accordingly, it is necessary that the nurse be involved in coping with ethical problems and in making joint decisions. Physicians have expertise in the diagnosis, prognosis and treatment of diseases.[22] Nurses have expertise in the patient's response to health problems. Both areas of expertise of the two essential professional health care provider groups are necessary for humane and competent ethical decision-making.

As nurses begin to disagree more with other health care professionals and institutions who reduce quality nursing care in the interests of cost containment, communication will continue to break down and litigation may result unless nurses are intimately involved in patient care and institutional decisionmaking.[23] In the past, nurses did not feel comfortable blowing the whistle, partly because of fear of losing their jobs, but mostly because it was difficult to determine which potential solution to a patient's problem would cause the least harm to that patient. How does a nurse humanely blow the whistle on unsafe institutional practices, unethical practices of other health professionals or honest harm-benefit ratio conflicts with regard to treatment? Should he or she tell the patient lying seriously ill in the intensive care unit or should he or she go through bureaucratic channels that will more than likely suppress the conflict? Answers are not clear, but it is likely that an ethics committee, where the nurse's input was valued, would be a preferable course.

REFERENCES

1. Hellegers, A., *Accountability in the Health Care System: To Whom is the Nurse Responsible?* CONNECTICUT MEDICINE 43(10): 5–6 (October Supp. 1979).
2. *Id.* at 6.
3. A. ETZIONI, MODERN ORGANIZATIONS (Prentice-Hall, Inc., Englewood Cliffs, N.J.) (1964); A. ETZIONI, READINGS ON MODERN ORGANIZATIONS (Prentice-Hall, Inc., Englewood, N.J.) (1969); B.S. GEORGOPOULOS, S.C. MANN, THE COMMUNITY GENERAL HOSPITAL (MacMillan, New York, N.Y.) (1962); GOSS, M.E.W., *Influence and Authority Among Physicians in an Outpatient Clinic,* AMERICAN SOCIOLOGICAL REVIEW 26(1): 39–50 (February 1961).
4. J.A. ASHLEY, HOSPITALS, PATERNALISM, AND THE ROLE OF THE NURSE (Teachers' College Press, New York, N.Y.) (1976) at 16.
5. *Id.* at 77.
6. Murphy, C.P., *Moral Reasoning in a Selected Group of Nursing Practitioners,* in PERSPECTIVES ON NURSING LEADERSHIP (S. Ketefian, ed.) (Teachers' College Press, New York, N.Y.) (1981) at 45–75.
7. Murphy, C.P., *Models of the Nurse-Patient Relationship,* in ETHICAL PROBLEMS IN THE NURSE-PATIENT RELATIONSHIP (C.P. Murphy, H. Hunter,

eds.) (Allyn and Bacon, New York, N.Y.) (1982) at 8–25.

8. *Id.* at 11.

9. *Id.* at 18.

10. J. NAISBITT, MEGATRENDS: TEN NEW DIRECTIONS TRANSFORMING OUR LIVES (Warner Books, New York, N.Y.) (1982).

11. *See Three New Studies Seek Reasons for RN Shortage,* AMERICAN JOURNAL OF NURSING 81(2): 264 (February 1981); Wandelt, M.A., Pierce, P.M., Widdowson, R.R., *Why Nurses Leave Nursing and What Can Be Done About It,* AMERICAN JOURNAL OF NURSING 8(1): 72–77 (January 1981).

12. Kohlberg, L., Scharf, P., *Bureaucratic Violence and Conventional Moral Thinking* (unpublished manuscript) (April 1972).

13. NURSING: A SOCIAL POLICY STATEMENT (American Nurses Association, Kansas City, MO) (1983) [hereinafter referred to as SOCIAL POLICY].

14. Brown, G., Feldsine, E., Piemonte, R., *Implementing the Definition of Nursing Practice,* JOURNAL OF THE NEW YORK STATE NURSING ASSOCIATION 6(1): 14–18 (1975).

15. SOCIAL POLICY, *supra* note 13.

16. Cassell, E.J., *Illness and Disease,* HASTINGS CENTER REPORT 6(2): 27–37 (April 1976); Forstrom, L.A., *The Scientific Autonomy of Clinical Medicine,* JOURNAL OF MEDICINE AND PHILOSOPHY 2(1): 8–19 (March 1977); Engle, G.L., *The Need for a New Medical Model: A Challenge for Biomedicine,* SCIENCE 196(4286): 129–36 (April 8, 1977); Veatch, R.M., *The Medical Model: Its Nature and Problems,* HASTINGS CENTER STUDIES 1(3): 59–76 (1973); A.R. FEINSTEIN, CLINICAL JUDGMENT (Krieger Publishing Co., Melbourne, Fla.) (1974); E.A. MURPHY, THE LOGIC OF MEDICINE (Johns Hopkins University Press, Baltimore, Md.) (1976); R. WU, BEHAVIOR AND ILLNESS (Prentice-Hall, Englewood Cliffs, N.J.) (1973); Hellegers, *supra* note 1.

17. Murphy, C.P., *Nurses' Views Important on an Ethical Decision Team,* THE AMERICAN NURSE 15(10): 12–14 (November/December 1983) [hereinafter cited as *Nurses' Views Important*].

18. CLASSIFICATION OF NURSING DIAGNOSES: PROCEEDINGS OF THE THIRD & FOURTH NATIONAL CONFERENCES (M.J. Kim, D.A. Moritz, eds.) (McGraw Hill, New York, N.Y.) (1982).

19. Murphy, C.P., *Ethical Dilemmas in Nursing Practice: A Typology* (article in progress).

20. *Nondiscrimination on the Basis of Handicap: Procedures and Guidelines Relating to Health Care for Handicapped Infants,* 49 Fed. Reg. 1622 (January 12, 1984) (to be codified at 45 C.F.R.§ 84); PRESIDENT'S COMMISSION FOR THE STUDY OF ETHICAL PROBLEMS IN MEDICINE AND BIOMEDICAL AND BEHAVIORAL RESEARCH, DECIDING TO FOREGO LIFE SUSTAINING TREATMENT (U.S. Government Printing Office, Washington, D.C.) (1983).

21. NAISBITT, *supra* note 10.

22. *Nurses' Views Important, supra* note 17.

23. Grand Jury Report, Supreme Court of the State of New York, *Report of the Special January Additional 1983 Grand Jury concerning "Do not Resuscitate Procedures at a Certain Hospital in Queens County"*; Kirsch, J., *Mercy or Murder: A Death at Kaiser Hospital,* CALIFORNIA, pp. 79–81, 166–175 (November 1982).

Let's Stop Calling Ourselves "Patient Advocates"

Kathleen Deska Pagana

Hospitals are moving to Wall Street. Not physically, of course. But thanks in part to prospective payment systems, hospitals *have* adopted the language, methods, and attitudes of business. And one thing they're coming to expect is corporate loyalty, or employee support of their goals.

We nurses, however, usually think of ourselves as "patient advocates," whose first loyalty is to the patient. Yet doesn't this imply that others in the health care system somehow don't support the patient's best interests? And doesn't it set us up as adversaries of doctors and administrators?

But the truth is, the goals of doctors, administrators, and other health care personnel aren't actually that different from ours. A hospital can survive only if it attracts patients, and patients won't be "satisfied customers" who come again unless they receive good care. Doesn't that common goal make us all patient advocates?

Remember, hospitals (and so their employees) have two types of clients, two sources of income: patients and doctors. Many times, a nurse who sees herself as the patient's advocate will complain directly to administration about a doctor, rather than approaching him first. What could happen? The irate doctor could send his patients elsewhere and the hospital could lose that revenue.

Under prospective payment, the number of nurses a hospital employs depends on how well the hospital performs as a whole, not just on how efficiently nursing does its job. Besides our patients' health, we must also tend to our hospital's fiscal health. To do that, we have to become team players, loyal to both our hospital and our colleagues.

"Joining the team" essentially means recognizing that the health care system is in transition. That's what's making many people very nervous. But it's no reason to resist change or the administration's cost-reducing and cash-producing efforts. Better to look for ways to make the changes go smoothly.

BLIND LOYALTY?

So are we suggesting, "My hospital, right or wrong"? No. While becoming more aware of the hospital's business goals, we have to try to steer it in directions that promote good patient care. Indeed, nursing can become the fulcrum that helps hospitals balance cost with quality.

Consider this example: Many hospitals are introducing "same-day" surgery units. Two patients at two different hospitals who underwent surgical procedures around 3 P.M. reported being almost "shoved" out of the hospital by 6 P.M., although they were still affected by general anesthesia. They had severe nausea and vomiting during discharge and over the next few hours.

In these cases, blind loyalty to the same-day surgery concept resulted in physical discomfort for the patients, lost business for the hospitals (both patients said they'd never return), and diminished professional pride for the nurses.

No doubt the nurses felt uneasy about the quality of care given. However, in a sense nursing has the most power here—the ability to find a way to prevent similar problems in the future.

Pagana, K. D. (1987, February). Let's stop calling ourselves "patient advocates." *Nursing, 17,* 51. Reprinted with permission of © Springhouse Corporation. All rights reserved.

Hospital administrators, seeing only the daily case totals, may think nothing's wrong. As team players, the nurses can let them know the real situation: "We have a problem that we need to resolve—if we want future referrals."

Together, the nurses, administrators, and doctors can arrive at a solution. For instance, if all the same-day surgical cases can't be completed before a certain time, perhaps the remainder can be rescheduled.

Compare this with the "patient advocate" approach. Suppose a nurse on a same-day surgical unit complains to a patient and his family about its poor organization. By pitting herself against the system, she's jeopardizing her job and increasing the patient's and family's anxiety. Hardly the best way to win over administration.

NO "NAY SAYING"

Not only will team playing help us win support for our care ideas, it can also benefit our patients more subtly. Presenting the image of a unified, competent team builds patients' trust and confidence in the care they receive.

To maintain that image, let's think—and look—before we speak. No more derogatory remarks about doctors, administrators, or other health care personnel that patients or families can overhear. After all, that's criticizing the product.

Such disloyalty isn't accepted elsewhere: When the computer company's representative is busy fixing the unit's computer terminal, doesn't he typically blame the breakdown on misuse, not on his company's equipment?

A hospital needs to improve its efficiency and productivity for its economic survival. And that can happen only if we cooperate with each other.

In today's economy, Wall Street is no Easy Street. If the hospitals where we work can't make it there, we may find ourselves out of a job.

Nobody's advocate.

SELECTED REFERENCES

1. Ellis, J., and Hartley, C.: *Nursing in Today's World: Challenges, Issues, and Trends,* 2nd edition. Philadelphia, J.B. Lippincott Co., 1984.
2. Feldman, J., and Goldhaber, F.: "Living with DRGs," *Journal of Nursing Administration.* 14:19, May 1984.

STUDY AND DISCUSSION QUESTIONS
PHILOSOPHICAL FOUNDATIONS OF NURSING PRACTICE

1. Is Sarah Dock's first law of nursing—obedience without question—still applicable?

2. What do you think her attitude might be toward providing comfort measures when the physician had ordered no treatment? Or the withholding of emergency treatment at the client's request?

3. Dock states that doctors should report nurses who fail to carry out orders, but recommends that if a doctor's conduct is offensive or violates conscience that the nurse withdraw from the case rather than report the situation. Is there a moral justification for such a double standard?

4. What are the essential components of Newton's image of the traditional nurse and do you think that she is right in claiming that this is what the public wants?

5. What is the public image of nursing? Is it a barrier to professional autonomy?

6. Newton claims that without the humanizing presence of the traditional nurse, hospitals will become mechanical monsters. To what extent is it the nurse's responsibility to humanize the hospital environment?

7. Part of Newton's defense of the traditional role draws on the meaning of the word *nurse*. Has that term outlived its usefulness? Is it a liability or asset?

8. As noted in the Introduction, Newton's proposed aims of the hospital as the "saving of life and health" were similar to the commitments announced in nursing's first professionally accepted code of ethics (1950). Since that time, however, both of these commitments have been modified in more recent codes. Why do you think this happened? Is it a change for the better?

9. A key premise of Newton's argument is that being professional excludes being emotional. Is this true?

10. Consider the Holfing experiment. Would such an experiment be approved by institutional review boards today?

11. How would you account for the fact that when presented with a hypothetical situation only 2 of 12 graduate nurses and 0 of 22 student nurses would give an overdose of an unfamiliar drug phone-ordered by an unfamiliar psychiatrist, but 21 out of 22 nurses would give the drug in an actual staged situation?

12. Discuss the norms and virtues associated with the two metaphors Winslow believes played a prominent role in the formation of nursing ethics.

13. How has the doctrine of respondent superior affected nurse–physician relations?

14. What are the factors Winslow identifies which make nurses ideal patient advocates? Do you agree?

15. Has the metaphor of advocacy influenced nursing role conceptions and practice as much as Winslow suggests?

16. What is your opinion of Winslow's assessment of the advocacy metaphor?

17. What do you think of Gadow's suggestion that nursing be defined by its basic philosophy and not by the specific tasks nurses perform?

18. According to Gadow, how does "existential advocacy" differ from paternalism and consumerism?

19. Why, according to Gadow, is it impossible to define a patient's "best interests" apart from the patient's own preferences? Do you agree?

20. Do you think it is possible for a nurse to assist a patient in decision making without the nurse's views having undue influence?

21. Newton believes that the expression of emotion is unprofessional. Gadow, on the other hand, defends a notion of professional involvement that includes the possibility of emotional involvement of a certain sort. What kind of emotional involvement do you think is open to the professional nurse?

22. Describe the two functions of an advocate according to Mary Kohnke?

23. What are the differences between Gadow's and Kohnke's version of advocacy? Is Kohnke's view consumerism? Does Gadow's professional involvement lead to what Kohnke calls "rescuing"?

24. Are nurses ever justified in acting paternalistically? If so, under what circumstances?

25. Why does Catherine Murphy believe nurses should have a greater role in ethical decision making?

26. What explains the shift, which apparently began in the late 1970s, from bureaucratic and physician advocate models of ethical decision making to patient advocacy?

27. Murphy cited a number of studies that attributes nursing attrition to a lack of meaningful decision-making power in the clinical process. Alice Ream, however, believes that nursing drop out might be more directly attributable to changes in nursing education and its decreased skills emphasis. What do you think?

28. Do you think Kathleen Pagana has accurately described patient advocacy?

29. Do you believe that maximizing the profits of the hospital and producing satisfied customers are always in harmony?

30. Should the provision of health care be viewed as a consumer item or is it somehow different and special?

31. Where does the ultimate loyalty of Pagana reside? With the client? The health care team? The employing institution? Where should it reside?

2

The Nurse as Advocate:
Concepts and Controversy

INTRODUCTION

The previous chapter introduced the concept of client advocacy as a philosophical foundation for nursing ethics, its historical evolution, and some criticism of it. This chapter continues that dialogue. In particular, we focus on the patient rights advocate as originally envisioned and the degree to which this idea can or should be incorporated into the nursing role.

The first article is an articulation of the concept of patient advocacy as it was originally developed in 1974 by two lawyers intimately involved in health care, George Annas and Joseph Healey. Annas, in the second and third articles, discusses the relationship of this idea to nursing and the scope of client rights to be protected.

It is no secret that patient representatives are one response to the patients' rights movement. The four articles selected (Gikuuri, Cote, McDonald, and Zusman) discuss the origin of patient representatives, their function, value, and their relation to nursing.

The articles by Abrams, Miller et al., the Trandel-Korenchuks, and Curtin discuss the relationship of patient advocacy to the role of the nurse. Abrams argues that nurses are not best suited for this role because of conflicting obligations and the risks the role may involve. Miller et al. and the Trandel-Korenchuks have similar conclusions and complementary analyses about why nurse advocacy of patients rights is more myth than reality. Finally, Curtin, although critical of some excessive formulations of advocacy, considers it part of good nursing practice.

A more detailed discussion of these articles follows.

THE PATIENT RIGHTS MOVEMENT AND NURSING

Two attorneys, George Annas and Joseph Healey, proposed a patient rights advocate system in their article "The Patient Rights Advocate." As they saw it, the problem was that patients had many interests (some of which were rights protected by law) that were either limited, unprotected, or went unrecognized by health care facilities. The solution they envisioned was an independent patient rights advocate system where the advocate is legally empowered to protect the rights and interests of the patient. Advocates would have such privileges as unrestricted access to medical records, consultations, participation on relevant hospital committees, the ability to lodge complaints with the hospital's director and executive committee, and access to all support services. The primary function of the advocate would be to assist the patient in protecting and asserting personal interests ("interests" and "rights" are used almost interchangeably here). Such a system, the authors believe, would alter the traditional doctor–patient relationship and give greater decision-making power to the consumer.

The central part of the article is devoted to outlining the interests that patients have and how an advocate system could work to acknowledge or protect them. The examples used to illustrate the failure of the present system revolve about failures to provide information, respect childbirth preferences, or respect privacy. These violations of patient interests may not lead to any physical harm, but they are nevertheless wrongs inflicted on the individual. The patient advocate system would provide for the protection, assertion, and redress of these violations.

In "The Patient Rights Advocate: Can Nurses Effectively Fill the Role?", George Annas further elaborates on the nature of the rights of patients and considers the title question. He suggests the main educational qualifications for the patient advocate are training in medicine, law, and psychology. Annas concedes that it would be easier for a nurse to obtain the needed legal and psychological qualifications than for someone with those qualifications obtaining the needed medical knowledge. But there are at least two barriers to nurses becoming patient advocates in his sense. The first barrier concerns how the nurse perceives the role. Annas believes qualities that define the "traditional" nurse are incompatible with patient advocacy—the nurse's first loyalty is not to the patient. The second barrier concerns the public image of the nurse. The nurse cannot function effectively as a patient rights advocate as long as the patient sees the nurse as the doctor's helper.

In "Patient Rights: An Agenda for the '80's," George Annas presents a five-point agenda for humanizing the hospital and respecting the right of self-determination. One of those five points is "an effective patient advocate." Annas has taken the view that it is likely that the only effective patient advocacy can be given by someone not financially tied to the employing institution. This short article, written seven years after Annas entertained the question,

"Can Nurses Effectively Fill the Role of Patient Rights Advocate?", stresses the independence of the advocate.

THE PATIENT REPRESENTATIVE AND THE ROLE OF THE NURSE—GIKUURI, COTE, McDONALD, AND ZUSMAN

The ANA Code for Nurses with Interpretive Statements states: "Each nurse has an obligation to be knowledgeable about the moral and legal rights of all clients and to protect and support those rights."[1] This is one of the roles of the nurse that coincides with the Annas and Healey conception of a patient rights advocate. The role of the patient representative, under some descriptions, also functions to implement and monitor patient rights. In their 1974 paper, "The Patient Rights Advocate," Annas and Healey gave a rather cool reception to this role. In their view, the term *patient representative* is misapplied because according to job descriptions he or she actually represents the hospital or employing institution and more often than not is restricted to non-medical "housekeeping" matters.

The patient representative has some of the same problems Annas finds objectionable about nurses. That is, patient representatives are employed by institutions and may be perceived by the public as acting in the institution's interest. Nevertheless, this idea deserves some exploration. The article by June Gikuuri, "The Role of the Patient Representative," describes the evolution and need for someone to protect the rights of clients.

Anne Cote, in "The Patient's Representative: Whose Side Is She On?", explains many of the same rights covered in Gikuuri but also relates them to the role of the nurse. Perhaps because Cote is a nurse herself, she sees the patient representative as an ally of nursing. Cote says "all we're doing is *specializing* in a job that's been a part of [nursing's] role for a long, long time." One way to do that is to call in a patient representative when the client's rights are being abused; the patient representative then will join the battle on the client's side and so the nurse need not suppose that he or she is in the battle alone.

Nancy McDonald, also a patient representative, makes an economic case for patient representatives in "Patient Rep Can be Viewed as Fiscal Asset." The case is based primarily on common sense assumptions about risk management, that is, if patients have no other recourse for their complaints except legal, they will use that avenue of redress more often than when the complaint can be solved internally. McDonald presents no statistical evidence to support this assumption, but if it is true it would also be an argument for why it is in the facility's best economic interests for nurses to fulfill this role.

Like Cote, Jack Zusman, a physician who is director of a patient advocacy training program, sees patient advocacy as both a responsibility of nursing *and* an independent function of patient representatives. It is unclear, however, whether he means to distinguish patient advocates created by law with certain legal authority from patient representatives, ombudsmen, and patient hostesses who have delegated authority from the employing institution. Nevertheless, Zusman, in his "Want Some Good Advice?: Think Twice About Being a Patient Advocate," differentiates two kinds of advocacy styles: adversarial and responsible.

Zusman prescribes a form of advocacy so qualified and conditioned by other factors that it hardly resembles the concept as described by Annas. The "responsible" style also seems quite different from Mary Kohnke's (previous chapter) where clients are entitled to support for their choices. In Zusman's view, what the patient wants and has a right to is only one point to be considered. A "responsible advocate" doesn't take everything a patient says at face value because in spite of what the patient may say the situation may suggest a different approach to the problem of protecting the patient's best interest. (This is traditional medical paternalism.) Thus, what a patient wants is sometimes restricted by what is in his or her best interest. Zusman further qualifies the actions on behalf of a patient by insisting that a responsible advocate must consider "everyone's welfare"—patients and other staff members. These considerations then significantly condition which actions a responsible advocate will advocate on behalf of the patient and how far the advocate will go in advocating them. However, Zusman does believe that if "something terrible" is going to happen to a patient an advocate should risk job and career for the patient.

PATIENT ADVOCACY: ASSESSMENTS AND CRITIQUES—ABRAMS, MILLER ET AL., TRANDEL-KORENCHUK, AND CURTIN

A philosopher, Natalie Abrams, in "A Contrary View of the Nurse as Patient Advocate," presents objections to the nurse being an advocate for the patient. After discussing five, possibly overlapping, models of advocacy and the need for them, Abrams particularly criticizes the idea that the nurse should act as spokesperson for the patient or as a defender of the patient's rights. Three problem areas are identified. The first concerns the kind of advocacy involved. That is, does the nurse serve the patient's wishes or act in the patient's "best interest" (paternalism)? The second concerns potential conflicts of interests and hazards to the nurse. Supposing that the nurse acts on the preferences of the patient, this may create conflicts with the nurse's own professional standards and obligations to the employing institution and other health care professionals. The third problem is related to the second. Since the nurse has divided loyalties, an independent advocate without such loyalties is preferable. Although Abrams admits it is naive to suggest that such advocacy is taking place within hospitals, she believes that patients have the right to as impartial and extensive advocacy as possible. No plan as to how that is to be accomplished is offered. Clearly, however, if nurses are unsuited for the role because of divided loyalties, it makes no sense to think that somehow the whole system serves as the patient's advocate. The system also has divided loyalties. Barbara Miller et al., in their article "Patient Advocacy: Do Nurses Have the Power and Authority to Act as Patient Advocates?", posed the main question in the title and answered it negatively. Here, the authors (all nurses) lament that although patient advocacy is part of the nurses' role, they do not have either the power or the authority to act in the patient's interest. A three-fold problem arises: some nurses are good caregivers but they are not risk takers; nurses have not cohesively united to support one another and nursing itself; and nurses do not have the formal authority to act in behalf of their patients.

The case of Jolene Tuma has been mentioned several times already in the articles contained in this anthology. Darlene and Keith Trandel-Korenchuk, a nurse and lawyer respectively, also highlight this case as emblematic of nursing's problems. Their article, "Nursing Advocacy of Patients' Rights: Myth or Reality?", finds advocacy more myth than reality.

According to the Trandel-Korenchuks, the Tuma case illustrates the problems of nursing as a whole. Tuma, they say, lacked respect for her own judgment, lacked authority to meet patients' needs, was treated as subordinate to the physicians, and lacked the autonomy to carry out nursing functions. It is the lack of these four qualities (respect, equality, autonomy, and authority) that hinders nurses in making appropriate moral decisions and protecting client rights. The article goes on to explore the reasons behind this predicament. Significant factors include the historical establishment of a male-dominated medical profession, a female-dominated nursing profession bound to traditional gender expectations, the socialization of females and nurses into certain role stereotypes, and the influence of those stereotypic role expectations on the nurse–physician and nurse–nurse relationships. Such stereotypes also include the manner in which the forces that maintain the system—nursing education, hospital bureaucracies, and even state nurse practice acts—are viewed.

Finally, Leah Curtin, a nurse with a background in philosophy, discusses and critiques a variety of conceptions of advocacy in her "The Nurse as Advocate: A Cantankerous Critique." In this article, many of the views and issues we have encountered are summarized. Curtin concludes that it is easier to say what advocacy forbids than what it demands, but it is nevertheless clear to her that nurses are advocates and that advocacy is an internal part of good nursing practice.

SUMMARY

This chapter has focused on the rights of patients and how best to protect them. Although the authors of the articles under discussion express a clear need for such protection, their proposals differ about how to accomplish this. Can nurses fill this role? Should there be a separate health care professional who fulfills this function? Would the existence of an effective patient advocate system relieve nurses of the obligation to protect the rights of patients as required by the code? How should nurses go about advocating patients' rights? Do nurses have the power and authority to act as patient advocates or is this an unrealizable ideal? Is advocacy something distinguishable from the role of the nurse?

It is possible for a variety of means to simultaneously protect patient rights—that is, nursing's commitment to protecting and preserving the moral and legal rights of clients can exist in harmony with both a legally authorized patient advocate scheme and patient representatives.[2] Some authors have thought that nurses would not be the best kind of patient advocates, but no one has argued that patient advocacy and nursing be totally divorced from each other. Indeed, the most disturbing aspect of these articles is the suggestion that, while advocacy has become an inalienable obligation, nurses are incapable of carrying out this obligation except at great risk and with enormous personal courage.

NOTES

1. American Nurses' Association, *Code for Nurses with Interpretive Statements* (Kansas City, Mo.: American Nurses' Association, 1985).
2. Still another possibility is the approach developed by Barbara Huttman, a nurse, in her book *The Patient's Advocate* (New York: Penguin Books, 1981). This is a handbook on patient's rights, hospital jargon and routines, and other information so that any intelligent person can secure the rights of a hospitalized patient.

The Patient Rights Advocate

George J. Annas and Joseph Healey

Medical advances have greatly increased the ability of physicians to cure patients and postpone death. While the medical profession has become technologically more proficient, it has increasingly tended to ignore the human qualities and rights of the patient. This trend toward increased inequality in health rights contradicts trends such as consumer/seller rights in other areas of human affairs. Hospitals currently provide few methods patients can use to safeguard their human rights and participate in a meaningful way in medical decision-making. The *patient rights advocate* is suggested as a mechanism to increase the ability of the patient to participate in medical decision-making regarding his care.

The Commission FINDS that the interest of health-care providers and the consumers are best served by effective consumer participation at the decision-making level.

Report of the Secretary's Commission on Medical Malpractice, U.S. Dept. Health, Education, & Welfare, January 1973.

Increased attention to the concept of the rights of a patient is a product of two trends prominent during this century: (1) progress within the American legal system toward redefining such previously protected legal relationships as landlord-tenant, buyer-seller, educator-student, warden-prisoner, administrator-committed mental patient and employer-employee. The emphasis in this process of redefinition has been on the need to correct the imbalance which the law enforced or protected by substituting a more equitable sharing of duties and rights, powers, and liabilities; and (2) the rise of the consumer movement as the attempt of an inquiring citizenry to compel equalization of bargaining power, participation in the selection and implementation of policy goals, and accountability for the quality of performance.

There have recently been rigorous exchanges concerning the sources of such new directions. Quite frequently, those who seek to encourage these trends rely on the concepts of human or personal rights. A good example of this has been the redefinition of the relationship between the buyer and the seller. Some go so far as to argue that it is no longer *caveat emptor*—let the buyer beware—but *caveat vendor*, in the wake of refined credit laws and products liability suits. Truth in lending laws, for example, are a product of the concept that the consumer has a "right to know" the true interest rate he will be charged. In the discipline of philosophy in general and legal philosophy in particular, there has been a great deal of discussion concerning the appropriateness of using the concept of "rights," and of the efficacy of so doing, even if appropriateness is conceded. We hope to avoid a concept of patient rights which does not require an investigation of the source of each of these rights, but begins with a basic recognition of certain personal interests. These interests are neither absolute nor summarily dismissible and form the basis of a series of problems in society as a whole and within the health care facility in particular, when in conflict with the interests of others. These conflicts among competing interests must be resolved if the health care facility is to function appropriately. The manner in which that resolution takes place is of maximum importance to the patient. His interests demand not only representation but protection. Decisions concerning him unavoidably affect the quality and often the length of his

Annas, G.J., & Healey, J. (1974, May–June). The patient rights advocate. *The Journal of Nursing Administration, 4,* 25–31.

life. We use the word *right*, therefore, to mean "personal interest," and as a concept which enables us to examine the conflict between competing interests and the resolution of such conflicts.

Generally speaking, the problem is twofold. The American medical consumer possesses certain interests, many of which are recognized within the American legal system, which he does not automatically forfeit when he enters a health care facility, and most health care facilities fail to recognize them, to provide for their assertion or protection, and limit their exercise without recourse for the patient. We suggest that a solution to this problem may be a patient rights advocate system.

THE NATURE OF THE RIGHTS

Four general areas of personal interests which we suggest are rights assertable in the health care facility context and are worthy of protection:

1. The right to the whole truth.
2. The right to privacy and personal dignity.
3. The right to retain self-determination by participation in the making of decisions regarding one's health care.
4. The right of complete access to medical records both during and after the hospital stay.

These four areas can be most understandably considered chronologically as they arise in the interaction between the patient and the health care facility. The first series of problems involves the selection of the health care facility by the patient. They can be stated as questions:

1. To what extent does the potential patient have a right to know the *available medical resources* within the community?
2. To what extent does the potential patient have a right to know what research and *experimental protocols* are being used within the health care facility and what alternatives for treatment exist?
3. To what extent is there a right to know one's "rights" as a patient?
4. To what extent is there a right to the "best medical treatment available" and the highest degree of care without regard to the source of payment for that treatment and care?

5. To what extent is there a right to complete *secrecy* concerning the source of payment for treatment and care?

The second series of questions arises at the time of entrance into the health care facility, whether as an outpatient, inpatient, or emergency case:

1. To what extent is there a right to be examined by a *qualified* medical practitioner?
2. To what extent is there a right to *prompt* attention, especially in an emergency situation?
3. To what extent is there a right to a *complete* and *accurate* diagnosis, especially with regard to avoiding the premature attachment of label?
4. To what extent is there, from the very first form that must be signed, a right to have each form carefully explained and the significance of consent clarified?
5. To what extent does a person who does not speak English have a right to an interpreter?

The third series involves questions that arise during the patient's stay in the health care facility:

1. To what extent does the patient have a right to a clear, *complete*, and accurate evaluation of his condition?
2. To what extent does the *family* of the patient have a right to a clear, complete, and accurate evaluation of the patient's condition?
3. To what extent does the patient have a right to his medical record and to discussion of his condition with a consultant-specialist, at his own request?
4. To what extent is such information (1–3) unavoidably linked to informed consent?
5. To what extent does a patient have a right to a detailed explanation of every diagnostic test, treatment, procedure, or operation, including alternative procedures, costs, risks, and especially including the identity and qualifications of the person actually performing the procedure?
6. To what extent does the patient have a right to know whether a particular test or procedure is for his benefit or for educational purposes?
7. To what extent does a patient have a right to refuse any particular drug, test, or treatment?

8. To what extent does the patient have a right to both personal and informational privacy with respect to
   A. Hospital staff
   B. Other doctors
   C. Residents, interns, and medical students
   D. Nurses
   E. Other patients

9. To what extent does the patient have a right to access to the "outside world" by means of visitors and the availability of a telephone; or to limit such access as he sees fit?

10. To what extent is there a right to leave the health care facility, regardless of physical condition or financial status?

The fourth and last series of questions arises after leaving the health care facility.

1. To what extent does the patient have a right to have a complete copy of his medical record?

2. To what extent does the patient have a right to continuity of care by means of access to the doctors who provided treatment?

Each of these rights represents an area of personal interest. Few, if any, involve clear-cut, absolute principles. All involve a resolution of conflicting interests and the delicate balance between the interests of the patient and the interests of the provider. The manner in which these conflicts have traditionally been resolved provides a starting point to understand the need for a Patient Rights Advocate.

The Traditional Resolution: The Doctor–Patient Relationship

Traditionally, resolution of the conflicting interests has been performed by the individual doctor. These important decisions, like all major medical decision-making, are rooted in the traditional doctor–patient relationship. This relationship has failed to keep pace with parallel historical contractual developments.

As recently as the turn of the century a random patient meeting a random physician had less than a fifty-fifty chance of benefiting from the encounter. Physicians were emerging from the era when they were essentially tradesmen, with little more to offer their patients than comfort and company. The principal causes of mortality were the infectious diseases against which they stood impotent. There were few medical schools, few diagnostic tests, no specific treatment of disease, and no specialization of physicians. In the words of former AMA president Dwight L. Wilbur, "It is difficult to accept that physicians of that day and this were even in the same profession"[1].

Medical progress has brought about a radical change in the doctor's ability to diagnose and treat disease. Infectious disease has been all but conquered and the chronic diseases, such as heart disease, have become the major killers. Hospitals have replaced "pest houses," and medical education has become increasingly demanding and exact. While the technology of medicine no longer resembles that of a century ago, physicians continue to argue that the "traditional doctor–patient relationship" must be maintained at all costs. In view of the tremendous changes in the content and context of that relationship over the past century, this argument would seem to be of dubious merit. The advantages of maintaining such a traditional relationship *in theory* if not in actual practice are many, however. Accountability for actions is likely to be restricted to peer review. Public scrutiny of medical decision-making is likely to be minimal. Autonomy of action is likely to be maximal. Patient-consumer influence on services rendered is not likely to be significant.

The problems generated by attempting to retain the traditional model of the doctor–patient relationship can be viewed as the characteristics of present day medical decision-making:

1. Ambiguous identification of the decision-maker.
2. Ambiguous identification of the person or entity that commands the decision-maker's loyalty.
3. Control of pertinent medical information by the attending physician.
4. Lack of reporting or review of the ultimate treatment decision.
5. Justification of the decision on the basis of public policy[2].

The questions of who actually makes the decision and whose interests command the decision-maker's loyalties have received a great deal of attention in the kidney transplant cases of *Strunk v. Strunk* and *Hart v. Brown* with respect to the action of a guardian giving consent on behalf of an incompetent and a minor respectively[3, 4]. Other aspects of characteristics 1 and 2 include the identity of the person paying the bill, the existence of research in which the decision-maker is involved, and the decision-maker's own biases. The third characteristic is self-explanatory. The fourth concerns the lack of any systematic review of medical decision-making. Present peer review mechanisms are unsatisfactory, and often the only way a person can determine relevant facts about a past decision is to institute a malpractice action. The fifth relates to the increasing frequency of discussions about "quality of life," resource allocation, and societal goals by members of the medical profession[5]. Decisions on these issues are usually best left to judicial and legislative bodies.

If any third party were to become involved in examining a medical decision (a relative or a patient rights advocate, for example) the first thing he or she would need to know would be the answers to the five questions posed by the characteristics of medical decision-making:

1. Who has the power to make a treatment decision?

2. Where do the decision-maker's loyalties lie?

3. Who controls the pertinent information?

4. Is there any review of the treatment decision? If so, by whom?

5. On what basis is the treatment decision justified?

To answer this set of questions the third party may need some help. For example, access to the patient's medical records and someone who can interpret them is essential. The only way to avoid the problem of monopoly over information is to make that information available to a knowledgeable representative of the patient. The four other characteristics might be similarly attacked. Such an attack cannot, however, be successfully mounted by a public relations person or a nurse or unit manager lacking autonomy or individual power. The Patient Services Coordinator for New York Hospital has described the person needed as, "someone who will greet the patient with a smile, listen to him, get to know him as a person and be his voice"[6]. While such a person may be needed, the role described is an extremely limited one and one which does *nothing* to resolve the five problems generated by modern application of the concept of the "traditional doctor–patient relationship." Other nurses have recognized this[7,8].

When individuals are sick, dying, or both they need more than a "placebo practitioner" to hold their hands. They need to know that they can count on the loyalty and judgment of a competent person who, at their direction, has access to their medical records and staff consultants and can and will give them straight, unbiased answers to their questions. Anything less means that both their health *and* their human rights are potentially in danger.

Some Examples of How an Advocate System Would Function

Case One: Outpatient

Patient 1 has been having intermittent chest pains for 3 years. One year ago he had a myocardial infarction and was hospitalized in a community hospital. At his last visit to his physician he got the impression that his continuing episodes of chest pain were causing the doctor concern. Under questioning the physician admitted that the patient had an abnormal electrocardiogram, but said he would recommend activity and dietary restrictions only. Patient 1 has a friend with a similar history. This friend has recently undergone an operation on his coronary blood vessels and has been doing much better since the surgery. Patient 1 wants to know more about this operation, its (1) indications, (2) cost, and (3) prognosis. His doctor will not discuss it with him.

Under the current system patient 1 could either get another doctor or go to a medical library or bookstore and try to find relevant materials. Under a patient advocate system with a community education program, patient 1 could call the patient rights advocate and get some of the information he desires. The advocate would *not* give medical advice, but would have a file on the types of operations performed at his health care facility, their indications, costs, and success rate. He could read summary information over the phone and refer the patient to a physician who would be willing to discuss it in detail. The advocate here would be performing the function of information broker. A variation on this theme is presently in effect at four Madison, Wisconsin, hospitals and enables patients to dial a number and listen to a 4- to 5-minute tape recording concerning various medical topics such as "your hysterectomy," "having a myelogram?" and "the pill in perspective"[9]. The public needs more information about health and the health care system, and one hopes the patient rights advocate could find ways to utilize mass media for such education.

Case Two: Breast Cancer

Patient 2 enters the hospital to have a breast biopsy. She is extremely nervous and upset. She is asked to sign a consent form that she doesn't understand. She is assured it is "routine" and signs it. When she sees her doctor she asks him about the alternative methods of treatment available if her tumor turns out to be malignant. He tells her that he does only radical mastectomies, but that she shouldn't worry before they know whether her tumor is malignant or not. The doctor then leaves the hospital for the day. Patient 2 continues to think about her condition and asks the nurse what will happen if her tumor is malignant or not. Specifically she wants to know if the doctor will immediately proceed with the mastectomy while she is still unconscious. The nurse says that this should be discussed with the doctor[10].

Under the present system the patient has little recourse but to either try to get her doctor on the phone or wait until the next day when she might see him again before the biopsy. As to the consent form, no one is presently available to explain it to her. Under an advocacy system a patient rights advocate would be on call to explain consent forms and their implications to all patients required by the hospital to sign them. She would also be provided with a card on which a list of questions is printed which she would be advised to ask anyone requesting her to sign such a form:

—What treatment does the doctor want to use and why?

—What alternative treatments are available and why is the method chosen superior to others?

—What are the risks involved of the procedure; of not having the procedure?

—Is the procedure experimental?

—Who will perform the procedure (name and status, e.g., doctor, intern, resident, medical student)?

—What are the side effects and how long will they last?

—How much will it cost?

—How long will it mean in terms of hospitalization?

—What will be the permanent effects?

—What are the possibilities of a complete cure?

Had patient 2 asked her doctor these questions initially, and had the doctor responded to them, the difficulties she is now experiencing would not have occurred.

Case Three: Childbirth

Patient 3 and her husband have attended classes on natural (Lamaze) childbirth. They have discussed the matter with the doctor in the outpatient clinic of the hospital where the child will be delivered. The hospital has a policy of allowing the husband in the delivery room "at the doctor's discretion." They enter the hospital and spend three hours together in the labor room. As she is being transferred to the delivery room the doctor (a resident) says to the husband, "Sorry, you can't come in, you make me nervous." In the delivery room patient 3, who has previously given birth by the natural method in England, demands that the stirrups be removed. The attendants laugh at her and hold her down as her wrists are strapped to the table by leather thongs[11].

Under the current system patient 3 and her husband have little, if any, recourse. Under a patient advocate system with an advocate assigned to the maternity ward, the advocate would be in charge of advising the medical personnel about the couple's desires concerning natural childbirth. He or she would make whatever preparations were deemed necessary, and be present at the parents' request to be sure both that the father was not denied access to the delivery room during birth and that the mother is not subjected to coercion or ridicule during birth (this latter function would probably not be necessary if the husband were allowed to be present in the delivery room as a matter of course). The advocate would function similarly in the emergency room when delays could be cut or when an interpreter was needed.

Case Four: Diagnostic

Patient 4 was admitted to the hospital for a series of tests to determine the identity of the condition he was suffering from. A neurologist and three medical students ran him through a neurological examination. In his words: "I got a reinforcement of the sense of not only am I a patient who is supposed to behave in a certain way, but I'm almost an object to demonstrate to people that I'm not really people any more, I'm something else. I'm a body that has some very interesting characteristics about it . . . . I began to feel not only the fear of this unknown, dread thing that I have, that nobody knows anything about—and if they know, they're not going to tell me—but an anger and a resentment of 'Goddamn it, I'm a human being and I want to be treated like one!' And feeling that if I expressed anger, I could be retaliated against, because I'm in a very vulnerable position"[12].

Some of the frustrations of patient 4 could find an outlet in the person of the patient rights advocate. The advocate would be a person that the patient could talk to without fear of retaliation. A person who could pull out his medical records and tell him whether or not a diagnosis had been made. A person who, on behalf of a busy medical staff, could take the time to explain the reason for the tests, why medical students were present, that he could have them excluded if he wished, that no matter what his attitudes toward the medical staff or his expressions of fear and resentment, no retaliatory action would be taken against him in any manner.

DISCUSSION

The reason cases like the four cited occur is that the present hospital system does not make provision for the exercise of the human rights of patients. Some hospitals are better than others, however, and some have made moves to improve. In a recent survey of 2,000 hospitals having more than 200 beds, 462 of the 1,000 responding said they had at least one employee whose primary job was "to serve as management's direct representative to patients"[13]. While they termed this person a *patient representative*, it is clear from the job description that the person is perceived as a "management representative." Most are restricted to non-medical "housekeeping" matters.

Some hospitals and consumer organizations have developed books or pamphlets that explain patient rights to the patients. Perhaps the most complete is *Your Rights as a Patient at Yale-New Haven Hospital*, which was prepared by the Dixwell Legal Rights Association, Inc. of New Haven, Connecticut. The strengths of this publication are that it gives the patient specific questions to ask the staff and the doctor as well as the name and extension of a *patient assistant* to call. Problems include incompleteness in terms of explaining rights, and the lack of authority of the patient assistant. The Martin Luther King Health Center of New York has a publication entitled

Your Rights as a Patient[14]. Unfortunately, it is more of a cartoon sketch of the predicaments of patients than a working document for the protection of patient rights. One innovation, however, is the inclusion of a patient complaint form in the pamphlet itself. The problem, again, is assertion of rights.

In Boston, the Beth Israel Hospital has published a one page brochure entitled *Your Rights as a Patient at Beth Israel Hospital*. The rights enumerated in this document come essentially from the Preamble of the standards of the Joint Commission on Hospital Accreditation published in 1970. No mention is made in this pamphlet of any person at the hospital in charge of seeing to it that these rights are not violated. While Massachusetts law specifically grants patients access to their medical records, the Beth Israel brochure fails to mention this fact. The 12-point "Patient's Bill of Rights" promulgated by the American Hospital Association on January 8, 1973, follows the pattern of the Joint Commission and Beth Israel statements in its vagueness and lack of an enforcement mechanism[15]. In the field of landlord–tenant law it would seem obviously anomalous to permit the landlord alone to determine tenant rights. In the hospital field, however, such provider dominance over the consumer is so commonplace that it seldom is even commented upon.

The collections of rights currently being promulgated by hospitals remind one very much of the free enterprise economic philosophy of Ayn Rand, restated to the medical profession by Dr. Robert M. Sade in a recent article[16]. Not being able to recognize the difference between medical care and the banking industry, Dr. Sade is incapable of going on to consider the human rights of his patients while they are under medical care. What is needed is *not* more lists from providers, but a well-reasoned and complete consumer-prepared catalog of the rights of hospital patients of at least the quality of the American Civil Liberties Union Handbook Series. The document will be the foundation of a Patient Rights Program.

THE PATIENT RIGHTS ADVOCATE SYSTEM

The goals of a program of patient advocacy are:

1. To protect patients, particularly those at a disadvantage within the hospital context (the young, the illiterate, the uncommunicative, those without relatives, those unable to speak

English) by making available a series of processes and procedures.

2. To make available to those who seek it the opportunity to participate actively with one's doctor as a partner in one's personal health care program.

3. To restore to proper perspective medical technologies and pharmaceutical advances, and to confront the exaggerated expectations of the modern American medical consumer.

4. To reflect in the patient–doctor relationship the reality of the health-sickness continuum and to reassert the humanness of death as inevitable and as natural as birth.

The advocate represents the patient. Therefore the powers of an advocate are those that belong to the patient. His purpose is to assist the patient in exercising his rights. To be effective a patient rights advocate must have at least the following: (1) Complete access to medical records and the ability to call in a consultant to comment, explain, or advise the patient (both at the direction of the patient). (2) Participation in those hospital committees responsible for monitoring quality care within the health care institution, especially utilization-review, patient care, and human experimentation. (3) Ability to exercise patient rights through the hospital's Executive Committee or other mechanism established to deal with patient complaints. (4) Access to support services for all patients who request them.

The patient/advocate ratio must also be such that the advocate is available to perform these services for all who request it. He would meet the patient shortly after admission, explain his function, and give the patient a pamphlet on his rights. Thereafter the initiative would generally be taken by the patient, but the advocate might also make periodic rounds.

This may seem a modest response to the problems of the doctor–patient relationship in the hospital, but it represents an important first step toward accepting and recognizing the central role of the patient in medical decision-making and providing him with the information he needs to participate in decision-making in an intelligent manner. There are many things the advocate cannot do and many problems he cannot solve. But the primary consideration in presenting this discussion model has been to create a proposal that is efficacious and practicable.

We call for the creation of a position to be filled by a person whose primary responsibility and loyalty is to the patient alone and whose function is to assist the patient in protecting or asserting personal interests. The difficulties in allowing the doctor to continue to make the decision have been pointed out. The difficulty in allowing a member of the administrative staff to serve as a patient rights advocate includes serious questions of conflicts of loyalties and interests since such a person often views as his primary responsibility the elimination of conflict in the hospital. This is often accomplished only by subordinating the patient's interest to those of the individual doctor and the health care facility. The result is unsatisfactory at best. The patient needs someone who can provide him with information and who has the ability to assert and protect his interests. While training in medicine, law, and psychology will be important, most training will probably be done on the job. We suggest that it is critical to decide who shall supervise the work of the advocate and who shall support his work. The most preferable situation would be support and supervision from *outside* the health care facility (e.g., Department of Public Health or Consumer Affairs, a statewide medical care foundation, or a health consumer group). If there is no alternative but to make the advocate a member of the hospital administrative staff, it is imperative that he be accountable only to the patient he services.

This proposal is designed to begin to redefine the doctor–patient relationship in the hospital. It is the first step toward creating appropriate procedures within the health care facility to make decisions which neither doctors, administrators, nurses, lawyers, or judges are exclusively competent to make. It is a start which we hope will serve as a basis for discussion and experimentation. The goal is not to create "another layer" between the doctor and the patient, but to attempt to get the doctor and patient to make medical decisions *together*, with the patient having the *final* word. When one is sick, one is willing to give up many rights if by so doing one can be cured of illness or injury. While this is a natural human reaction, it is neither desirable nor necessary, and the patient rights advocate can help insure that human rights do not become the victims of medical progress.

REFERENCES AND NOTES

1. D. Wilbur, D. Let's lead rather than be led. *J. Tenn. Med. Assoc.* 62:607, 1970.
2. Annas, G. Medical remedies and human rights: Why civil rights lawyers must become involved

in medical decision-making, *Human Rights* 2:151, 1972.

3. 445 S.W. 2d 145 (Ky., 1969).
4. 289 A. 2d 386, 29 Conn. Sup. 368 (1972).
5. Duff, R., and Campbell, A. Moral and ethical dilemmas in the special care nursery. *N. Engl. J. Med. 289:890, 1973.*
6. Cote, A. The patient's link. *Trial* 9:30, 1973.
7. Nations, W. Nurse-lawyer is patient-advocate. *Am. J. Nurs.* 73:1039, 1973.
8. Koski, S. Patient advocacy or fighting the system. *Am. J. Nurs.* 72:694–698, 1972.
9. M. Bartlett, M., Johnston, A., and Meyer, T. Dial access library—patient information service. *N. Engl. J. Med.* 288:994, 1973.
10. Campion, R. *The Invisible Worm.* New York: Macmillan Co., 1972.
11. Based on the experience of Joan Haggerty. *Ms.* 4:16, 1973.
12. Hanlan, A. Notes of a dying professor. *Pa. Gazette,* March 1972, p. 21.
13. Thompson, F., et al. Patient grievance mechanism in Health Institutions, Appendix to U.S. Department of Health, Education and Welfare; Report of the *Secretary's Commission on Malpractice,* Govt. Ptg. Office, 1973, DHEW Publication No. (OS) 73–88, p. 760.
14. Reprinted in Medical Committee for Human Rights, *Patient Rights Advocacy.* Boston: Medical Committee for Human Rights, 1972.
15. *New York Times,* Jan 9. 1973, p. 1.
16. Sade, R. Medical care as a right: A refutation. *N. Engl. J. Med.* 1288, 1971.
17. For example, Ennis, B., and Siegel, L. *The Rights of Mental Patients.* New York: Avon, 1973. One of the authors, G. Annas, is writing a volume entitled *The Rights of Hospital Patients* for this American Civil Liberties Union series.

The Patient Rights Advocate: Can Nurses Effectively Fill the Role?

George J. Annas

Upon her return from the Crimean War, Florence Nightingale wrote: "The very first requirement in a hospital is that it should do the sick no harm." It was not until the early 20th century that a patient was likely to gain from a stay in a hospital. As hospitals have increased their ability to deal with injury and disease, their purposes have also multiplied. Today it is usually agreed that the major goals of a large hospital are:

—To care for the sick and injured;

—To provide an educational facility for doctors, nurses, and other health care personnel;

—To promote public health in the community; and

—To encourage active research.

As these latter three goals have been adopted, potential conflicts within the hospital have proliferated. In some cases, for example, the goals of education or research may eclipse the goal of caring for the sick. In attempting to maintain care as the primary goal, and in promoting the medical dictate of "do no harm," the nurse's role in the hospital context is unique.

It is the nurse, for example, who is most often responsible for the moment-to-moment and hour-to-hour management of the patient. It is the nurse who bears the responsibilities of patient monitoring, accurate observation, and medical care. It is the nurse to whom patients most often turn with their questions and concerns. These considerations give the nurse a unique opportunity to develop the skills needed by a patient advocate. There are other forces at work in large hospitals, however, that tend to discourage the nurse from becoming an activist on behalf of the rights of an individual patient.

It is instructive to compare the lines of command and authority in a large hospital to those of the armed forces. Doctors deliver "orders." Patients who do not complain, who obediently follow the doctor's orders, are described as brave and courageous. Patients who complain, who do not take orders well, are labeled trouble-makers. The entire enterprise is often described in battlefield terminology. One "fights" or "combats" disease, "knocks out" infections and uses an "arsenal" of drugs. Difficult medical decisions are described as "front line" decisions. Extreme or extraordinary measures are "heroics." Young staff physicians are house "officers." In this scheme nurses are likely to be viewed by the medical staff as "good soldiers," most likely with the rank of private or corporal. The battle is waged in the patient's body, with the aim of destroying the disease that has "invaded" him.

The movement toward promulgating patient bills of rights is a direct result of what is viewed by many as the dehumanizing experience of hospitalization. These bills are the first step in defining patient rights and educating both patients and hospital personnel to the fact that such rights exist; but many problems persist. One is that many of the bills, like the A.H.A. proposal, are often so vague that they are almost meaningless.[1] Comedian Johnny Carson has parodied the A.H.A. effort by adding the following items to it:

A patient who is in a coma has a right not to be used as a door jamb;

Annas, G.J. (1974, July). The patient rights advocate: Can nurses effectively fill the role? *Supervisor Nurse, 5*, 20–23, 25.

No patient who has been given an autopsy may be denied the right to seek further medical consultation;

No matter what the extenuating circumstances, no patient can be forced to take a sponge bath with Janitor-in-A-Drum.

PROPOSED BILL OF RIGHTS

The following bill of rights is proposed here both to address this problem and to include other items that are of importance to patients.

Preamble[2]

As you enter this health care facility, it is our duty to remind you that your health care is a cooperative effort between you as a patient and the doctors and hospital staff. During your stay you will have a Patient Rights Advocate available. The duty of the advocate is to assist you in all the decisions you must make and in all situations where your health and welfare are at stake. The advocate's first responsibility is to help you understand who each of the people are who will be working with you, and to help you understand what your rights as a patient are. Your advocate can be reached at any time of the day by dialing _____. The following is a list of your rights as a patient. Your advocate's duty is to see to it that you are afforded these rights. You shall call your advocate whenever you have any questions or concerns about any of these rights.

Your Rights

1. The patient has a legal right to informed participation in all decisions involving his health care program.

2. We recognize the right of all potential patients to know what research and experimental protocols are being used in our facility and what alternatives are available in the community.

3. The patient has a legal right to privacy respecting the source of payment for treatment and care. This right includes access to the highest degree of care without regard to the source of payment for that treatment and care.

4. We recognize the right of a potential patient to complete and accurate information concerning medical care and procedures.

5. The patient has a legal right to prompt attention, especially in an emergency situation.

6. The patient has a legal right to a clear, concise explanation, in layman's terms, of all proposed procedures, including the possibilities of

any risk or mortality or serious side effects, and the probability of their success.

7. The patient has a legal right to a clear, complete and accurate evaluation of his condition and of his prognosis without treatment before he is asked to consent to any test or procedure.

8. We recognize the right of the patient to know the identity and professional status of all those providing service. All personnel have been instructed to introduce themselves, state their status, and explain their role in the health care of the patient.

9. We recognize the right of any patient who does not speak English to have access to an interpreter.

10. The patient has a legal right to all the information contained in his medical record while in the health care facility, and to view the record upon request.

11. We recognize the right of a patient to discuss his condition with a consultant specialist, at his own request and his own expense.

12. The patient has a legal right not to have performed on him any test or procedure designed for educational purposes rather than for his direct personal benefit.

13. The patient has a legal right to both personal and informational privacy with respect to: the hospital staff, other doctors, residents, interns and medical students, any researcher, nurses, other hospital personnel, and other patients.

14. The patient has a legal right to refuse any particular drug, test, procedure or treatment.

15. We recognize the patient's right to access to people outside the health care facility by means of visitors and the telephone. Parents may stay with their children, and relatives with terminally ill patients, 24 hours a day.

16. The patient has a legal right to leave the health care facility regardless of physical condition or financial status, although he may be requested to sign a release stating that he is leaving against the medical judgment of his doctor or the hospital.

17. A patient has a right to be notified of discharge at least one day before it is accomplished, to demand a consultation by an expert on the desirability of discharge, and to have a person of the patient's choice so notified.

18. At the termination of his stay at the health care facility we recognize the right of a patient to a complete copy of the information contained in his medical record.

19. We recognize the right of all patients to have 24 hour-a-day access to a patient rights advocate who may act on behalf of the patient to assert or protect the rights set out in this document.

DISCUSSION

Adoption of such a bill of rights by the hospital is the first important step toward guaranteeing human rights to patients. By itself, however, a bill of patient rights is only a public relations gimmick, often providing lip service but no substance.

It is to address this second problem that the patient rights advocate program is proposed. Specifically, the role of the patient rights advocate would be to insure that the rights enumerated in the document were guaranteed to all patients.

The powers of the advocate would be precisely the legal powers of the patient. An advocate is necessary because the patient is sick and his main concern is to regain his health. Under these circumstances, the exercise of human rights will be dispensed with if the patient perceives that this might in some way compromise his likelihood of being cured or properly treated. The relinquishing of basic human rights, however, is neither necessary nor desirable in the hospital context. It is, after all, the patient who is sick. It is the patient and the patient alone who has the legal authority to determine what is to be done with his body. This right of "self-determination" is fundamental to Western man's view of himself. To help the patient retain this right in the hospital, the patient rights advocate must be given at least the following *unrestricted* powers on behalf of individual patients upon their request:

—complete access to all medical records;

—the ability to call in qualified consultants;

—ex-officio participation in those hospital committees responsible for monitoring health care quality;

—the power to lodge complaints directly with the hospital's Director and Executive Committee;

—immediate access to all chiefs of services;

—access to all patient support services;

—the ability to delay discharges.

The first thing that should be clear from both the bill of rights and this list of minimum powers is that unit manager or patient representative systems, which confine duties to housekeeping matters, completely miss the point of patient autonomy. They are almost irrelevant to the patient's major concerns. *The patient, regardless of staff perception, is primarily concerned with health, not housekeeping.* By creating an atmosphere in which the concept of patient rights is only mouthed, the management system of advocacy simply postpones progress towards the recognition of patients' rights in the hospital and as such may do more harm than good. Another significant weakness of such a management system is that the patient representatives are viewed by themselves as part of the hospital administration and are thus likely to see their job as "smoothing over" problems rather than solving them. It is probable that only independent financing of advocates (e.g., through a government agency) will solve this loyalty problem.

THE NURSE AS ADVOCATE

Before concluding that an entirely new professional is called for, serious consideration should be given to the use of specially-trained nurses as patient advocates. In this regard, I would make a number of suggestions. The first is that a nurse's experiences in the hospital context provide an exceptionally valuable background for being an advocate. The nurse's knowledge of medicine, medical terminology, and hospital administration are all traits that any patient advocate should possess. These qualities alone, however, are insufficient for a functioning patient rights advocate. The advocate, for example, needs some clear understanding of the law as it relates to the rights enumerated in the bill of rights, a speaking knowledge of its language, and a knowledge of the community. The advocate also probably needs some training in psychology and patient interviewing.

Of course, it would be easier for a competent nurse to achieve these other qualifications than it would be for another individual to gain both the medical knowledge and other qualifications necessary for an advocate. This fact alone, however, may not make the nurse the most natural candidate for the post of patient rights advocate. The nursing profession, for example, is saddled with the images of helpmate and willing assistant to the doctor, so well depicted in the 30 volumes of *Cherry Ames, Student Nurse.* Nor has the more modern M*A*S*H image of Hot Lips Houlihan added to the prestige of the profession. As one nurse has described the nurse's relationship to the doctor: "He's God almighty and your job is to wait on him." Nursing schools have also often helped to perpetuate this attitude by inculcating subservience and by discouraging defiance and any signs of independent judgment in their students.[3]

It may be needless to say, but a nurse who has taken any of these "traditional" qualities seriously cannot be an effective patient advocate since the person to whom many patient demands will be directed is the patient's physician. The job will often require, for example, the open questioning of diagnoses, prognoses, prescriptions, dosages, treatment suggestions, explanations of risks and alternatives to surgery, etc.

In addition to the nurse's perception of her or his role in the hospital, the patient's perception of the nurse's role is also critical. If most patients have accepted the traditional view of the nurse's role, a patient advocate that either is a nurse or was a nurse may not be viewed by patients as someone who can be trusted to fight for their rights. Insofar as nurses are seen by patients as partners in medical care rather than doctor helpers, the patient may view the nurse as advocate as a type of "double-agent." For example, the nurse may be seen as more concerned with obtaining information *for* the doctor than in helping the patient obtain information *from* the doctor. If so, the nurse cannot function effectively in this role.

While these problems are real, they are not insurmountable. Indeed, a general movement by nurses to aid patients in asserting the rights outlined in the proposed bill of rights would both improve the position of the patient in the hospital and enhance the image of the nurse in the eyes of the public. Nursing schools also owe it to their students to train them in the art of advocacy. Nurses so trained can act not only as independent practitioners, but can also move into the direct care of patients as partners of doctors rather than servants to them.

Florence Nightingale's injunction to "do no harm" should be read not only to include the patient's physical condition, but also the patient's human rights. In promoting these rights the nurse as patient advocate has the *potential* of playing the key role.

REFERENCES

1. Annas, G.J., *The A.H.A. Bill of Rights,* 9 Trial 59–63 (Dec., 1973).
2. Annas, G.J. and Healey, J.M., *The Patient Rights Advocate: Redefining the Doctor-Patient Relationship in the Hospital Context,* 27 Vanderbilt Law Review 243, 266–268 (1974).
3. Stein, L.I., *The Doctor–Nurse Game, Arch. Gen. Psychiat.* 16:154 (1967).

Patient Rights: An Agenda for the '80s

George J. Annas

Most nurses not only accept the notion that patients have rights, but also stand ready to help patients assert them. But how far will nurses go? Will they be willing allies as patients press for more recognition of their individuality and autonomy? At the National Conference on Patients' Rights held in Nashville in late September, 1980, I outlined for patient rights activists a five-point agenda for the '80s. Since then I have presented this agenda to nursing audiences in Kentucky, Massachusetts, New York, California, and Michigan. The reception has varied, but many nurses are uncomfortable with the proposal. The purpose of this column is to present the agenda in written form to give *Nursing Law & Ethics* readers an opportunity to comment on it.

As with all major patient bills of rights, this proposal is based on two premises: (1) citizens possess certain rights that are not automatically forfeited by entering a health care facility; and (2) most health care facilities fail to recognize these rights, fail to promote them, and limit their exercise without recourse.[1] Whether the patient rights movement turns inward—toward the health care provider—or outward—toward more governmental regulation—will in large measure be determined by the response of nurses and physicians to reasonable patient demands. The hospital environment can be humanized and patients' right of self-determination can be respected in the '80s if we attend to the following five-point agenda:

1. **No Routine Procedures:** It is all too common for nurses and others to respond to the question "Why is this being done?" with "Don't worry, it's routine." This should not be an acceptable response. No procedure should *ever* be performed on a patient because it is routine; it should only be performed if it is *specifically* indicated for that patient. Thus routine admission tests, routine use of johnnies, routine use of wheelchairs for in-hospital transportation, routine use of sleeping pills, to name a few notable examples, would be abolished. Use of these procedures means patients are treated as fungible robots rather than individual human beings. These procedures are often demeaning and unnecessary.

2. **Open Access to Medical Records:** While currently provided for by federal law and many state statutes and regulations, open access to medical records by patients remains difficult, and a patient often asserts his right to see his record at the peril of being labeled "distrustful" or a "trouble-maker."[2] The information in the hospital chart is about the patient and properly belongs to the patient. The patient must have access to it, both to enhance his own decision-making ability and to make it clear that the hospital is an "open" institution that is not trying to hide things from the patient. Surely if hospital personnel are making decisions about the patient on the basis of the information in the chart, the patient also deserves access to this information.

Patient Rights Agenda

1. No Routine Procedures
2. Open Access to Medical Records
3. Twenty-Four-Hour-a-Day Visitor Rights
4. Full Experience Disclosure
5. Effective Patient Advocate

Annas, G.J. (1981, April). Patient rights: An agenda for the '80s. *Nursing Law & Ethics*, 3. Reprinted with permission of © American Society of Law & Medicine, Inc. All rights reserved.

3. **Twenty-Four-Hour-a-Day Visitor Rights:** One of the most important ways to both humanize the hospital and enhance patient autonomy is to assure the patient that at least one person of his choice has unlimited access to him at any time of the day or night. This person should also be permitted to stay with the patient during any procedure (*e.g.*, childbirth, induction of anesthesia, etc.) so long as the person does not interfere with the care of other patients.

4. **Full Experience Disclosure:** The most important gain of the past decade has been the almost universal acknowledgment of the need for the patient's informed consent. Nevertheless, some information that is material to the patient's decision is still withheld: the experience of the person doing the procedure.[3] Patients have a right to know if the person asking permission to draw blood, take blood gases, do a bone marrow aspiration, do a spinal tap, etc., has ever performed the procedure before, and if so, what that person's complication rate is. This applies not only to student nurses, but also to board certified surgeons—we all do things for the first time, and not every patient wants to take such an active role in our education.

5. **An Effective Patient Advocate:** While a patient bill of rights is necessary, it is not sufficient. Rights are not self-actualizing. Patients are sick and desire relief from pain and discomfort more than they demonstrate a desire to exercise their rights; they are also anxious, and may hold back complaints for fear of retaliation. It is critical that patients have access to a person whose job it is to work *for the patient* to help the patient exercise the rights outlined in the institution's bill of rights. This person should sit on all major hospital committees that deal with patient care, have authority to obtain medical records for patients, call consultants, launch complaints directly with all members of the hospital medical, nursing, and administrative staff, and be able to delay discharges. While there appear to be some successful "patient representatives" that are hired by hospitals, it is not fair to give them this title since they must represent the hospital, and it is likely that ultimately effective representation can only be obtained by someone who is hired by a consumer group or governmental agency outside of the hospital in which the representative works.

These steps must be taken if we are to effectively safeguard patient rights. I hope that readers will accept the invitation to comment on and criticize this proposal.

REFERENCES

1. *See generally* G.J. Annas, *The Rights of Hospital Patients* (Avon, New York, 1975); G.J. Annas, *How to Make the Massachusetts Patients' Bill of Rights Work, Medicolegal News* 8(1):6 (February, 1980).
2. *See, e.g.*, Altman *et al.*, *Patients Who Read Their Hospital Charts, New England Journal of Medicine* 302:169 (January 17, 1980).
3. G.J. Annas, *The Care of Private Patients in Teaching Hospitals: Legal Implications, Bulletin of New York Academy of Medicine* 56(4):403–11 (May, 1980).

The Role of the Patient Representative

June P. Gikuuri

What is the cause of all the interest in patient's rights? Where did it originate and what were the precipitating factors? I believe it was the civil rights movement in the late 1950s and early 1960s. At that time, the consciousness of the American public arose to try and fulfill the commitment of the constitution to "the right to life, liberty and the pursuit of happiness." Presently, the only statement of commitment we have to health care can be found in the 1966 preamble to the Comprehensive Health Planning Act, which states "the fulfillment of our national purpose depends on promoting and assuring the highest level of health," and this issue is what we are concerned with today.

NEED FOR PATIENT'S BILL OF RIGHTS

What are some reasons that lead us to believe that perhaps patients have been abused, or their rights have been infringed upon? For one thing, many patients have not been told of the medical alternatives for treatment of their illness. For instance, one of the patients who came to my attention had a fractured vertebrae. The physician told the patient that he would have to have corrective surgery. However, when the physicians went on rounds, the patient overheard them discussing alternatives. The orthopedist conducting rounds told the other physicians outside the patient's door that this problem could be treated medically, but because they would soon leave the service, he wanted to give them some experience in surgical procedure and that the patient would be scheduled for

surgery. You can imagine how upset this made the patient. His family came to the community board office and asked if the patient had heard the physician correctly. Was it possible that he could be treated medically, in neck traction for a period of weeks as an alternative to surgery? We spoke to the physician and asked him if there was a medical alternative to treating this patient. Reluctantly, the physician answered yes, but the fracture would be better treated surgically. We asked the physician if this information was shared with the patient. This question resulted in some hostility and prickling; eventually, however, it was explained to the patient that there was a medical alternative to the surgical procedure, and he was put into neck traction for six weeks. Luckily, for the patient, he did not have to have the surgical procedure. This is an example of one of the rights that has been infringed upon—the right to know treatment alternatives for a given diagnosis.

THE PATIENT REPRESENTATIVE

In 1974 The American Hospital Association's Patient's Bill of Rights was approved by the medical board, community board, and administration of my hospital. Through the encouragement of the community board, the first patient representative for the hospital center was hired in that same year. It was my job to handle patient complaints or requests for services that were being diverted for one reason or another. I attempted to confine myself to problems that cannot be dealt with in any other department. I do not take over any one else's job.

Gikuuri, J.P. (1978). The role of the patient representative. In E.L. Bandman & B. Bandman (Eds.), *Bioethics and human rights* (pp. 281–284). Boston: Little, Brown and Company. Reprinted with permission of © Little, Brown and Company. All rights reserved.

I am not a social worker; I am not an administrator. Whenever a problem comes to my attention that should be handled by another department, I route that problem to the appropriate department.

Patient's rights must continue to evolve and grow. A statement of rights that is applicable in 1976 may not be applicable in 1986. We are now concerned with the right to information, the right to medical records, a discharge summary, and the right to health education. Although we think we have passed the early stages of basic human decency and respect, we must constantly implement and monitor them. There must be someone in every institution who monitors these rights. Someone must be responsible in all settings. A patient representative could be an administrator, who along with other duties is responsible for patient rights, or it could be a provider whose primary responsibility is for patients rights. It could even be a volunteer. It depends on the institution, the volume of patients, the type of patient population, and the type of staff available. In my hospital, there is a paid person to implement and monitor patient rights, and this person is paid by the hospital. The person must be able to cross departmental lines and have the authority to carry out recommendations.

INFORMED CONSENT

One of the largest problem areas of the American Hospital Association's Patient's Bill of Rights is the area of informed consent. Within this sphere is obviously a very large area for potential and actual abuse. A patient has to sign a consent for every procedure that is done, but many times he is not informed of the procedure, the risks involved, and again, the medical alternatives. We have had patients who were given a paper to sign but were not given an explanation as to what the procedure entails. For example: I have had patients and relatives call me and say, "My husband is going for an operation tomorrow and neither he nor I have been informed of what it is. Can someone explain this operation to us?" When I asked a physician about the procedure he intended to do the following day, he answered, "I told the patient that he is having an exploratory laparotomy." I asked, "Is that what you said to the patient?" He said, "Yes. I've told him several times. I don't understand why he doesn't understand what I'm talking about." Here is another area of concern—explanation of the procedure to be performed in language that the patient

can reasonably be expected to understand. Physicians are insulated during their premedical and medical schooling, and tend to forget the everyday language that most people use. Of course, a patient should learn the medical terminology specific to his illness, but he certainly should receive explanations in language that he can reasonably be expected to understand. This is the only way a person can give *informed* consent. Consent can be obtained but it may not be *informed*.

Another example: I had a mother come to my office very upset because her son, age nine, was scheduled for surgery the following day. She had signed the consent for surgery but still was not aware of what type of procedure was to be performed. I called the physician and he told me that the patient had diverticulitis and they were going to correct the problem. I asked him if he had explained it to the mother. He answered me, "Yes, I told her that the patient had diverticulitis and we were going to correct it." That was all. The mother said to me, "Yes, that sounds familiar, but I still do not know what that is." I asked the doctor to explain to the mother what this procedure was in language that she could understand. The physician became very upset and couldn't understand why this mother was so retarded that she did not understand the terminology he used. I felt that this mother was in such a nervous state that I opened the dictionary and let her read the definition for herself. She then felt a little more comfortable with understanding the procedure her son was to have. I did not want to relieve the physician of his responsibility so I sent her back to him for an adequate explanation, which was done much to the physician's chagrin.

HUMAN EXPERIMENTATION

A patient has the right to participate or not to participate in human experimentation and research according to his own information and his own consent. A flagrant example of infringement in human experimentation is the situation in Tuskegee, started in the 1930s with patients who were diagnosed as having syphilis. Treatment was withheld to enable the researchers to observe what would happen to these patients as the syphilis germ invaded the body [1].

Other areas of infringement on patient's rights are experiments done on fetuses and care of the terminally ill who are often unable to protect themselves. How many of us have seen terminally ill cancer patients in whom the physician insists on finding the primary site of the disease, as if finding it will cure the patient? Doctors often continue to draw blood, order x-rays, and persist in putting the patient through all types of rigors in order to advance the knowledge of medical science. Barber reports a study on human experimentation and research and concluded that stricter curbs on medical research were necessary because a significant number of researchers were found to be very permissive or more willing to accept an unsatisfactory risk-benefit ratio [2]. In other words, the risks to patients were higher than the benefits. We also must be concerned with patients who cannot refuse treatment: prisoner, the fetus, the incompetent, the terminally ill, and children.

PHYSICIAN–PATIENT RELATIONSHIP

We have been dealing with physicians as deities who have promoted superior–inferior relationships between physicians and patients, but we are about to break through that traditional role and develop, instead, cooperative relationships. As we become better educated concerning health and our rights, physicians will be compelled to relate to us in an intelligent cooperative manner.

Another personal experience concerns a patient who was in the coronary unit and signed himself out against medical advice. Everyone spoke to this man about the dangers: the physician, the nurse, and even the psychiatrist. The psychiatrist stated that the patient was mentally competent and could not be held against his wishes. As a last resort, they brought him to my office in a wheelchair. The nurse did not want to leave him. I spoke to the patient and found that he had many emotional burdens and much guilt. Some very tragic things had happened in his life. Because of his guilt, he just could not stay confined in a hospital. He had to be home, he had to be able to cry, and he had to be able to grieve for the many tragic things that had happened. He revealed many things

to me that the staff did not know because I took the time to listen to him. I was very fearful about him being home and called him every day afterward to find out how he was doing. Attempts have been made to get him back into the hospital. He feels that he cannot return to the hospital after he signed himself out. I have told him to return at any time as we are here to take care of him. He cannot be forced to accept treatment unless the illness is contagious or unless he is judged mentally incompetent or dangerous to other people or himself.

THE LAW AND PATIENT'S RIGHTS

In 1975 the New York State Health Department issued the State Hospital Code (chapter V of title 10, section 720.3), which is another patient's rights statement that is law for New York State and must be implemented in all health facilities in the state. The New York City Health and Hospitals Corporation is also formulating another patient's rights statement. Each document is more progressive than the previous one.

In the past when a patient came to the hospital, his rights were suddenly in escrow; they were frozen. The patient could no longer exercise his rights. We are trying to break through this tradition and give the patient back his rights and responsibilities because rights and responsibilities are linked together. A person should not have to abdicate his civil and common law rights in order to obtain quality health care.

REFERENCES

1. Barber, B. The ethics of experimentation with human subjects. *Sci. Am.* 234:25, 1976.
2. Linton, O. American study of lifetime effects of syphilis ends in 1.8 billion dollar lawsuit. *Can. Med. Assoc. J.* 109:410, 1973.

The Patient's Representative: Whose Side Is She On?

Anne A. Cote

"I'm going to sue you." It's hard to believe how often I hear this from an irate patient or member of his family. When I became a nurse, back in the sixties, a threat like this was unheard of. Now it seems as though I hear it daily. And hospitals, my own included, *are* being sued weekly.

Not only are hospital patients, like all consumers, becoming more demanding, but some people think litigation is the only way to solve a problem. Others just want to get attention, and at the price of settlements today, they usually succeed. As a result, part of my job as a patient's representative is to try to resolve patient/family grievances before they wind up in a court of law. I can do that best by seeing that our patients' rights are respected and upheld by every service and agency of the hospital.

Whenever a patient feels he's not being treated properly, we intervene as quickly as possible. More often than not, his problem is an administrative or clinical one that can best be settled right here in the hospital—not in a court of law 3 years from now. For this reason, we depend heavily on our nursing staff to let us know when problems occur. They have to be sensitive to their patients' rights and be ready to call us when the need arises. Nurses are the patient's advocates and our front line.

PATIENT'S BILL OF RIGHTS

If you read a Patient's Bill of Rights, either the American Hospital Association's (AHA's), your state's, or your hospital's, you're not going to find anything bizarre or radical. It's simply a statement of what a patient can expect from the institution. (And what sad commentary on health care delivery that anything so simple had to be put into black and white.) I'm sure you don't need the AHA, the legislature, or me to tell you that patients should be treated with courtesy and respect. But your role in upholding *other* patients' rights might need some clarification. Although your state or institutional laws and policies may differ from ours, learning how the nursing staff handles these matters at The New York Hospital might shed some light on your position.

INFORMED CONSENT

The New York Hospital Patient's Bill of Rights was begun in 1973 and approved in 1975—right in the middle of the malpractice crisis. Then and now, virtually every suit filed against any doctor or hospital alleges a lack of informed consent. Attorneys claim that the patient hadn't been given adequate information and wouldn't have agreed to the operation or treatment if all the risks had been explained and understood. There's even been a major case in California in which no negligence or malpractice was alleged, just the lack of informed consent. This should tell all health professionals how strongly the law feels about a patient's right to know and make informed decisions.

Well, Article 2 in our patient's rights pamphlet bites the bullet on informed consent. We don't just tell patients what they have a right to know. We tell them exactly what questions they should ask and whom they should be asking.

With all this spelled out, the patient has a tool to help him get the information he's entitled to, if the doctor doesn't volunteer the appropriate information. Also, it's a lot harder for a patient to say no one told him anything when he's been given the tool to get the information.

Will the patient use a tool like this? Good question. We know that a lot of patients get tongue-tied when their doctors come into the room. They may want to ask, but they're shy, or they forget, or they're afraid. They're afraid the doctor will view the question as an insult to his skills. But after the doctor leaves, they ask everybody else—nurses, orderlies, janitors, anybody.

RESPONSIBILITY FOR INFORMED CONSENT

In New York State, informed consent is the doctor's responsibility, but nurses—as always—are right in the middle of any problem that pops up. You've always had to interpret the doctor's information to your patients. Sometimes they haven't understood the technical language. Sometimes they're just not sure what to think, and they want to bounce it off another person. In any case, if the patient doesn't understand what's happening to him, you'll probably be the first to hear about it. Naturally, you'll try to clear up any misunderstanding and answer as many general questions as possible. However, if in your judgment as a professional nurse you feel the patient really hasn't a clue as to what the procedure is about, you have an obligation as a nurse and as the patient's advocate to inform the doctor that the patient does not have a clear picture of what's about to happen.

For example, a patient says "I'm getting an X-ray tomorrow." Suddenly, an alarm bell goes off in the nurse's mind because *she* knows he's getting an angiogram. She talks to him a little more and discovers that, like most laymen, this patient thinks all X-rays are like chest X-rays: You walk in, have your picture taken, and go home. No risks.

In a case like this, the nurse has clearly established the patient's lack of understanding of the risks involved in angiography. So she has an obligation to find his doctor or *some* doctor—and let him know the patient needs a better idea of what's going to happen to him. No matter that the patient has signed a consent form; if he doesn't understand what he's consented to, the form isn't valid. Somebody has to get a doctor into that room to clarify the risks.

If the nurse can't get a doctor to cooperate with her, she should alert her head nurse or call our office. It's our job to run interference for both patients *and* staff when necessary. Often we can step in where staff nurses feel they can go no further.

As you can easily guess, some doctors aren't going to welcome a nurse's involvement here. Surgeons sometimes have a patient premedicated, then look at the X-rays and decide they want to do a different operation than the one the patient consented to. They don't always see why they can't just take another form in and have it signed then and there. Well, no way. A premedicated patient is not competent to give consent. The surgeon doesn't always like to hear about *that*, but it's most hospitals' policy because of the legal ramifications. Again, nobody wants to be the bearer of bad tidings, but with our office on call, a nurse doesn't have to feel she's in this battle alone.

WHEN THE PATIENT DOESN'T WANT TO KNOW

Patients have a right to know what's going on, and they also have a right *not* to know if they don't want to. Some will say, "I'll sign anything, just don't talk to me about it."

In a case like this, the nurse uses her professional judgment to decide if this patient is crying out for help or if he truly does not want to know.

If he truly doesn't want to know, the nurse covers herself and the hospital by noting the patient's attitude on his chart. If the record says, "Tried to explain procedure to patient, and he said he didn't want to know," we'll have some protection if he later decides to sue the hospital on the grounds that nobody told him anything.

THE RIGHT TO DECLINE TREATMENT

A consent form is nothing more than proof that a particular conversation took place at a particular time between a particular patient and a particular physician. It is *not* a contract, a point that's often hard to get across to some doctors and nurses.

"But he signed the consent form," they complain.

Tough. A *contract* obligates the signer to go through with the terms of the contract. But the fact that a patient has signed a *consent form* doesn't obligate him to anything. He can change his mind at the operating room door, and the consent form is invalid. In that case, the doctor has to go back to square one and get consent all over again. It's the patient's right and it's the law. The touching of another person without his consent is called battery. If the patient says "No" or "I've changed my mind," that ends all previous consent—written or verbal.

Just as a patient has the right to understand his treatment, he also has the right to refuse it—even if he'll die as a result. Cases like this have received a great deal of publicity in the past few years. But as I'm sure you know, most patients who refuse treatment aren't refusing lifesaving measures. They're more likely to be refusing a third barium enema in 3 days. In the 14 years I've been in health care, most of the patients I've seen refuse treatment have done so because they're frightened, confused, or just plain tired. They've had all the tests, preparations, clean-outs, or what have you they can handle right then, and they simply don't want anymore.

Rather than lecture the patient on why he ought to have the treatment, we take the time to find out why he's refusing. We usually find that a sympathetic talk, an explanation, or a schedule change that allows him a night's rest will turn him around. You've got to be imaginative and flexible enough to help this patient make a rational decision—not one determined by fear, confusion, or fatigue. We really have no choice, because when you get right down to it, rational or irrational, he *doesn't* have to have the treatment. And nobody can force him.

A CASE IN POINT

We once had a man come in with an abscess the size of an orange on the back of his neck. He had not previously been known to our hospital, and he denied any health problems. After being admitted on a Tuesday, he went to surgery on Wednesday for an incision and drainage (I&D). All was expected to go well; instead, he developed a hypotensive episode and an arrhythmia. The surgeons elected not to proceed with the I&D until the patient had a medical evaluation. Medicine did a workup and cleared him for surgery on Friday.

Friday morning at 9 A.M. the man's wife flew into my office screaming, "I'm going to sue you if you send my husband to surgery."

She got my attention. I put my coffee down. We talked for a while and then went up to see her husband. When we walked into the room, there he was, lying on his side, with an I.V. in his arm and a monitor attached to his chest. He looked terrified—scrunched up in his rumpled bedclothes, staring at the monitor, clearly afraid to move. "I'm too sick to go to surgery," he moaned. "I walked in here a well person on Tuesday, and now I'm dying. They've got this thing in my arm and this cardiac thing here. I must be dying. I can't go to surgery today."

With that, the surgical resident arrived. For those of you who've worked in an operating room, picture the grief the resident was getting because he was holding up a room . . . where was his patient . . . what was going on . . . blah, blah, blah. No wonder he came on like a fire-breathing dragon. Why was the patient refusing surgery . . . holding up the schedule . . . other patients to take care of . . . blah, blah, blah. In spite of his anger, I could see the resident was honestly concerned about this patient. He spelled out the risks of not having the surgery: The abscess could go to the patient's brain, and so on.

Finally, the man said, "Okay, you can do what you want to me tomorrow, but I just can't take it today. I'm too sick." This was Friday. Saturdays they don't do elective surgery.

The resident threw up his hands. "If that's the way you want it, go home," he said, and stalked out of the room.

I went after him and asked if he *really* wanted us to pull out this man's I.V., disconnect his monitor, and put him on the street. He took a few deep breaths and said maybe he'd get another opinion. Great idea. How about the attending doctor?

The attending doctor arrived, looked at the patient, and ordered hot wet packs. The abscess opened and drained, and the patient went home Saturday morning on oral antibiotics.

So the moral is this: Any patient is capable of refusing treatment if he feels overwhelmed. If you treat the refusal as an either/or proposition, the patient will probably go right on refusing. But if you use your head, you can usually find some alternative. They're not all as easy as wet packs and antibiotics, but the solutions are there if you just keep seeing the patient as an individual and not as another case.

PRIVACY

Protecting the confidentiality of the medical record can be a real challenge in a hospital. Actually, it's not just the physical record that has to be protected. The information it contains is confidential as well. That's something people tend to forget. In a teaching hospital especially, there's a tremendous amount of case discussion going on all the time—and in all the wrong places. Ride the right elevator at the right time, and you can find out anything. The cafeteria is even worse. I suspect the people from the neighborhood eat in our cafeteria because the gossip's so terrific. When the Shah of Iran was hospitalized here, you could barely get a seat.

Actually, if your hospital is built anything like ours, there aren't a lot of places where staff members can conveniently and privately discuss their work. So it all goes on in hallways, nurses' stations, even at bedsides. Here you have an environmental problem that contributes to an ethical problem. All we can really do is encourage the staff to remember where they are before they start exchanging information about patients.

The Shah's stay here raised the whole issue of a patient's right to privacy and the public's right to know. A lot of important and well-known people are treated here. We had the Pope's medical history in case anything happened to him while he was in New York. So this is a pretty high-powered place, and the staff's often pressured to reveal information that they shouldn't. In general, we follow the rule of thumb that if a patient's presence here is not a matter of public record, he's not here. We don't talk about him, period. If it's a matter of public record, a staff member may talk about almost anything *except* the patient's condition and treatment.

WHOSE RECORD IS IT?

In New York State, a patient's medical record is the property of the institution. Some states let patients have their records after treatment is completed, and in Massachusetts a patient can see his chart any time. If he gets bored waiting in X-ray, he can read his chart. Our policy, however, is that patients may not see their charts.

Of course, under the Patient's Bill of Rights, they're entitled to the *information* contained in the charts. But they should get this information only from appropriate clinical personnel. Patients can get very upset by terms they don't understand or by references to diagnoses that have been ruled out. I'll never forget one elderly gentleman who was enraged when he saw a copy of his emergency

department record and thought the resident had called him a son of a bitch. He calmed down after I explained that SOB meant shortness of breath.

Under our policy on patients' records, the nurse can find herself in the middle. If a patient asks for his chart, she's forbidden by hospital policy to show it to him. On the other hand, she may not refuse him the information he wants. Either she or the doctor should keep the patient informed. There are certain items of information, e.g., diagnosis, I feel quite strongly should first come from the doctor. After that, the nurse should use her professional skills as counselor and educator to keep her patients up to date. If a patient in our hospital still insists on seeing his chart, he may be referred to a patient representative. Usually, the problem is not so much one of wanting to read the chart but of having lost faith in the care givers. Sometimes we can help to restore that faith.

NURSING IMPLICATIONS

The patient's rights issue has undoubtedly added some extra burdens to your job. You may have to determine whether or not a patient has received enough information to give informed consent—strictly a professional judgment on your part, and not always one you'll be rewarded for. And you might have to deal with some pretty impatient doctors when the patient hasn't given consent. You'll have to think up alternative approaches to patients who refuse treatment. You might have to spend time explaining complicated medical terms to patients who ask for their charts.

Nobody has to tell you that patients are no longer passively accepting whatever we health care providers, in our wisdom, have deemed best for them. But for any of you who may view the patient's representative as someone working *for* the patients and *against* you, look again. All we're doing is *specializing* in a job that's been a part of your role for a long, long time. With the growth of technology and the numbers of people your patients come in contact with, it may no longer be fair to ask you to do it all. Still, it's your responsibility to make the system work for your patients, and one way you can discharge that responsibility is by letting a patient representative know when your patient needs help. None of us can do it alone, but together with other health professionals, we can make health care a whole lot better.

Patient Rep Can Be Viewed as Fiscal Asset

Nancy McDonald

Patient representative programs began to appear in hospitals during the late 1950s, and since the early 1970s their numbers have steadily increased. Charged with responsibility for patient problem solving and for humanizing health care, patient representatives offer hospitals the benefits of improving patient relations and quality of care.

In this era of cost containment, however, it cannot be overlooked that, superficially, a patient representative may be seen as not being essential to patient care or compatible with cost containment objectives. From this perspective, it is unlikely that the patient relations benefits alone will continue to be enough to justify establishment of new programs. Therefore, a thorough understanding of the relationship of patient representatives to cost containment is critical to the growth and development of hospital patient representation.

BENEFITS AND SAVINGS

One of the most visible and significant cost savings a patient representative can contribute is in the area of risk management. By communicating directly with patients, acting as their advocate and problem solver, the patient representative is in a position to identify potential liabilities quickly and work expeditiously toward reaching a solution. In this regard, fiscal advantages would include saving the time of administration, legal counsel, and other staff members to whom a patient would ordinarily have to explain his problems. By providing a centralized and consistent grievance mechanism, the patient representative decreases the chance that, because of frustration and dissatisfaction, the patient will seek legal recourse. Another indirect benefit in such cases would be the possibility of decreasing malpractice insurance premiums.

Even in instances where litigation is involved, the patient representative can effect cost savings by facilitating communication and cooperation between the patient and his family and legal counsel, insurance carrier, or risk management team. This will likely result in lessening settlement and administrative costs and possibly result in eliminating court costs as well.

Because part of the patient representative's responsibility is to monitor patients' impressions and perceptions of the hospital, a natural extension of the function would be to elicit cost-saving ideas. Patients are certain to be favorably impressed with such an effort to contain costs, and valuable suggestions stand to be uncovered and implemented. The patient representative might discover that patients are supplied with items for which they have no use or that there are services being provided that patients do not feel are beneficial. The patient representative is also in the advantageous position of coming in direct routine contact with patients, their families, physicians, and staff and can work to assimilate hospital-wide cost-saving ideas and benefits into programs and recommendations.

There are other cost benefits that the patient representative provides because of having primary responsibility for patient advocacy and patient relations. Because the patient representative can cross

McDonald, N. (1980, May 1). Patient rep can be viewed as fiscal asset. *Hospitals, 54,* 44, 47. Reprinted with permission of © American Hospital Publishing. All rights reserved.

departmental lines and has the time and commitment required to invest in problem resolution, a great burden is lifted from other direct care staff members. These are frequently the employees who, rather than supervisors or department heads, are presented with problems that they do not have the time or the expertise to solve. However, when a responsible and dependable problem solver is available to them, their time can be more effectively used in patient care. Hence, these staff members are not plagued by unresolved difficulties and it is not necessary for them to contact their department heads for minor concerns. The patient representative takes responsibility for seeing that a problem is resolved and contacts supervisors, department heads, or administration only when circumstances warrant their involvement. Ultimately, this kind of organization results in increased accountability and efficiency.

Because the patient representative is available to handle patients' institutional problems, the stress under which nurses and physicians must perform is reduced. The result is increased productivity for highly trained staff members.

There are also advantages to be gained when the patient representative undertakes a staff education program to promote better patient relations throughout the hospital. First, staff training programs designed to increase awareness of patients' needs can improve overall patient care by enhancing staff's sensitivity to patients. Increased sensitivity in turn contributes to personalizing the hospital environment. Second, whether through formal or informal training, the patient representative can advance the philosophy and practice of patient representation. Finally, the fundamentals of patient relations are incorporated into other staff members' jobs so that good relations are intensified without the hiring of additional staff.

SUMMARY

An effective patient representative can save an institution money in unnecessary expenditures for patient products and services and in reduced legal fees, court costs, and malpractice insurance premiums. A patient representative can also be instrumental in increasing efficiency and productivity of other staff members by serving as a consistent grievance mechanism, advocate, and problem solver. Therefore, a patient representative represents a fiscal asset rather than a fiscal liability. In view of the money-saving components of the job, it is not unreasonable to believe that the patient representative may even make money for the hospital.

Patient representatives are not unique in their ability to contain and reduce costs, but they can work to enhance cost containment programs while at the same time working to improve the quality of patient care. In this way patient representatives and cost containment ideals are compatible, uniting to ensure that hospitals are subscribing to excellence in patient care and holding down costs.

Want Some Good Advice?
Think Twice About Being a Patient Advocate

Jack Zusman

Advocacy is a popular term these days. Many people claim to be advocates for some group or other. Many nurses, for example, claim they're patient advocates—or think they should be.

The revised code of nursing ethics reinforces that thinking. It defines a nurse's responsibility as "protecting the patient from incompetent care." The 1950 code, you may recall, considered nurses to be "doctor advocates," responsible for carrying out doctors' orders and protecting their reputations.

The shift in philosophy is clear, but the shift in responsibility isn't. What is a patient advocate? Should you be one? And when? Before answering those questions, let's define our terms.

WHAT IS ADVOCACY?

In our advocacy training program at the University of Southern California, we defined patient-care advocacy as an organized effort to ensure that a patient gets the appropriate social or medical benefits with minimum cost—in terms of money, human rights, and personal comfort. Of course, an advocate's ability to ensure these benefits requires a great deal of authority. Yet much can be done without formal authority, by just using persuasion.

For many reasons, patient-care advocacy has progressed furthest for psychiatric patients. Several important lawsuits have established the rights of psychiatric patients. And states such as New York, New Jersey, and Michigan require (or financially support) a network of advocates in public psychiatric agencies. In California, every county has a mental-health advocate.

These full-time advocates inform agencies of psychiatric patients' legal rights and facilitate joint efforts by several agencies to help patients. They also inform psychiatric patients of available services and use their legal authority to protect patients' legal rights.

Many general hospitals employ full-time patient advocates, sometimes called patient representatives, ombudsmen, or patient hostesses. But these employees have no legal authority to represent patients' rights. Their authority is delegated to them by the hospital administration and is limited to dealing with little things that other staff members may forget. They handle the small problems that can loom so large to a patient; arranging for special visiting hours for a family that can't come during regular hours; helping the patient check on health-insurance coverage; smoothing out misunderstandings between the patient and a doctor or staff member.

YOUR ROLE AS A
PATIENT-CARE ADVOCATE

The nurse's role as a patient-care advocate isn't usually described in hospital policy manuals; nor is it explicitly dealt with in law or in the nursing code of ethics. But both the law and your code of ethics are moving toward increased nursing responsibility for quality care and for independent decision making.

What does this mean to you? If you see an important gap in your patient's care, do you have the freedom and responsibility to step in?

Probably you already step in sometimes. You may assume the task of enhancing communication, for example. When a patient doesn't seem to understand the treatment planned, you may mention the problem to the doctor or attempt to explain the treatment to the patient. When a patient admits being afraid to ask the doctor a question, you may mention this problem to the doctor.

But what do you do in situations where feelings run high and nurses have traditionally backed off? Should you intervene when you suspect a patient is being charged an unreasonable fee by his doctor? Should you intervene when you think a patient is being improperly advised about treatment? Should you intervene when a patient doesn't know he has been injured through the negligence of a staff member?

The decision to get involved in such complicated situations requires a careful understanding of the advocate's responsibilities and of the elements in the individual case.

WHAT ARE AN ADVOCATE'S RESPONSIBILITIES?

Some people use the common perception of the lawyer's role as a model for advocacy. They see the advocate in what we'd call an "adversarial" role— an adversary to other health-care professionals.

If you use this model of advocacy, your goal is to obtain whatever the patient wants and has a right to have. You will completely and wholeheartedly pursue this goal—even if it might be destructive to others or to the patient. You'll put yourself completely on the patient's side and let him establish the boundaries.

I don't think you can serve anyone's best interests using the adversary model of advocacy. You'll jeopardize your relationships with the staff members in the inevitable battles of pitting one patient's wants against everything else. And you may harm the patient because you can't be sure you're serving the patient's overall needs by meeting just one of them.

In our training program, we proposed *responsible* advocacy.

CHARACTERISTICS OF A RESPONSIBLE ADVOCATE

Responsible advocacy means having a concern for the patient's total situation, rather than for just one facet of it, such as an isolated legal right.

If you accept this responsibility, you'll recognize that people under stress are changeable and often shortsighted. The patient who wants something today—such as immediate discharge from the hospital before treatment's completed—may regret that decision tomorrow. So you won't take everything the patient says at face value.

Instead, you'll face the difficult problem of trying to figure out what the patient needs—or will want when he can consider the situation calmly.

Another hallmark of responsible advocacy: recognizing the widespread effects a change in the patient's situation may have on others. A better situation for that patient may produce a worse situation for other patients or staff. For example, more nursing care for one patient may decrease the care available to other patients who need it equally.

So you must take everyone's welfare into account and balance the patient's needs against everyone else's needs. Then, meet the patient's needs partially or gradually. Recognize that everyone must share injustice—as well as justice—and that change must come slowly lest the whole system collapse.

Finally, recognize the importance of good working relationships and communication with others. Knowing that advocacy will be hampered—if not defeated—without staff cooperation, you'll work hard to negotiate and compromise rather than *fight* for goals. You'll work hard to convince other staff members that your advocacy is an asset rather than a liability.

Sometimes, of course, "the other side" may not budge, even when something terrible seems about to happen to a patient despite all your efforts to prevent it. In my experience, this is rare—most health professionals are trying hard to do their best for patients and are willing, when properly approached, to consider another view. But if necessary, you must speak up—risking your job or even your career if you have to. In such cases, involve your supervisor or an advocacy-type agency, such as a licensing board or ethics committee. Neither you alone nor a patient can accomplish what a designated official or group can.

WEIGHING THE ELEMENTS OF AN INDIVIDUAL CASE

Even the most responsible, capable advocate can get into a situation where people take sides and an intense battle results. This may be particularly likely if you act as a patient's advocate and perform your regular staff nurse duties at the same time.

How do you know if the possible negative effects outweigh the positive? How should you act if you decide to get involved? Here are some guidelines to help you analyze a particular situation.

1. *Analyze the need—and probable results—of getting involved before you take the plunge.* Some people may see your advocacy as an unwarranted invasion of the doctor–patient relationship, as trouble making, or as trying to help where no help is needed. Recognize this risk and weigh the probable outcome:

- How serious is the damage or inconvenience to the patient without your intervention?
- Who else is available to act as the patient's advocate?
- Will the advocacy role enhance your relationships with other staff members or damage them?
- Will a negative effect jeopardize your future effectiveness as a nurse and advocate or simply inconvenience you temporarily?

2. *Decide in advance what result you want to achieve. Then decide what you want to do.* For example, what should you do if a patient doesn't understand the likely results of impending surgery? That depends on your goal.

If you want to help the individual patient, ask the doctor to explain the surgery again, or get permission to do this yourself. If you're generally concerned about patients not understanding surgery, look into some of the excellent patient-education material now being published.

3. *Consider alternative ways to meet your goals for the patient.* As you sift through alternatives, examine how much potential each one has for success; for antagonizing or disturbing other patients, supervisors, or colleagues; for backfiring and damaging the patient's situation; and for producing long-term improvement.

For example, what should you do for a patient who doesn't seem to be receiving adequate treatment? Consider these possibilities:

- If you talk to the patient, will he believe you— or think your intervention is improper? Will you destroy a long-term doctor–patient trust that's possibly more beneficial than alternative treatment?
- If you talk to the doctor, will you alienate him or convince him to discuss other options with the patient?
- If you talk to the patient's family, will you help the patient or create guilt and fear because the family can't afford other options? And so on.

4. *Distinguish between honest disagreement and dishonesty, neglect, and incompetence before you involve a patient in controversy.* Valid treatment choices exist for almost any condition, and many patients—even in this day of informed consent— choose to accept their doctors' recommendations without question. Don't interfere with that relationship until you've tried first to work with the doctor or other staff members to resolve a controversy.

5. *Ask a colleague's opinion.* All of us—no matter how experienced or sophisticated—can misjudge a situation, particularly when we have strong feelings about it or are closely involved with the patient. To avoid misjudgment, describe the situation to a colleague who isn't involved—who can examine your proposed solution in a dispassionate way.

6. *Look for ways to be unobtrusive.* Sometimes you can achieve your goal by making information available to interested parties without emphasizing their mistakes. For example, if you think a treatment is ill-advised, you might be able to delay it, without comment, until others can evaluate it and make a decision.

7. *Try asking questions.* Sometimes you can stimulate someone to change an order or resolve a problem simply by asking questions. This informal approach can lead to the results you want without fuss or anxiety.

WHEN NOT TO ACT AS A PATIENT ADVOCATE

Sometimes, your best advocacy role is to refer your patient to a full-time patient advocate, who has more time, authority, and expertise to follow a problem through until it's resolved.

If your hospital has an advocate, I recommend that you refer these problems to her:

- a patient's complaints that his legal rights aren't being respected. The advocate knows the patient's legal rights and can inform the hospital and the staff without risking her job.

- a patient's need for help from other departments or agencies.
- the need to coordinate efforts of several agencies or departments in a patient's behalf.

Mrs. Apple is an example of a patient with such complex needs. An 80-year-old coronary patient about to be discharged from the hospital, Mrs. Apple doesn't seem capable of caring for herself.

Her nurse knows she hasn't even applied for food stamps and other social benefits she's eligible for.

The nurse has been in close contact with Mrs. Apple, her daughter, and her doctor. Is the nurse the best advocate?

The nurse could function effectively with the people involved—with little or no antagonism likely. But what nurse has time—or the necessary contacts—to see the problem through to completion? If the nurse wants to try, she should probably discuss the situation with Mrs. Apple, her daughter, and her doctor, and give Mrs. Apple's daughter the names of agencies that might be able to help her mother.

If Mrs. Apple and her daughter get lost in the bureaucracy, the nurse should refer them to a full-time patient advocate.

Unfortunately, decisions about advocacy aren't usually clear or easy to make. Even situations that appear to cry out for intervention may be far less clear after all the facts are known. Yet without intervention, all the facts wouldn't have become known.

You're in a position to observe and learn a lot about patients' problems, but your involvement to help patients can be extremely costly in terms of time and work relationships. Following the principles of responsible advocacy can help you decide the extent of your involvement. It's the surest way to gain confidence and protect your patient's best interests.

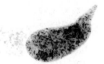

A Contrary View of the Nurse as Patient Advocate

Natalie Abrams

The trend to encourage the professionalization of nursing and the assumption of more individual responsibility usually includes the claim that one of the functions of a "professional" nurse is to assume the role of patient advocate. My concern in this article is to examine that concept and the particular suitability of the nurse for assuming the role of patient advocate.

First, why should there be a patient advocate, i.e., what is there about being a patient that suggests the need for an advocate? Second, what responsibilities should a patient advocate have? What should be his or her functions? Third, is the nurse best suited to fill this role and perform these functions?

The need for a patient advocate is generally thought to emanate from the unfortunate but inevitable physical and psychological state of being a patient as well as the overwhelming complexity of the hospital structure. (Here, and for the remainder of this article my attention is focused on nursing practice and patient care in a hospital context. However, by restricting my consideration to hospital-based situations, I do not mean to imply the primacy of the hospital context over other very interesting and difficult ▓▓▓▓ in which nurses function.)

The picture of the hospitalized patient ha▓ become a classic. In addition to the fear and uncertainty that naturally accompany illness, upon entering a hospital one frequently experiences feelings of loss of autonomy or control over one's life, loss of initiative, and a loss of a sense of identity. In many instances an active, independent, and responsible "person" is transformed into a passive, dependent, and obedient "patient." As a patient, the individual is necessarily separated from family and friends and frequently is burdened by worries about this separation, about absence from work responsibilities, financial difficulties, care of children left at home, and so on. These concerns are, of course, in addition to those centered on the particular health problem which led to the hospitalization. Usually, these are the features of hospitalization that suggest the need for a patient advocate.

Given this picture, what responsibilities or functions would a patient advocate have? What would be his or her role vis-à-vis patient care? Numerous alternatives initially appear plausible. First, a patient advocate's role might be that of a counselor or lay therapist whose function would be the alleviation or reduction of fear, consolation, re-establishment of feelings of autonomy and self-control, recognition of one's feelings, and finally, but not of least importance, companionship and attention.

A related but slightly different model is for an advocate to help a patient reach decisions about his or her health care. For example, the advocate would discuss alternative therapies or treatment plans in order to help the patient decide which option is most in accordance with his or her lifestyle, plans, and values. The advocate would not impose decisions or choices on the patient, but would reason through the various options to enable the patient to make decisions which are consistent with his or her own beliefs.

A third model is to view the advocate as a patient's "rights" advocate who serves the function of

Abrams, N. (1978). A contrary view of the nurse as patient advocate. *Nursing Forum, 17,* 258–267. Reprinted with permission of © Nursecom Inc. All rights reserved.

an information provider and "watch-dog." According to this view, it would be the advocate's responsibility to inform the person about his or her rights as a hospital patient. In addition to providing the person with what has become known as the "Patient's Bill of Rights," the advocate would insure that he or she fully understands these rights and how to exercise them. The advocate would also make certain the patient's rights were respected, and would serve as the one to whom the patient would report any known, suspected, or anticipated violations of rights in order to secure their recognition and the correction or prevention of any violation.

A fourth model is to view patient advocacy as representation. According to this view, the advocate would be a spokesman for the patient or a representative of the patient in those contexts in which it is not possible for the patient to speak for himself or herself. Although this function might certainly be appropriate even for competent adult patients (owing to the nature of the particular illness or the context of hospital care), it is an especially significant function for those classes of patients who cannot speak for themselves, namely, some patients in emergency situations, the comatose, the mentally ill, and children.

Finally, a fifth possibility is to view patient advocacy as the securing of or checking on quality health care. It would be the advocate's responsibility to make certain that the patient is receiving the best possible care. This function could assume many forms. For example, the advocate might try to compensate for the lack of continuity of care in many teaching hospitals by making sure that necessary information is transmitted either verbally or in the chart from one group of hospital staff to the next, or by serving as the constant or steady contact between patient and staff or between family and hospital. The advocate might even double check such items as blood type, drug type and/or dosage, conformity of food to diet restrictions, and even report new symptoms or changes to the appropriate personnel. The advocate might be sensitive to inappropriate staff behavior, language, and subtle forms of communication, and suggest changes. For example, talking about a patient in his presence as if he or she were not there ought not to occur, and it might be the advocate's role to be sensitive to such incidents and bring them to the attention of the staff.

I do not mean to imply that these models of advocacy are mutually exclusive, or that other models are not possible, but, for the remainder of this article, I would like to concentrate on the implications of these five approaches for the nurse's role. In my discussion I will suggest some of the problems inherent in the nurse's assumption of the advocacy role. I suggest that because of these inherent problems it might be more appropriate for someone other than the nurse to perform patient advocacy functions. Furthermore, I suggest that although it might be desirable, it does not seem possible, to leave the choice of the advocacy model up to the patient. It is sometimes suggested that this is possible in terms of the general nurse/patient relationship; i.e., that the individual patient can choose whether or not the nurse assume the role of "parent-surrogate, physician-surrogate, healer, patient advocate, health educator, or contracted clinician." It is unrealistic, however, to believe that the patient can "choose" in any rational sense how he or she will interact with the nurse. The psychological state of the patient, as well as general characteristics of both patient and nurse are significant in determining the type of interaction or relationship which develops between them.

Consider the first and second models presented, the advocate as a counselor or advisor. It is sometimes argued that because the nurse has such intimate and daily contact with a patient, the nurse is the ideal one to understand and relate to the patient as a unique person and help the patient regain a sense of autonomy and think through his or her feelings and values. Those who hold this view, see the nurse as the best person to fill the role of counselor/advisor. Intimate and daily contact has other implications, however, which may frequently be overlooked.

In our ordinary dealings and relationships with people, we are usually not as physically dependent on them as a patient often is on a nurse. A patient's fear and pain, as well as forced dependency, exposure, and physical contact can make it extremely difficult for the nurse (who is usually a total stranger) to understand or appreciate the individual as a patient but as a person. In our ordinary relationships we usually have the right and the ability to share with others only those aspects of our body and personality as we desire and at the moments we desire. This right or ability is completely removed from the patient, and the inherently "coercive" nature of the nurse/patient relationship at least makes it questionable whether the nurse is the appropriate person to understand and relate to the patient as a unique individual.

There is another difficulty in assuming the nurse to be uniquely suited for the role of counselor; i.e., the general educational background of most nurses.

Obviously, this is a contingent factor which might easily be remedied by modifying the nursing curricula to require sufficient preparation in such fields as psychology, counseling, and the humanities.

The fifth model of patient advocacy, which views the advocate as the check on quality health care, appears considerably less problematic and probably would not even be considered an addition to the nurse's role but as already part of it.

Perhaps the most significant difficulties of advocacy are highlighted by the third and fourth models, the advocate as patient's rights advocate and as patient representative. Of central importance is the question of whether the advocate, as a representative of the patient, should argue as the patient would argue, were he or she capable, or in the best interest of the patient, as interpreted by the advocate. In other words, should the advocate be viewed as a spokesman for the patient and as a defender of his or her wishes or as a protector of the patient's interests, whether or not this is desired? Furthermore, if the advocate is to act paternalistically as a protector of the patient, how is it to be determined what is in the patient's best interest? Simply because it is a hospital context, should health always reign supreme? Should all other interests and values be considered subservient to increased physical or even mental well-being?

This issue takes on special significance in the hospital context, although it is not unique to this situation. A congressman or senator is one's representative, yet there is the question as to whether a political representative should vote according to what he or she believes is in the state's best interest or as the constituents would want. However, the political representative at least has been chosen by the constituency. The patient advocate, on the other hand, is in no way chosen by the patient. For this reason, paternalism on the part of the advocate would seem totally inappropriate. An advocate would seem bound by a stricter interpretation of representation and should function solely as a spokesman for the patient.

But how does this approach relate to the underlying principles of nursing practice? Are there certain actions or decisions which a nurse could not recommend because they would run counter to his or her professional standards, even though they were desired by the patient? Does patient advocacy imply the supremacy of a rights-based theory of morality over one based on duty—in other words, patient's rights over nursing duties? It would seem that a possible conflict exists between the advocate's role of representing the patient's wishes and the nurse's role of always acting in the best interest of the patient. In addition, the nurse already has built-in potential conflicts with protecting the patient, namely, multiple obligations to physicians, the nursing hierarchy, and hospital administration.

This raises a further question about institutionalizing patient advocacy. To ensure that the advocate's sole concern is the patient, should not the advocate be financially independent of the hospital? Should not the advocate be paid by an outside source or even by the patient and be accountable only to the patient? But if this were so would it not imply that the patient could reject the advocate's services and possibly secure the services of another? If this is the implication, nurses would obviously not be appropriate advocates, at least the way hospitals are currently structured. The need for nursing care, apart from advocacy, makes it impossible for the patient to do without a nurse, even though he or she may reject the nurse as an advocate.

Viewing patient advocacy as part of the nursing function seems to be fraught with difficulties. In my view, patient advocacy should not become the prerogative or the sole responsibility of any particular health professional, but rather should be part of the responsibility of all health professionals. Isn't the whole health care system and hospital structure organized for the benefit of the patient and in a sense to serve as advocate between the patient and society?

It is undoubtedly naïve on my part to suggest that such advocacy exists. In fact, it may even be argued that the need for patient advocacy is the result of the failure of the health care structure to function as it should. If this is the case, it is also the case that nurses, both as individuals with human frailties and as functionaries in a less than ideal system, at times fail to "advocate" for their patients. Because of the multiple obligations and pressures on the nurse, advocacy might be necessary even between the patient and the nurse. It might be necessary for someone to argue for or represent the patient to the nurse and possibly to the nursing hierarchy. I believe that another person who does not have additional loyalties and obligations within the hospital structure itself, would be the best person to advocate for the patient.

An analogy might be drawn between the nurse/patient relationship in the hospital context and the parent/child relationship. Although nurses and parents should and usually do act as patient/child advocates, there are situations in which conflicts of interest make it necessary for another person to represent either the patient or the child. In the parent/child situation, this conflict is sometimes thought to exist in the case of defective newborns. Because of the enormous financial, emotional, and psychological burdens the family might have to bear, it has been argued that the usual child advocates, namely the parents, might not be the appropriate ones to fully consider the interests and rights of the defective child. Similarly, owing to potential conflict with the nursing hierarchy, the possibility of loss of job or benefit as a result of

disobedience in certain situations, the nurse may not be the appropriate person to represent or defend the rights or best interests of a patient. Therefore, since it is in situations of conflict that certain types of advocacy are most needed, it is the premise of this article that the nurse may not be the one best suited to fill this role. In such situations, it would seem that all patients have the right to as impartial and extensive advocacy as possible.

Patient Advocacy: Do Nurses Have the Power and Authority to Act as Patient Advocate?

Barbara K. Miller, Thomas J. Mansen, and Helen Lee

Traditionally, nursing is pictured as being a profession dominated by physicians on one side and institutions on the other, each dictating what nurses should do. At the turn of the century nursing within institutions encompassed the care of the patient who was placed there to die. However, nurses were not performing the discarded functions of physicians at that time but were practicing independently.[1] Those nurses utilized aseptic technique which helped to control infectious diseases, thereby lowering the mortality rate. Thus, through the effective nursing care that was given, the focus of the hospitals changed from care of the dying to care of the acutely ill.

In the past few decades, the emergence of bureaucratic organizations and the growth and development of technological knowledge among other changes have had a dramatic impact on nursing. Today, many nurses within hospitals are concerned with carrying out, directly and indirectly, task-oriented functions. Thus the performance of skills is highly valued, and authority is delegated to those in administrative positions.

In addition, the public, or consumer, has viewed the physician as the sole authority and primary provider of health care, a perception that continues today. It is the physician whom the consumer considers to be the decision maker, and although nurses are publishing more extensively and participating in research, it is the ideas of those in the medical profession and their articles in the medical journals which are quoted and reiterated.[1] Moreover, the consumer does not differentiate nursing from medicine but rather perceives nursing to be dominated by medicine and related to the traditional male-female roles associated with medicine and nursing, respectively.

Consumers do not recognize the nurse as an initiator of health care nor do they separate nursing activities from medical treatment. They are generally unaware of the many independent activities of the nurse. Consequently, consumers envision the physician as the person to whom they turn for changes in health care and for protection of their rights; the nurse is seen as the care giver and not the advocate.[2] Nurses traditionally have been the mediator between the institution and the patient, but they often supported the institution, thereby failing to initiate any changes in the provision for health care delivery.

Donnelly, Mengel, and Sutterly[3] have differentiated the nurse into the care giver and the risk taker. The care givers are task oriented with a command of nursing skills which are highly valued in the institution. They conform to group norms and do not differ with their superiors. Care givers expend their energies developing cooperative and collaborative relationships. However, a patient advocate must not only be a care giver but a risk taker. Leininger suggests that too many of our leaders in nursing have been satisfied with the status quo and have not become risk takers for nursing.[4] It is the risk takers who initiate changes that must be made. They are not comfortable with mediating nor with conforming to the mold but more important, they uphold their values and principles. They not only support the patient in his decision-making process but become influential in upholding the patients' decisions. The risk taker has the motivation to enact change and be a patient advocate.

Because there is disagreement and confusion concerning the nurse's role in advocacy, the purpose of this article is to delineate the concept of patient advocate and its relationship to power and authority and to present one of the issues involved in the interaction between advocacy and nursing practice so that nurses may become more cognizant of the dimensions of the role of patient advocate.

An advocate, according to Webster, is one who "pleads another's cause" or speaks in favor of an individual.[5] Advocacy is the act of defending, supporting, or protecting an individual. These definitions are apparent in items 3, 4, and 6 of our Nurses Code, 1976.[6] Item 3 states, "The nurse acts to safeguard the client and the public when health care and safety are affected by the incompetent, unethical or illegal practice of any person." Item 4 states, "The nurse assumes responsibility and accountability for individual nursing judgments and actions," and item 6 states, "The nurse exercises informed judgment and uses individual competence and qualifications as criteria in seeking consultation, accepting responsibilities and delegating nursing activities to others."[6] Another definition of advocacy is offered by Kohnke, who states that advocacy is "the act of informing and supporting a person so that he can make the best decisions for himself."[7] This interpretation closely resembles one of the rights stated in the Patient Rights Code issued by the American Hospital Association in 1973. Annas and Healey suggest that the advocate is a representative of the patient, a person who assists the patient to exercise his rights.[8]

There is no disagreement that the nurse becomes an advocate of the patient in order to give good nursing care since the care may involve questioning of orders or pursuing other avenues to promote patient comfort. Such advocacy may involve advancing through the hierarchy of the nursing or the medical staff in pursuit of effective nursing care. Patient advocacy, however, is more encompassing and pertains to the patient's participation in making decisions regarding his health care. Since these decisions may include the health care delivery in any of the services or medical regimen protocol, the nurse's power and authority within the system to be an effective patient advocate has been questioned. In order to determine whether the nurse has the necessary authority it is well to examine the concept, authority.

Authority, as well as advocacy, is an elusive concept having many definitions and related terms.

Yura and Walsh, citing numerous and varied definitions for authority given by experts in the various disciplines, conclude that the experts cannot agree on this term.[9] Yura and Walsh have reviewed authority as a component of leadership; however, Field has recently classified the components of authority.[10] She defines authority as a select power with its own nature, one which comprises three constituent powers: personal, invested, and delegated, all of which interact and are interdependent. On the basis of Field's definition, a nurse should have personal, invested, and delegated powers which in turn will give her authority.

The nurse who has personal power is competent in her field of expertise, has confidence and self-esteem, and is able to communicate effectively and listen skillfully. Such a nurse keeps up with progressive changes in nursing practice and is held in high regard for her skills and logical thinking by her peers and co-workers.

Invested power is given by the person (such as the nurse) who places her trust and confidence in an agent or an institution (such as a hospital). She trusts that the institution will support her autonomy and the accountability of her position, and she in turn will give effective nursing care. Some of the nurses depicted in the film, "Nurse, Where Are You?" (CBS Reports, TV Documentary, Marlene Sanders, Correspondent, 1981) expressed this constituent of authority when they declared that the hospital administration would listen to them concerning their needs and problems. Other nurses in the film placed their trust in the American Nurses' Association when they wished the professional organization to represent them to meet the problems and nursing needs at the hospital. There were also some of the nurses who were thinking of leaving nursing since they could not give their trust to the ANA or the institution. Invested power may endure for a short or long period of time; nevertheless, the receiver gains power through the support given. For example, the ANA would be one of the most powerful organizations in the nation if the more than one million working Registered Nurses would invest their power to it. Similarly, the institution of employment gains power by virtue of the nurse's support—her invested power (trust). Another area of invested power is that of society, a powerful influence that nurses and nursing have not fully utilized. Although public opinion is elusive, should consumers invest their power in nursing, the nurse's role as patient advocate would gain impetus.

The third power, delegated power, is formal and intentional. Delegated power is the power given to an individual, such as the staff nurse, and which is perpetuated in the policies, rules, and regulations of the agency. This power would be recognized in job descriptions. Delegated power would be necessary for the enactment of specific duties, which may differ from one position to another. For example, the staff nurse would have duties different from those of the supervisor or the clinician. In some hospitals, the critical care nurses have patient care policies different from those of nurses on the medical-surgical units or in the obstetrical department. In some hospitals, job descriptions are so lacking in specificity that it may be difficult to ascertain the delegated power or authority that the nurse may have.

Ultimately, however, it is the interaction of each of these powers, personal, invested, and delegated that is unique to authority. A nurse may have any one of these powers without authority, such as the nurse who has invested trust in the hospital and is competent and admired by her co-workers, yet has little delegated power to enact any changes. Conversely, a nurse may be in a position of authority, yet lack personal power and has not invested power in nursing. In other words, the nurse has advanced through the hierarchy by virtue of her seniority in the system and her loyalty to the institution. That nurse may then be delegated the authority to enact beneficial changes for the patient and the health care system; however, she is more concerned with task-oriented skills than with the autonomy of the nurse or the advancement of nursing practice. She is not a risk taker. This lack of power and failure to invest power in nursing while holding the position of authority maintains the status quo.

Using the concept of authority and power as presented, the question or issue is, "Do nurses have the authority to act as the patient's advocate?" The issue is not *should* nurses have the authority but *do* they have the power? Many of our noted leaders in nursing have stated that nurses are the patient's advocate and should act in that manner in order to give effective nursing care.[11] Many writers indicate that nurses have expertise and educational background to explain and assist the patient with his decision making. Nurses are prepared and educated using the nursing process to assess and inform according to the patient's needs or problems. These illustrations of expertise enhance the personal power of the nurse, and by being accountable and responsible for nursing actions the nurse gives effective nursing care. However, without the delegated power to intervene or to institute nursing measures incongruent with the physician's care, the nurse's personal power

is negated. Even when the nurse believes certain measures would enhance the patient's well-being, the physician must concur. In many institutions, patient teaching must be ordered by the doctor (i.e., diabetic teaching, cardiac rehabilitation information) before the planning for teaching may proceed.

In order to illustrate the many varied factors that may involve patient advocacy, the following situations are offered.

A patient has numerous diagnostic x-rays ordered and decides after many hours in the x-ray department that he wants no more tests and returns to his room before they are completed. He states the x-ray department was cold and the personnel unfeeling, and now wants his breakfast and the doctor called. He also states that he has been subpoenaed to be in court tomorrow and must be there.

A patient has been told by his physician that he must have surgery. Surgery has been scheduled for the next morning, but he is now having misgivings and wants more information concerning the complications, the number of this type of surgery that is done in this institution, and how many surgeries of this type have been performed by his surgeon. He has asked the nurse for this information.

A patient complains that the doctor has only been in to see him for about two minutes each day without giving time for questions, and now the patient wants this information. He also wants his wife in the room when his physician comes to visit. The patient in the next bed complains about the nursing care that he has been given. He states that the nurse was rude to him and won't allow him to do anything for himself. He wants another nurse to care for him.

A patient with diabetes states that he wants more information about blood glucose self-monitoring and about diet to control his allergies. He also states that he is concerned about his retarded daughter who is staying with a neighbor. He says he thinks she has diabetes, too, but his physician states that it is more important for him to get better and follow the orders he has given. The patient is now questioning how much his internist knows about diabetes care; perhaps he should see a specialist.

These situations are not presented so that the reader may attempt to solve the patient or nurse's dilemma nor devise a solution for the problems. The situations are offered to illustrate the mutiplistic aspects of patient advocacy. In each of the situations, if the patient's rights are to be protected, some action must be taken. In each of these situations, other departments or other medical or nursing personnel are involved. The procedure to assist the patient and support his right to make decisions would involve the nursing process. The nurse would collect needed data, assess and plan, but the intervention of the plan would depend upon the authority of the nurse.

Most institutions do not give authority to the nurse to intervene in care in which she is not directly involved, nor is this authority written in the job descriptions. Although nurses have the code of ethics, the statements are broad and subject to misinterpretations. The most renowned example is the Tuma case wherein this RN was accused of intervention between patient and doctor. Tuma gave information to a patient concerning alternative modes of treatment upon the patient's request without obtaining the permission of the patient's physician. The nurse was cited for intervening without the authority to do so.[12] The Idaho Board of Nursing, acting in response to a complaint filed by the hospital, suspended Ms. Tuma's license for six months for interfering in a physician–patient relationship. The decision was later reversed by the Supreme Court of Idaho. While the situation raises questions regarding team work and communication, it also directs the nursing profession to the larger issues of nursing, such as informed consent, the nurse's right to practice nursing, and the role of the nurse as patient advocate.

There have been many articles written on patient advocacy espousing the right and obligation of every nurse to act as a patient advocate. It has been reiterated that nurses are professionals who have autonomy and who, therefore, should be acting to protect the patient. However, in order to suggest and intervene for the patient it is necessary to have the authority to do so. Within the hospital, the nurse serves both the medical and the administrative authority. Nurses have become involved in advocacy; however, when they have been admonished or punished for intervention, they turn back to the care giver role and no longer become involved.[13]

There are too few risk takers in nursing: moreover, a crucial factor inhibiting progress in nursing practice is that nurses do not speak out and support nursing colleagues when they have dared to become involved.[14,15]

One writer suggests that as nurses become more educated and more articulate (personal power) the relationship between nurses and administration may become more collegial in nature. However, unless the professionals unite into a cohesive group (invest in nursing) the bureaucratic organizations will retain the power.[15] It is well to note how very few hospital policy-making boards include nurses and then to note the number of physicians who sit on these boards.

The patient-advocate role is becoming one of patient representative in many hospitals, with well-specified written policies and descriptions for this role. It has been suggested in some hospital journals that the patient advocate should be someone outside the realm of nursing.[16] This person would have specific duties to assist the patient if a problem occurs during his hospitalization. It should be considered, however, that if the hospital is paying the representative, the representative may well have invested her power in the hospital. The main concern may not be to the patient but to assist the hospital to have complacent, noncomplaining and nonsuing patients. In other words, she could become an advocate for the hospital if a choice were made between patient and hospital.

One such patient representative and non-nurse states that nurses do not have the time to care for all the patient's needs and problems; moreover, they do not have the authority to intervene between departments. In one hospital in New York, the patient representative is a nurse in an administrative position who attempts to resolve patient/family grievances. She expects the nursing staff to be "front line patient advocates" and notify her when problems arise. She explains that she specializes in a job that has been a part of the nurse's role for a long time and will "step in when the staff nurses can go no further."[17] It has also been suggested that a patient advocate must know the patient's rights in addition to having a background in law. The writer of this suggestion has a position in a psychiatric setting. She states that some patients may be hospitalized due to stresses resulting from problems that can only be resolved through legislation.[18]

Philosphically and traditionally, many nurses have been assuming the role of patient advocate to a certain degree. We react emphatically and emotionally that we are advocates for the patient and that we must continue to support the patient physiologically and psychologically. However, the issue, "Do nurses have the power and authority to act as an advocate," will not be resolved by verbal reactions and possessive territorial assumptions. As long as we do not possess the authority to make changes for the benefit of the patient, then we are not acting as patient advocates. We may indeed be giving good nursing care but only in the realm of our immediate care giving tasks.

In summary, most nurses believe that they are advocates for the patient; however, if they do not possess delegated powers from the institution nor have power invested in them from either the medical profession or the consumer, then their personal power of competence and expertise will not be sufficient to give them the authority to act as patient advocate. It will become the position of the nurse in the institution which will dictate the degree of autonomy and responsibility to the patient.

Perhaps this issue of patient advocacy will be a factor to entice all nurses to act as professionals, be risk takers, and demand the authority and autonomy of the professional. Or perhaps we will remain only a care giver, but only to the extent we are allowed.

REFERENCES

1. Ashley J: *Hospitals, Paternalism and the Role of the Nurse*. New York, Teachers College Press, 1976.
2. Hughes L: The public image of the nurse. *Advances in Nursing Science* Feb 1980, pp 55–70.
3. Donnelly G, et al: *The Nursing System: Issues, Ethics and Politics*. New York, Wiley Medical, 1980.
4. Leininger M: The leadership crisis in nursing: A cultural problem and challenge. *J Nurs Admin* Sept–Oct 1972, pp 62–68.
5. *Webster's Dictionary*, ed 2. The World Publishing Co, 1974, p 20.
6. *Nurses' Code of Ethics*, Kansas City, American Nurses' Association, 1976.
7. Kohnke M: *The nurse as advocate. Am J Nurs* Nov 1980, pp 2038–2040.
8. Annas G, Healey J: The patients' rights advocate. *J Nurs Admin* May–June 1974, pp 25–31.
9. Yura H, Walsh M: Concepts and theories related to leadership. *Nursing Dimensions* Summer 1979, pp 75–86.
10. Field E: Authority: A select power. *Advances in Nursing Science* 1980; 31(1):69–82.
11. Letters—Feedback on The Right to Inform. *Nursing Outlook* Dec 1977, pp 738–743.
12. Lewis E: The right to Inform. *Nursing Outlook* Sept 1977, p 561.
13. Kelly L: The patient's right to know. *Nursing Outlook* Jan 1976, pp 26–32.
14. Smith C: Outrageous or outraged. *Nursing Outlook* Oct 1980, p 624.
15. Kudzma E: Patterns for effective nursing action within health bureaucracies. *Nursing and Health Care* Feb 1982, pp 68–72.
16. McDonald N: Patient rep can be viewed as fiscal asset. *Hospital* May 1, 1980, pp 42, 47.
17. Cate AJ: The patient representative: Who's side is she on? *Nursing 81* Jan 1981, pp 74–78.
18. Nations W: Nurse lawyer is patient advocate. *Am J Nurs* 1973; 73(6):1039–1041.

Nursing Advocacy of Patients' Rights: Myth or Reality?

Darlene Trandel-Korenchuk and Keith Trandel-Korenchuk

The specific environment in which the nursing practice takes place often limits the ability of nurses to perform and make moral decisions. The clinical setting may be seen to constrain and cripple the nurse in protecting and advocating the rights of patients. The case of *Jolene Tuma v the Idaho Board of Nursing*[1] reminds the nursing profession of its limited ability to support the rights of the patient while practicing in a setting where the nurse is subordinate to the hospital administration and medical staff and is obligated to meet the needs and goals of the institution. It remains difficult for nurses to make moral decisions which serve the individual needs of the patient and protect patient rights in a practice environment where conflicting loyalties exist.

Tuma made a decision to meet her patient's needs by sharing the information personally requested by the patient about the chemotherapy currently being received by the patient and an alternative form of treatment, laetrile. Shortly thereafter, Tuma was charged with "unprofessional conduct." For these actions said to "interfere in the physician–patient relationship," Tuma's nursing license was suspended for six months by the Idaho Board of Nursing.

The patient's right to self-determination is assured through the legal and ethical doctrine of informed consent.[2,3] This doctrine includes, but is not limited to, a description of the therapy recommended to the patient, the benefits and risks of such therapy and the available alternatives to the suggested treatment, including no treatment. According to the facts found in the case, Tuma discussed chemotherapy, which had been initiated, and natural products as an alternative treatment. She did not say that the alternative treatment would cure the patient.[1] This information

about the chemotherapy and alternative treatments could reasonably be deemed elements in the informed consent process. Although the current trend in law gives the responsibility for obtaining informed consent prior to the initiation of therapy to the attending physician, the law does not specifically prohibit other professionals from contributing to and assisting in the process of informed consent. It is therefore reasonable to conclude that Tuma, in sharing information about alternative forms of treatment which *was specifically requested by the patient*, was contributing to the process of informed decision making.

Meeting patients' needs is part of the caring process in nursing. One important need of patients is to be informed about what is happening to them in the hospital and what is being done to their bodies.

The patient in the Tuma case could have easily requested the information from her doctor or she could have sought other available resources for such information, for instance, printed material. The patient, however, chose to obtain the information not from her physician and not from other resources, but from Tuma. Clearly, the patient had a right to this requested information and because the patient made the request, she seemingly also had a need. Because Tuma responded to the patient's need for and right to such information, she was charged instead with interfering in the physician–patient relationship labeled as unprofessional conduct. It would be interesting to speculate what would have occurred if the patient chose instead to obtain her information from printed materials concerning medical therapy rather than seeking the information from Tuma. Would such literature have been seen as interfering with the physician–patient relationship?

The Idaho Board of Nursing found Tuma guilty and its decision was supported by the Idaho State Nurses' Association.[4] According to the facts cited in the case, answering patients' inquiries about their conditions and possible treatment alternatives is part of nursing practice and in conformity with what a reasonable nurse would do.[1] Nurses might therefore be led to question why the board of nursing and the state nurses' association condemned rather than supported Tuma's actions.

Other factors may have precluded Tuma from receiving protection in her decision to talk to the patient and to promote the patient's right to self-determination. Such factors may have included Tuma's own personal feelings (recorded in the case report) that what she was doing was "unethical." According to the case, she questioned the "correctness" of her nursing judgment and action. In addition, it appears from the case record that the attorney(s) for the defense defended Tuma's action from a negative posture rather than approaching Tuma's performance positively as appropriate and reasonable nursing procedure.[1]

In summary, it appears in this case that Tuma lacked respect for her own nursing judgment, she held no authority to serve the patient's needs and rights to information concerning treatment, she was treated as a subordinate to the physician and she did not possess professional autonomy to carry out her nursing functions. These issues exemplified in the *Tuma* case seem to revolve around four important concerns of nursing: autonomy, equality, respect and authority. It is these concerns which may be seen to hinder nurses from making appropriate moral decisions regarding patient care.

In the current practice situation, nursing often suffers from a lack of respect, an insufficient amount of authority, inequality and an inadequate amount of respect in the position it occupies in the health care bureaucracy. Social, economic and political environmental variables historically and contemporarily have affected the nursing profession creating and sustaining such a situation. Multiple environmental factors affect and are affected by the information and maintenance of the characteristics of the profession which in turn affect and are affected by the ability of the nurse to make moral decisions and protect patients' rights.

Environments, like people, have unique personalities.[5] From that assumption one can inquire into the personality traits (i.e., variables) present in the health care setting which affect the nursing profession in obtaining autonomy, respect, equality and authority. The remainder of this paper will explore this question.

Moos conceptualizes three basic types of dimensions which may be salient characteristics in a variety of different social milieus: 1) personal development; 2) relationship dimensions; and 3) system maintenance and system change.[5] These categories, with an additional fourth category, will be utilized as the framework for analyzing nursing's environmental variables. The fourth category, labeled "developmental dimensions," is added to the categories suggested by Moos since the historical development of nursing has greatly affected the contemporary characteristics possessed by this profession.

The categories used in this analysis sometimes overlap and each category considers multiple dimensions including social, political and economic forces. The developmental dimensions will be considered first, then the personal development and relationship dimensions will be examined. The final category discussed will be system maintenance and change.

DEVELOPMENTAL DIMENSIONS

The evolution and establishment of the nursing and medical profession, as a progression of historical variables, has had a great impact upon the development of nursing characteristics. Women have always been healers. Over time, women have, however, been removed from their primary role as independent healers and placed in a subordinate, dependent position as caretakers. Health care became the near-exclusive domain of the male professionals and the male-dominated health care industry. These two factors have had a tremendous negative influence upon the development of nursing autonomy, respect, equality and authority.

Establishment of Male-Dominated Medical Profession

The exclusive control of the health care system by males was effectively won in the early part of the twentieth century. According to Ehrenreich, witches of the Middle Ages, as lay women healers, represented a political, religious and sexual threat to the church and the state. The new male medical profession, under the sponsorship of the wealthy ruling class, executed well-organized, well-financed witch-hunt campaigns under the guise of the church and state. These hunts effectively destroyed women healers.[6]

Ehrenreich's historical account articulates the strategies employed by the male medical profession to acquire and maintain prominent status and dominant power over the art and science of healing. By serving the elite ruling class, medicine received status and power. The lay women healers, on the other hand, served poor peasants. According to Ehrenreich, such a situation resulted in the persecution of the "witches" by the all-powerful church and state and the legitimization of the doctor's professionalism.

The establishment of medicine as a profession requiring university training made it easy to prohibit women from becoming trained physicians. By the 1800s, regular doctors (physicians who were formally trained) became the prominent medical establishment. These "regulars" continued to be closely tied to the upper class and carried legislative strength. By 1830, 13 states licensed "regular" doctors and outlawed any other "irregular" practice.[6]

The popular health movement, appearing on the scene during the 1830-'40s represented both a class and feminist struggle.[7] This women's movement was particularly concerned with issues related to women's health and with the discriminating practices against admitting women into medical training. The AMA, as a professional stronghold formed in 1848, was able to defend against the demands of this popular health movement. The chilling blow to this feminist position occurred in the early 1900s when the Flexner report was issued.[6] With the objective of improving medical education, this report closed the smaller poor schools that educated blacks and women medical students. This report closed the medical profession to the poor, the black and the female population.

According to Ehrenreich, the medical profession became distinguished not because it was scientific, but because it was associated with the wealthy ruling class in the Middle Ages and, later, with the business establishment rising in the United States.[6] Medicine gained more power and prestige was won by the intervention of the Carnegies and the Rockefellers who, with massive wealth and organized philanthropy, created a respectable and scientific medical profession. In addition, by serving the upper class and gaining legislative clout, the medical

profession established a professional monopoly. This monopoly gave the physicians authority in law to select their own members and regulate their practice. Ehrenreich states the physician became the "man of science: beyond criticism, beyond regulation and very nearly beyond competition."[6]

The last stronghold of independent women health care providers was the midwives. Brack claims the displacement of midwives by male physicians was due to a series of cultural factors. First, the medical profession, growing in power and autonomy, could protect their own interests. By utilizing legislative clout, they restricted the opportunities for midwifery practice and imposed legal sanctions on midwives through state licensing laws. In addition, by redefining birthing as pathological and socially sanctioning the attendance of a male during labor and delivery, the medical profession monopolized the practice of "obstetrics."[8] Other factors which contributed to the displacement of midwives included the lack of established training schools for student midwives, the taboo placed on women in American society entering a high prestige profession and a high physician-to-consumer population ratio.[8]

Establishment of Nursing as Traditional Women's Role

The only remaining health occupation for women was nursing. Ehrenreich describes the situation in nursing as a product of the oppression of upper class Victorian women.[6] The "ideal lady" was transplanted from home to the hospital. Nursing was called a "natural, instinctive" vocation for a woman. In the hospital setting, Aroskar and Ashley describe the nurse as playing the role of devoted wife to the male physician and selfless mother to the patient.[9] The occupation of nursing presented no threat to the perpetuation of feminine virtues. Furthermore, nursing attracted women from the lower middle class segment of society. Upper class values were thereby imposed on the working class women in nursing training, transforming them into "virtuous and respected Victorian ladies."[6]

Nursing was forced to contend with the sexism of individual physicians and the medical profession as well as with sexual exploitation from the hospital institutions where nurses were trained. As described by Ashley, it was a whole class system which supported male power and dominance in American society. In the early 1900s hospitals were a lucrative business, and since nursing care was the main service the hospital offered to the public it was the nursing service that produced the high revenues from which hospitals profited.

When nursing schools were first established, the schools faced financial problems. Unlike the medical schools which received private and public monies and support, the nursing schools had no subsidizing source of revenue. To overcome these monetary problems, nursing schools agreed to give free nursing service to hospitals that would in turn provide clinical experience to the student nurses.[10] This arrangement, according to Ashley, allowed the hospital to continue its lucrative business by using this cheap source of nursing labor. The commercial value of the student to the hospital was the root of many problems in nursing.[10]

Ashley describes this hospital apprenticeship training as a paternalistic system where individuals of a superior nature watch over those of an inferior nature. All policies and procedures were formulated to support the overall interests of the institution.[10]

Not only were nurses exploited by serving as cheap labor under the guise of "nursing education," but the public was unknowingly sold by the hospitals the services of a young apprentice in the name of a fully trained professional nurse, according to the report made by Ashley.

Perhaps as a means of maintaining dominance and control over the nursing profession, physicians as well as hospitals continued to advocate apprentice-style nursing training. The "born nurse" theory was used as an argument to keep nursing training to a minimum.[10] Medical text books and popular literature were fraught with warnings about the physiological and emotional dangers of education to women.[11] Physicians were heard to express fears that nursing would gain its independence and compete with the medical profession.[10]

One must be careful of interpreting historical situations in terms of contemporary norms. For instance, a situation which today might be labeled as "sexist" or "paternalistic" might be interpreted as the appropriate role and treatment of women in the context of past traditional cultural norms.

In this environment, the nursing profession was born. Such a climate has had a significant impact on the characteristics of today's nursing profession— one that possesses little authority, respect, equality and autonomy. But while this historical account makes the physicians and hospital institutions appear like the "bad guys," they cannot carry the full responsibility for hindering the nursing profession from attaining authority, respect, equality and autonomy. It seems legitimate to question why nurses allowed the physician and hospital to create such a situation for the practice of nursing.

PERSONAL DEVELOPMENT

Every society ascribes different psychological attributes, tasks and duties and modes of living to males and females. In American society, boys are socialized with different attitudes and behavioral characteristics than are girls. Although roles are changing, women in American society are stereotyped. In the past, the most important role for a woman to fulfill was thought to be her natural and nurturing role of wife and mother. Anthropological studies report that in most societies the woman's work has mainly been associated with food gathering and preparation, clothing manufacture, crafts and home maintenance.[12] In contemporary American society, however, many women are attempting to combine motherhood with a career.

Attitudinal Characteristics

Women are often characterized as emotionally unstable, passive, dependent, weak, unscientific, subjective and overly sensitive. Men, on the other hand, are characterized as aggressive, independent, confident, competitive, stoic, objective and rational. American society generally values the traits attributed to men while the traits attributed to women are less socially desirable. Broverman found that a double standard of health exists for men and women. In his study, the concepts held by mental health clinicians regarding healthy mature men did not differ significantly from their concepts of healthy mature adults. Their concepts of healthy mature women, however, differed significantly from those of men and adults.[13] For a woman to be judged "healthy" in our society she must display the behavioral attributes for the female sex, even if they are less socially desirable.

Behavioral Characteristics

The socialization of little boys is different than that of little girls. At an early age, boys learn to develop a sense of self-worth and independence.

Little girls, on the other hand, are socialized in a manner that delays their search for identity, development of autonomy and self-esteem.[14] According to Spengler, since one of the main goals in life for the woman will be to please others (i.e., husband and children), she must become, in some sense, passive. In so doing, she renounces her autonomy.[14] These behavioral sex differences, observed in infancy and childhood and considered by some to be natural and predetermined, seem more likely to be promoted and reinforced in the socialization process by parents, between peers and in school.

Closely associated to the stereotyped female is the stereotyped nurse. The sex-linked nurse stereotype, commonly embodying obedience, warmth, caring and nurturing is the image cast by the media and the literature.[9] Fagin contends that this nursing image may discourage "the career minded more aggressive woman from choosing nursing."[15] This statement implies that the nursing stereotype may be effectively changed by recruiting more agressive personality types into the nursing profession. Murphy suggests, however, that personality characteristics may be a preselection factor in choosing nursing as a career.[16] According to Murphy's statement, one can view the nurse stereotype as perpetuated by the "traditional" woman who enters the profession.

The female is therefore seen to be socialized into a passive rather than an independent autonomous role. Furthermore, the characteristics possessed by the female are less socially desirable and hence less respected. In addition, she is taught to please men and be their subordinate rather than their equal. The female's authority is found in the household rather than in the outside world. Such traditional conditioning of a female to her role in life is therefore unsupportive of the personal as well as the professional characteristics of autonomy, authority, respect and equality.

The third category of variables consists of the relationship between the nurse and physician and the nurse and other nurses.

NURSE–PHYSICIAN

Evidence has been accumulated which indicates that the physician–nurse relationship can be characterized by medical authoritarianism on the one hand and nursing's acceptance of dependence on the other.[17] This has led some nursing leaders to suggest that the biggest problem facing nursing is its status as a woman's occupation in a male-dominated culture.[18-19]

One type of communication that occurs in the relationship between doctors and nurses is described by Stein. The object of the "doctor–nurse game" is that the nurse should be assertive and responsible for making decisions concerning patient care while appearing passive and subordinate at the same time. In this manner, the decision appears generated by the physician. Disagreement between the two personalities is to be avoided at all costs and the reward of this game is a successful and smooth operation as a doctor–nurse team.[20] This game indicates that the autonomy and independence of nursing actions is generally prohibited in relation to the physician. This doctor–nurse game supports and protects the authority of the physician.[20]

Another communication pattern that supports the authority of the physician over the nurse is information control.[21] The physician, as the person most knowledgeable about and ultimately responsible for the treatment and cure of the patient's pathology or disease, controls all information regarding the diagnosis and treatment of the client. At times nurses are only given the kind and amount of information concerning their patients that the attending physician wants the nurse to know. A collaborative exchange between the doctor and nurse may not occur; rather, the pattern of interaction may subordinate the nurse to the authority of the physician and emphasizes the inequality of these two professionals.

The social and economic differences between physicians and nurses also contribute to the inequality between these professional groups.[23] While the first nursing schools did their best to recruit upper class women as students, before long, most schools were attracting only women from the lower and working classes of society.[22] In addition, the apprentice-style nurse training, with minimal educational requirements, kept these student nurses ignorant of the arts and sciences.[10] Nurses remained largely from the lower class and uneducated. On the other hand, the medical profession was accessible only through a long and expensive course of university training.

The educational and class bias between nursing and medicine still exists and is another source of inequality. Ladd pointed out that the present day oppression and exploitation of nurses can, in a large measure, be explained historically by this social class differential. He speculates that by becoming professionals, nurses will be able to enter the middle class and so achieve social parity with other middle class professionals, including physicians.[23]

Physicians have had in the past and continue to have authority over nurses. Ladd suggests that authoritarianism is not necessarily sexist or economically exploitative.[23] One may question the nature of the authoritarian relationship which exists between the doctor and nurse.

When examining the nature of authority, a distinction between power and authority should be made.[23] Authority always carries the connotation of legitimacy, whereas power does not. Power is the capacity to make oneself be obeyed.[28] Authority calls for respect rather than fear, and it is accepted voluntarily because it is reasonable to obey commands. One might ask whether the authority physicians have over nurses is authority or power.

To accept authority means there exists a good reason to do so. If the authority physicians exert over nurses is either spurious or exceeds its limits, nurses should question whether a duty to obey the doctor exists.

Ladd distinguishes between two types of authority, belief and conduct. The authority of a physician is often in the category of belief authority which characterizes a type of intellectual or expert authority. If one has belief or intellectual authority, it is not necessarily assumed, however, that one has conduct authority. Conduct authority concerns the authority to command the behavior of an individual in a certain manner.[23] While it is obvious individuals must take the word of expert authorities (i.e., the physician), no one who is in authority automatically assumes the right to make decisions for other people.[23] Regarding moral decision making, Ladd suggests "anyone who wishes to base a doctor's right to command on his superior knowledge must be prepared to show that doctors know more about ethics than others and are more virtuous than their nurses or their patients."[23]

One reason for the acceptance of an authority figure is the recognition that a particular authority structure is a means to an end. When the goal is shared by the person in authority as well as by the individuals they command, the validation of the authority is based on the shared goals. When goals diverge, however, validation for that authority is more difficult and must come from some external source. In health care settings, it is common to have a multiplicity of goals; the physician may be concerned about the cure, the nurse about the care of the patient. According to Ladd, because of these multiple goals, a valid authoritarian relationship is difficult to justify. Mutual accommodation and persuasion should take the place of one person issuing commands to others.[23]

NURSE–NURSE

Nurses, as women and as professionals, face problems in their relationships with each other. The women's movement, begun in the early 1960s, helped develop a sense of sisterhood and relatedness among women which helped to overcome the sense of isolation felt by many women.[11] Spengler characterizes the problems in women's relationships as: a sense of privatism; a lack of group cohesiveness and solidarity; pressure to conform to traditional behavior through peer review; competitiveness from a lack of trust; fear of success; and lack of support for other women in their fight for or achievement of success.[14]

Similar problems to those noted above exist when examining the relationship between nurses. One problem faced by nurses is that often nurses do not form cohesive groups, leaving individual members without a sense of support. Nurses greatly outnumber physicians. The nursing profession has the potential to be powerful with their large numbers, but because nurses are seldom well organized, they are influenced and swayed by outside interests instead of their own nursing needs.

Spengler suggests that nurses, as women, need to develop an inner feeling of self-love and respect, for only through these feelings will women learn to love, value, trust and respect other women.[14] Perhaps if nursing attains unity and influence it will be better able to meet medicine and the hospital bureaucracy on equal ground in a collaborative relationship with mutual respect for the contribution each provides in administering patient care and cure.

SYSTEM MAINTENANCE AND SYSTEM CHANGE

The last category of variables consists of the hospital, education and legal systems. These systems will be examined regarding the influence they exert upon the characteristics of the nursing profession.

Nursing Education

Ashley documents how the paternalistic hospital and medical system exploited the labor of students and led nurses to believe that they were inferior and that they must remain subordinate to the medical and hospital hierarchy.[10] The early nursing education system did not encourage students to question but rather to accept the status quo. The conditions of nursing education still communicate to nursing students their inferior status. Spengler speaks of the impoverished facilities used in nursing education as compared to the facilities of the medical school. For example, nursing laboratory space and facilities are commonly inadequate and inferior to the laboratory facilities accommodating medical students.[14] Spengler says this situation may suggest to student nurses that the environment and tools necessary to prepare men (physicians) are more important than the tools and environment needed to prepare women (nurses) for their work.

The educational environment in nursing has been portrayed as rigid and authoritarian, reflecting teaching styles that impart a sense of subservience and a need to appeal to authority for approval.[24] Several research studies have examined the characteristics of nursing education. The findings of Stein and Stone indicate that nursing students did not feel free to express their opinions nor did they feel that the faculty treated them as autonomous independent persons.[25-26] Olesen reports that nursing students who did not possess the values of modesty and humility were branded as "overconfident" and considered "potentially unsafe" by the faculty.[27] In addition, the dropout students scored higher on a nonauthoritarianism scale than did the nursing students who remained.[27] According to the findings of Davis, profiles of student nurses in the late 1960s showed a tendency to be submissive, to sustain a subordinate role and to be more self-abasing than nonnursing students.[28] In contrast, the education of medical students instills confidence and pride in their special knowledge and skills, and prepares them to act independently and develop a demeanor that calls forth respect from others.

It appears that obedience and conformist attitudes are emphasized in nursing training. Those students who are found not to possess such attitudes or are unwilling to become dependent are soon weeded out and labeled as poorly suited for nursing. Aroskar contends that these characteristics are changing in baccalaureate prepared nursing students.[9]

Care and cure may not be equally valued in the health care system. Nursing, as a caring, nurturing process, is both historically and contemporarily considered to be a natural feminine attribute, and, as such, it is thought to be primarily an intuitive process[14] that requires little knowledge or skill to perform. Therefore the practice of nursing as well as the educational content is often devalued. Giving precedence to the tasks of the physicians as opposed to the tasks of nurses allows medical tasks to take on more significance than nursing tasks.

Bureaucratic Hospital System

Although essential for coordination of care as well as for the sake of efficiency, the hierarchy of authority in a bureaucracy produces among the lower echelons feelings of inequality and apathy toward the goals of the organization. The hospital bureaucracy concentrates authority in the hands of individuals (usually men). Because women are not generally considered partners of the men who are managing the health care institution, sex stratification commonly results.[14]

The hospital system may be seen to constrain the ability of the nurse to make decisions. The administrative hierarchy centralizes the decision-making process. Such arrangements require that nurses accept the conclusions of the individuals in power while preventing the workers from weighing competing considerations.[21] The system further confines nurse decision making by means of information control mechanisms and through the indoctrination of conforming values and attitudes. While the hospital bureaucracy places the nurse in the position of having a tremendous amount of responsibility, it effectively denies the nurse the decision-making powers necessary to appropriately carry out the responsibilities.

Many conflicts arise from the complexity of the nurse's role. Jameton calls this the "nurse in the middle" syndrome.[29] The nurse has a commitment to meet the individual needs of her patient. On the other hand, the nurse, as an employee of the hospital, is subordinate to the administration and must uphold the utilitarian goals of the institution: the greatest good for the greatest number.[16] In such a situation, the needs of the individual patient may be sacrificed for the greater good of all other patients in the institution. Furthermore, not only is the nurse responsible to the institution, but he/she is also responsible to the physician. The nurse is therefore subordinated to two lines of authority at one time.

The *Tuma* case illustrates this well. The authority figures, dismayed over Tuma's conduct, expressed their disapproval in the form of a lawsuit, charging Tuma with "unprofessional conduct."[1] When the nurse is forced to adhere to hospital and physician commands as opposed to serving the best interests of the patient, the delivery of health care is guided by loyalty to authority figures and institutions rather than to the process of caring.

Harding suggests there exists a contradiction between social value of nursing and the public recognition of this value.[30] The value of health is hardly questioned: "Society wants it and the more the better."[30] The statistics show that eight percent of health care workers are physicians compared to 50 percent who are nurses. The contribution of nurses to health care is therefore as crucial as any other health care worker, yet the nurse has relatively little status in the hospital hierarchy. In addition, gaps exist between what nurses are trained to do and what they are capable of performing, on the one hand, and what the hospital hierarchy allows them to do on the other.[30] Harding points out that the high social value of the large contribution nurses make to health care is not rewarded in commensurable income, appropriate social status or control over the conditions of nursing or manner in which health care is delivered.

Brown's analysis of the status of women in the health care system suggests that "health service is women's work but not women's power."[31] Woods cites six factors that seem to maintain the current distribution and low status of women in health care occupations. First, the determinant of the division of labor in the U.S. economy is the roles men and women assume in the family; that is, men are producers, women are reproducers and maintainers.[22] Second, women who go into and out of the labor force to raise families serve as a readily available reservoir of workers. Third, women have relatively limited professional opportunities in the health care system. For years women are discriminated against in admission into medical schools as well as into managerial positions in the hospital. In addition, the public and private sectors of society have not socialized significant parts of the women's work (i.e., child care) which has resulted in limited involvement in certain segments of the health labor force. Fifth, the nature of scientific medicine appears to reproduce social stratification by sex, class and race because of the intensive, long-term training required. Last, women have not been involved nor represented in policy-making groups at the hospital or national level.[22]

In total, the hospital organization perpetuates the subordinate and powerless position of nurses

by means of the bureaucratic hierarchy; it grants little respect and value to nursing skills; it places a tremendous amount of responsibility on nursing personnel with little decision-making power; and it fosters obedience and loyalty to the institutional goals as opposed to the individual needs and rights of the patients.

Legal System

The legal system has contributed as much to the oppression of nurses as the medical and educational system. While it was through legislative power and action that the medical profession obtained a monopoly over the practice of medicine, the legal recognition obtained by nurses gave that profession limited freedom and autonomy to practice as professionals. The laws regarding nursing practice served only to legalize the subservience of nurses to the physician.[10] In addition, the nurse practice acts gave legal sanction to medical sexism: Men were to supervise women whether or not they were in the presence of these women.[10] The fact is, many nurses function independently. Physicians are rarely present when nurses give patient care. Hence, while nurses are forced to make independent decisions concerning patient care because of the nature and provisions of the clinical setting in which they practice, they make many of these decisions illegally. The nursing profession remains in a "Catch 22": Nurses are given a tremendous amount of responsibility in patient care by physicians and hospitals, yet these same groups of individuals are often seen to hinder nurses from obtaining legal sanction of independent nursing practice. It appears that nurses remain legally exploited by the hospital and medical establishments.

The new definitions of nursing appearing in many of the state practice acts have been heralded as a triumph for the nursing profession. Such a reaction is unfounded. As of 1980, 15 states still maintained the tradition definition of nursing in the nurse practice act. In this definition, the nurse continues to be dependent on the direction and supervision of the physician for functions concerning diagnosis, prescription and treatment.[32] Some states have attempted to recognize the extended or expanded role of the nurse, but the autonomy such practice acts attempted to obtain seems more theoretical than real. The trend in defining nursing in these revised nurse practice acts is toward physician involvement/supervision of expanded nursing functions as evidenced by the common use of three strategies in the practice acts: 1) formulating and promulgating nursing rules and regulations by joint boards (i.e., medicine and nursing); 2) designating that certain procedures be performed under standing orders, policies and procedures, protocols, etc.; and 3) necessitating a written agreement between the nurse and the attending physician concerning supervision.[33] It is unlikely that a collaborative relationship as opposed to a superior-subordinate one will be achieved in light of the language of most state nursing statutes.

In summary, the nursing profession has not effectively attained respect, autonomy, equality and authority because of the presence of multiple environmental factors impinging on nursing practice. Until the nursing profession effectively possesses these characteristics, moral decision making and advocacy for patients' rights on the part of the nursing profession will continue to remain difficult if not impossible. In the current health care environment, nursing advocacy of patients' rights seems more of a myth than a reality.

REFERENCES

1. *Tuma v Idaho State Board of Nursing*, 593 P2d 711 (1979).
2. Trandel-Korenchuk, K. and Trandel-Korenchuk, D.: "Legal Implications of Informed Consent," *Nursing Administration Quarterly*, 1981, 5, pp. 101–105.
3. Trandel-Korenchuk, D. and Trandel-Korenchuk, D.: "Ethical Implications of Informed Consent," *Nursing Administration Quarterly*, 1981, 5, pp. 101–105.
4. Annas, G. et al.: *The Rights of Doctors and Nurses*, New York, Avon Books, 1981.
5. Moos, R.: "Conceptualizations of Human Environments," *American Psychologist*, 1973, 28, pp. 652–65.
6. Ehrenreich, B. and English, D.: *Witches, Midwives and Nurses: A History of Women Healers*, Old Westbury, New York, The Feminist Press, 1973.
7. Marieskind, J.: "The Women's Health Movement," *International Journal of Health Services*, 1975, 5, pp. 217–20.
8. Brack, D.: "Displaced—The Midwife by the Male Physician," *Women and Health*, 1976, 1, pp. 18–21.
9. Aroskar, M.: "The Fractured Image: The Public Stereotype of Nursing and the Nurse," in *Nursing Images and Ideals*, S. Spicker and S. Gadow (Eds.), New York, Springer Publishing Co., 1980, pp. 18–34.
10. Ashley, J.: *Hospitals, Paternalism and the Role of the Nurse*, New York, Teachers College, Columbia University, 1977.
11. Ruzek, S.: The Women's Health Movement, New York, Praeger, 1978.
12. Murphy, J.: "Changing Social Roles of Women," class lecture, MCHA 211b, *Health Care of Women*, Harvard School of Public Health, Nov. 25, 1981.
13. Broverman, I. et al.: "Sex-Role Stereotypes and Clinical Judgments of Mental Health," *J. Consult. Clin. Psych.*, 1970, 34, pp. 1–7.
14. Spengler, C.: "Conditioning of the Female to Her Role in Life," in *Woman Power and Health Care*, M. Grissum and C. Spengler (Eds.), Boston, Little, Brown and Co., 1976, pp. 1–15.
15. Fagin, C.: "Professional Nursing—The Problems of Women in Microcosm," *J.N.Y. State Nurses' Assoc.*, 1971, 2, p. 7.
16. Murphy, C.: "The Moral Situation in Nursing," *Bioethics and Human Rights*, E. Bandman and B. Bandman (Eds.), Boston, Little, Brown and Co., 1978, pp. 313–20.
17. Bates, B.: "Doctor-Nurse: Changing Roles and Relations," *NEJM*, July 16, 1970, pp. 129–34.
18. Cleland, V.: "Sex Discrimination: Nursing's Most Pervasive Problem," *AJN*, Aug. 1971, pp. 1542–47.
19. Davis, A. and Aroskar, M.: *Ethical Dilemmas and Nursing Practice*, New York, Appleton-Century-Crofts, 1978.
20. Stein, L.: "The Doctor-Nurse Game," *Arch. Gen. Psych*, 1967, 16, pp. 699–703.
21. Donovan, C.: "Impediments to Ethical Nursing Practice," *Oncology Nurs. Forum*, 1980, 7, p. 4042.
22. Woods, N.: "Women and the Health Care System," *Health Care of Women*, St. Louis, C.V. Mosby Co., 1981, pp. 40–55.
23. Ladd, J.: "Some Reflections on Authority and the Nurse," in *Nursing Images and Ideals*, S. Spiker and S. Gadow (Eds.), New York, Springer Publishing Co., 1980, pp. 160–75.
24. Mauksch, I.: "Let's Listen to the Students," *N.O.*, 1972, 20, p. 103.
25. Stein, R.: "The Student Nurse: A Study of Needs, Roles and Conflict, Part II," *N.R.*, 1969, 18, p. 433.
26. Stone, J. and Green, J.: "The Impact of a Professional Baccalaureate Degree Program," *N.R.*, 1975, 24, p. 287.

27. Olesen, V. and Whittaker, E.: *The Silent Dialogue*, San Francisco, Jossey-Bass, 1968.
28. Davis, A.: "Self Concept, Occupational Role Expectations and Occupational Choice in Nursing and Social Work," *N.R.*, 1969, 18, pp. 137–40.
29. Jameton, A.: "The Nurse: When Roles and Rules Conflict," *Hastings Center Report*, Aug. 1977, pp. 22–23.
30. Harding, S.: "Value-Laden Technologies and the Politics of Nursing," in *Nursing Images and Ideals*, S. Spicker and S. Gadow (Eds.), New York, Springer Publishing Co., 1980, pp. 49–75.

31. Brown, C.: "Women Workers in the Health Service Industry," *International Journal of Health Services*, 1975, 5, pp. 173–84.
32. Trandel-Korenchuk, D. and Trandel-Korenchuk, K.: "State Nursing Laws," *Nurse Practitioner*, Nov./Dec., 1980, pp. 39–41.
33. Trandel-Korenchuk, D. and Trandel-Korenchuk, K.: "Current Legal Issues Facing Nursing Practice," *Nursing Administration Quarterly*, 1980, 5, pp. 37–55.

The Nurse as Advocate:
A Cantankerous Critique

Leah Curtin

As though the problems faced by the modern nurse were not difficult enough, a "new" role has been added: the nurse as patient advocate. Presumably, whatever it was that nurses were doing before, they weren't being patient advocates. To assume this new role, then, we must first determine what it is that we should be doing for patients that we haven't been doing. In my innocent fashion, I turned to the nursing literature for enlightenment. There, I found the nurse-as-patient-advocate depicted as a combination lawyer-theologian-psychologist-family counselor and dragon-slayer wrapped up in a white uniform. I might add that an ordinary mortal like me felt depressed—even oppressed—by this vision of super-nurse.

To alleviate an incipient feeling of inadequacy, I diligently searched for a more modest definition of the nurse as advocate. Unfortunately, my search simply added frustration to inadequacy: the various explanations left me more bemused than when I began.

A SPIRITUAL ADVOCATE?

Some commentators seem to define advocacy in spiritual terms. A few months ago, I sat in an audience and listened to a speaker suggest that oncology nurses who *care* for patients (rather than merely treat them) must help them find meaning in their cancer and in their suffering and dying. As I sat there, I mentally reviewed different patients and families whom I had met:

- A young father who had just been told he had cancer of the liver. Bright, well-educated, loved—with so much to do and so little time left in which to do it.

- A three year old child suffering from lymphosarcoma. Not understanding her pain. Choking. Tears in her eyes. Tears in the eyes of her parents.

- A gentle grandmother with fulminating leukemia. Ulcers on her lips, in her mouth and nose. Her frail hand clutching tightly to mine. Her determination not to cry or complain in front of her children. The pain in her daughters' eyes.

I nursed them to the very best of my ability. I eased their suffering where I could. I touched them gently. I listened to them. I held them. Sometimes I even cried with them. Yes, and I carried out their treatment regimen. But never once was I able to find some reason why they suffered while others did not. Sometimes, things happen to people and there aren't any reasons why. In my experience, they were very *extra-ordinary* "ordinary" people. I learned from them. I was humbled by their courage. I had enormous respect for them. Certainly, I could see no reason why they should be singled out for suffering.

Looking for meaning where there is none is cruel and destructive—of self, of relationships to and with others, of faith itself. I suppose I'm not much of a patient advocate because I can see no reason in patients' suffering, so there's no way I can help *them* find meaning in it. And that's precisely why I expended so much energy and time in trying to mitigate their suffering and ease their dying. What comfort I gave was in providing *excellent* nursing care—and in sharing some measure of their burden. But that's not new, that's as old as nursing.

Curtin, L. (1983, May). The nurse as advocate: A cantankerous critique. *Nursing Management, 14,* 9–10. Reprinted with permission of © S-N Publications. All rights reserved.

THE NURSE AS LEGAL ADVOCATE

Other commentators seem to define patient advocacy in an almost purely legal context. They define the role as primarily one of informing patients of their legal rights and defending the patient's legal rights from all marauders (usually, the institution, physicians, and/or families). Quite aside from the adversary relationship that this definition infers, it poses other problems. First, nurses, of course, must know a great deal about the law and its application in specific circumstances. Presumably, then, nursing curricula ought to include, at the very least, three or four courses on law.

Although law is usually a good deal clearer than philosophy and nursing theory and things like that, the position of legal advocate can be quite ambiguous at times. For example, an Ohio nurse recently refused to administer anesthesia to a patient in the following situation:

Mrs. Jones was admitted to the hospital for chest pain. During the course of her hospitalization, she went into atrial fibrillation. Medical methods of treating her were not successful and her physician determined that the insertion of an atrial pacemaker was the only viable alternative. Mrs. Jones, still in atrial fibrillation, refused to have the pacemaker inserted. The physician and nurses in the cardiac care unit conferred with her family and explained her condition and its dangers. They also pointed out that atrial fibrillation could cause cerebral anoxia—which might explain why Mrs. Jones refused the pacemaker.

Finally, family members and health professionals decided that they could wait no longer, and Mrs. Jones was taken to the operating room. There, the nurse anesthetist, fulfilling her role as patient advocate, refused to administer the anesthesia. Eventually, another nurse anesthetist administered the anesthesia. Once inserted, the pacemaker returned Mrs. Jones' heart rhythm to normal. Mrs. Jones is now enjoying a near normal life and does not remember having refused the pacemaker.

Which nurse actually was the patient's advocate? Certainly, Mrs. Jones had a legal right to refuse treatment. However, she also had a legal right to treatment—and we had an obligation to provide it, particularly if her condition interfered with her ability to make decisions. To fail to treat her also could violate her rights. The question for those who would define advocacy purely in legal terms is, "Are there never exceptions?" What does one do when one right conflicts with another?

As soon as one admits to exceptions, the question arises, "Who determines the exceptions?" Clearly, the patient cannot determine the exceptions, so one is faced with the fact that others will decide for the patient what is in her best interests and that, quite frankly, is the definition of paternalism.

THE NURSE AS AN ADVOCATE FOR AUTONOMY

Still other commentators espouse a narrow definition of patient advocacy that seems to concentrate solely on patient autonomy. In this definition, the best interests of the patient are defined as *self-interest* which interest, moreover, can be determined only by the patient. The health professional, then, assumes an obligation to do what the patient decides is in his self-interest. Based on the principle of liberty and the right to self-determination, this approach has much appeal. However, when subjected to close scrutiny, many problems arise. For example, the cocaine addict may well include the continued use of drugs to be in his self-interest. Must one predicate a duty on the part of health professionals to obtain for and to administer cocaine to the addict—or, at least, to do nothing to prevent him from obtaining drugs? The suicidal patient similarly may define death as in his best interest. Do the health professionals then have a duty to help him kill himself—or, at least, to do nothing to prevent him from killing himself? To carry the argument further, the sadist may define his self-interest in terms of inflicting pain on others. Do health professionals have a duty to help him find victims to abuse—or, at least, to do nothing to prevent him from hurting others to fulfill his self-interest?

The definition of patient advocacy solely as a duty on the part of health professionals to do what the patient decides is in his self-interest denies professional responsibility and accountability for decisions made and actions taken. Certainly, advocacy cannot require avoidance of responsibility and accountability. Surely, the law expects professionals to use their knowledge and experience.

ADVOCACY AS DISINTEREST

Still other commentators seem to define advocacy in terms of disinterest. That is, health professionals are to provide all information for a patient and to clarify various options for the patient, but they must not indicate a preference for one course of action over another. Nurses must be neutral; detached, disengaged.

Such a position seems to me to be the antithesis of a fiduciary relationship which is based on the assumption that the professional *is* concerned about the well-being of the patient. It forces a patient to make a decision alone whether or not the patient thinks he needs advice, counsel or input.

Indeed, I do not claim that forcing a patient to make his own decision *alone* is always wrong; it is just that I am not sure that it is *always* right. It seems to me that it is arbitrary, unkind, and perhaps even irresponsible in some circumstances. People seek the advice and counsel of professionals precisely because professionals have spent many hours of study and have many years of experience in a particular field. Clearly, the patient wants to know what the professional thinks, particularly if he asks the professional for an opinion. This is not to claim that the professional should attempt to coerce the patient. It is simply to claim that sharing a considered opinion with a patient may be appropriate professional practice.

THE NURSE AS ADVOCATE:
A SUGGESTION

Clearly, nurses should respond to patients' spiritual needs. We also should respect the legal rights of patients, safeguard their autonomy and, at times, keep our opinions (however well founded) to ourselves. Quite honestly, it is easier to say what advocacy forbids rather than what it demands. Advocacy precludes coercion, exploitation or manipulation. Must we, then, define the nurse's role as patient advocate solely in negative terms? I don't think so, but I do think that the role of the nurse-as-patient-advocate must connect clearly to the role of "nurse."

Webster's Collegiate Thesaurus offers the following definitions of *role*—"(1) characteristic external properties and aspects, and (2) an atmosphere in which something intangible is discerned ≤ the moral *role* of the legislature ≥." I suggest that the second definition of "role" is most applicable. That is, the *role* of the nurse as patient advocate is a moral role—one in which something intangible is realized. *Webster's New World Dictionary* provides the following definitions of *advocate:* "(1) one who pleads the cause of another in a court of law; a counsel or counselor; as, *he is a learned lawyer and an able advocate;* (2) one who defends, vindicates, or espouses a cause by argument; or (3) one who is friendly to; an upholder; a defender; as, an advocate of peace, or of the oppressed." I suggest that the third definition *Webster's* offers is most applicable to nursing's concept of patient advocacy.

In a recent statement, the American Nurses' Association said that nursing practice includes "the diagnosis and treatment of *human responses* [emphasis added] to actual or potential health problems . . ." If this is true, then the nurse-patient relationship is determined by the patient's needs and the nurse's response to them.

The foundation of the relationship *is* advocacy in the sense that the nurse ". . . defends, vindicates, . . . is friendly to, . . . upholds . . . " The purpose of the relationship is, among other things, to maintain or to return control of his life to the patient. However, the form of the relationship varies. A relationship, by nature, is dynamic—a living interaction that changes, grows, contracts and, in this instance, ends. The needs of the patient, the knowledge and ability of the nurse, and environmental circumstances all influence the form of the relationship. So, a nurse *is* a patient advocate when her practice helps return a patient to independence or when her practice helps alleviate suffering or when her practice promotes respect for patients as persons.

In short, the role of the nurse as patient advocate is to create an atmosphere in which something intangible (human values, respect, compassion) can be realized. From where I sit, that is plain, not-so-simple, good nursing practice. *This, I understand.*

STUDY AND DISCUSSION QUESTIONS
THE NURSE AS ADVOCATE: CONCEPTS AND CONTROVERSY

1. What, according to Annas and Healey, has led to increased attention to the rights of patients?

2. Consider the four cases used to illustrate how a patient advocacy system would work. Are the problems cited as frequent and acute today as they were when this system was first proposed?

3. Why do Annas and Healey reject patient representatives as a solution to protecting the rights of hospital patients?

4. What are Annas and Healey's opinion of hospital produced pamphlets on patients' rights?

5. What is your opinion of Annas' proposed bill of rights?

6. Annas contends that Florence Nightingale's admonition to "Do no harm" ought to be extended to include protection against violating the human rights of clients even if no physical harm results. Do you agree that nurses should be concerned about both kinds of harm?

7. Do you think nurses could be advocates in Annas' sense of the term?

8. Do you agree with Annas' patient rights agenda?

9. June Gikuuri views the position of the patient representative as a protector of patients' rights but not as taking over anyone's job. Do you agree?

10. Anne Cote claims that patient representatives are allies of nursing. Do you agree?

11. How would you classify the patient representatives you are familiar with? Are they like those that Gikuuri and Cote describe or are they management representatives concerned with housekeeping and trivial problems, as Annas fears?

12. Nancy McDonald argues that patient representatives can actually save the hospital money. Do you agree? Supposing they do not save money, should hospitals have them anyway?

13. Is Jack Zusman's version of advocacy compatible with the conceptions we have seen from Gadow, Kohnke, and Annas?

14. Do you agree with Zusman that a patient's need must be balanced against everyone else's needs?

15. Natalie Abrams believes that nurses are inappropriate to console, counsel, and help patients with decision making because nurses do not know the patients well and therefore the relationship is inherently coercive; and nurses do not have the educational background in such fields as psychology, counseling, and the humanities. Do you agree?

16. Abrams sees a conflict that can result if nurses nonpaternalistically represent the wishes of their patients because those wishes may conflict with professional duties and hospital administration. Is this a problem? If so, how might it be solved?

17. Do you think the divided loyalties of nurses disqualifies them from being effective client advocates?

18. Both Miller et al. and the Trandel-Korenchuks conclude that nurses lack the power and authority to be patient advocates. Do you agree?

19. Consider the distinction Miller et al. uses to differentiate among nurses—caregivers and risk takers. Which more closely describes your nursing philosophy? Do you agree with Miller et al. when they say, "There are too few risk takers in nursing?"

20. The Trandel-Korenchuks cite the socialization of women as a major contributing factor to nursing's lack of autonomy and power. Do you agree? Would nursing be different if nursing had been male dominated?

21. Do you see allusions in Curtin's article to the positions on advocacy contained in this anthology?

22. According to Curtin, why can't nurses always act as spiritual advocates?

23. Curtin seems to favor acting paternalistically when there is doubt about the client's decision-making capacity. Do you agree?

24. Curtin cites some difficult cases for an all out advocate of autonomy—drug addicts, suicides, and sadists. Do you agree with Curtin on this issue? Can you think of other client decisions that would be difficult or impossible to support?

25. Curtin says, "sharing a considered opinion with a patient may be appropriate professional practice." She also says nurses should "at times, keep our opinions (however well founded) to ourselves." Do you see any guidance for knowing when it is appropriate and when it is not appropriate to share an opinion?

26. What is your opinion of Curtin's concept of advocacy? Is it more realistic for clinical practice than some other positions?

3

Nurses' Rights

INTRODUCTION

The readings in the last two chapters highlighted client rights and the role of the nurse in protecting those rights. However, nurses presently lack sufficient authority and autonomy in advocating client rights. Proponents of client advocacy, in all its emphases, acknowledge that acting as an advocate requires courage and risk taking. But why should this be so? Why should it be so difficult to protect client rights when many of those rights are protected by the doctrines of informed consent and prescribed by the ANA Code for Nurses? One feels like asking, "Don't nurses have any rights?"

The present chapter deals with this question. As the following articles indicate, *rights* is a complex and controversial topic that, in part, revolves around semantic issues. The article by Claire Fagin introduces the issue of nurses' rights. Bertrand and Elsie Bandman debate the issue of whether nurses have rights specific to their profession. Bertrand Bandman does not believe that nurses qua nurses have any special rights (and neither do doctors). What nurses and physicians have are privileges and duties. His position is elaborated in "The Human Rights of Patients, Nurses, and Other Health Professionals." The final article by Michael Bennett is "A Proposed Bill of Rights for Nurses."

The following presents a discussion on these articles.

FAGIN

Claire M. Fagin, a nurse educator, criticizes the statements and resolutions concerning nurses' rights that appeared in the early 1970s. Her article, "Nurses' Rights," argues that these statements confuse rights with duties and responsibilities. Fagin turns to the definitions of "rights" and its synonyms to define "right" as follows: "A just claim to anything to which one is entitled such as power or privilege."

With this notion in mind, Fagin compares manifestoes on human rights and the rights of women (the latter produced by the National Organization of Women) to derive her own list of what she considers the "special rights" of nurses as professionals. These rights are "special" in the sense that they are granted by society in exchange for something society values.

In Fagin's view, nursing has something of value—nursing speaks to an essential human need. The new definitions of nursing that define it as the diagnosis and treatment of human responses to actual or potential health problems is a fulcrum for power and leverage in seeking the recognition of nursing rights.[1] Fagin sees nursing as being a group in quest of rights that ultimately must be granted by society in recognition of the value of nursing to that society. But an array of sociological obstacles has prevented this recognition. Historically, nursing was a vocation; presently its services are often invisible to the general public; and nurses themselves have acted in socialized roles of women—submissive, dependent, indirect, and frightened. There needs to be a revision in this socialization process and concerted political action for nurses to gain control over their profession. Fagin believes nursing has adequately defended the right of the nurse to conscientiously refuse to participate in procedures that the nurse finds morally objectionable or beyond the competence of the particular nurse.[2] Now, nursing needs to go beyond this negative right of refusal to secure more positive rights that will enable nurses to carry out their roles. Fagin believes that if the public knows what nursing delivers then they will validate the rights nurses seek.

THE BANDMAN DEBATE

Bertram Bandman is a philosopher who argues that nurses, or any other professional for that matter, have special rights by virtue of their professional role. His position is stated in brief in "Do Nurses Have Rights?: No" and elaborated and qualified in "The Human Rights of Patients, Nurses, and Other Health Professionals." For the sake of clarity and convenience, we will consider Bertram Bandman's position as developed in these two articles.

Concentrating on the aspect relevant to the issue of the existence of professional rights, we can summarize Bandman's argument as follows:

First, nurses by virtue of their profession do not have any "special" rights. This is not to say they have no rights. They have human rights, legal rights, and employee rights, but these are held in common with other classes of persons. Rights attach themselves only to individuals, not to professions or any other collective group.

Second, so-called "professional rights" fail one or both of two important tests for being a right. First, they fail the test known as the correlativity thesis. This is the observation that for every right there is an imposed duty on someone to see that this right is exercised. (It is this sort of consideration that leads to the rejection of assertions of "the right to health," for example. Who can enforce such a right?) Second, while this test does not have a well-recognized name, we will call it "the prerogative thesis." This is the idea that if one has a right, one can exercise it or not without injustice—it is a prerogative. If something is one's duty, however, refraining from doing it creates an injustice or is morally wrong.

When these two tests are applied to so-called "nurses' rights," it is clear that they will not pass. For example, in the case of experimental treatment, does the nurse have the right to see that clients are so informed? Suppose the nurse does not exercise this right. Does the nurse fail in a duty? If so, it is not a right. It fails the prerogative thesis test.

What about the nurse's *right* to conduct research or to administer some drug or treatment? Although such talk seems natural and derived from the nursing role, does it pass the correlativity thesis test? Can we say that research subjects have a duty to participate in nursing research or to accept treatment? No. At best, we have a conflict of rights. Clients have fundamental human rights to refuse participation in experiments and they may refuse treatment. Since human rights are more fundamental than "nursing rights," these would "override, cancel, and annul" these putative special rights.

What nurses do have, and what accounts for their special authority, according to Bandman, is what are called privileges—a revocable, exceptionable, or extraordinary power or exemption. This is granted by the rights holder. It is a special power or license granted to the health profession by the client. A doctor has no "right" to treat a person except by the consent of that client (or surrogate). In other words, the client is always in the position of being able to revoke the license or privilege granted the doctor or nurse.

Bertram Bandman is adamant that nurses have no professional rights that impose correlative duties on clients, but he does allow for one rare exception where nurses may have rights that impose duties on other health care professionals (and also the reverse). He also says that what may have started out as a privilege can convert into a transferred right. This can happen when the health professional is protecting the "rational vital interest" of the client who knowingly and voluntarily transfers these rights in an atmosphere of deep trust. The analogous model for this relationship is the foster parent who gains legal rights as a result of deep and beneficial involvement with the foster child.

Elsie Bandman is a nurse educator who disagrees with her husband on this issue. In her article, "Do Nurses Have Rights? Yes," she claims that the role responsibilities given to nurses also carry with them the rights to carry them out. She does not directly assess the arguments of her husband but she does raise a consideration not sufficiently discussed by him. Bertram Bandman focuses primarily on revocable privileges issued at the discretion of individuals. Elsie Bandman, on the other hand, views nursing in a larger societal context. First, she notes the content of the role of the nurse and the fact that society imposes legal constraints on this sort of professional activity. If society desires professional nursing care, it must also legitimize and sanction the conditions necessary to discharge such role obligations via special rights granted to the profession.

To continue the argument, it can be seen that Bertram Bandman's analysis does not go far enough when viewed in light of some of the professional rights claimed by Fagin concerning the right to control professional practice and set standards for excellence. It is a fiction to believe that any individual client is granting privileges to a whole profession. Rather, all a client can do is refuse or consent to a nurse acting in the professional role on his or her behalf. The professional role is something that has been defined antecedently to any particular nurse–client relationships.

A BILL OF RIGHTS FOR NURSES

Michael Bennett, a lawyer, has proposed a bill of rights for nurses. Like the American Hospital Association's "A Patient's Bill of Rights," it summarizes many rights already protected by law. In view of the above readings, we can say that some of these "rights" are really duties and that many of the others are not peculiar to nurses alone but govern employee–employer relationships generally. Also absent from this list are the special professional rights claimed by Fagin and Elsie Bandman that concern the control and regulation of practice and the right to secure conditions that enable nurses to carry out their role responsibilities.

SUMMARY

The issue of rights in general poses questions more complex than can be addressed here. However, we can offer some commentary on the issue of whether nurses have special rights as professionals.

Bertram Bandman's claim that rights attach only to individuals is not supported by any argument and is not reasserted in his second article. It is a debatable issue as to whether only individual persons can have rights. Legal rights have been extended to ships and corporations. It has been seriously suggested that moral rights should be acknowledged for such things as animals, species, and ecosystems. The intelligibility of such talk and practice would place the burden of argument on Bertram Bandman to show why professions cannot have special rights.

The two tests mentioned by Bertram Bandman—the corollary thesis and the prerogative thesis test—are more persuasive. No supposed nursing right can impose a duty on a client—the human rights (and often legal rights) of the client take precedence over the so-called professional right. Also, many suggested nursing rights involve actions that nurses *must* do and are accountable and blameworthy if they do not. A right can be exercised or not, but a person is blameworthy if he or she fails in a duty. Nursing rights fail one or both of these tests.

Even if Bertram Bandman is correct about this, it still leaves unaccounted those privileges granted by society to professions. If these privileges are "rights on a loan," it is clear that they are not issued by individuals. Nevertheless, a key question can be asked about them: If nursing fails to fulfill these special professional "rights," is it blameworthy? If it is, then these so-called rights are really duties. But it is also interesting to note that some obligations concerning the control and welfare of the profession do not fall to each individual nurse to fulfill. For example, nursing has the privilege to expand its distinctive body of knowledge by doing research, but not every nurse need be a researcher.

As a powerful rhetorical tool, the appeal to rights is also indispensable in contemporary ethical debate. In our view, however, what has often passed for nursing rights is, on more careful review, special professional privileges. Nurses have certain authority and legal privileges that some wish to equate or make synonymous with the term *rights*.[3] Although our sympathies lean toward the more proper use of the term, popular usage, if it continues, could erase the distinctions we have relied on.

Perhaps more important than whether we wish to call special professional authority "privileges" or "rights" is the sociological issue raised by Fagin— why haven't nurses been successful in achieving recognition of these rights or privileges? The next chapter highlights this issue.

NOTES

1. This definition is from the New York State Nurse Practice Act but it was shortly to be adopted into the 1976 ANA *Code for Nurses with Interpretive Statements* (Kansas City, MO.: American Nurses' Association, 1976).
2. Fagin may have been a bit too sanguine about the right to refuse to participate in certain treatments. For example, this issue was raised in *Warthen v. Toms River Community Memorial Hospital*, 199 N.J. Spuer. 18, 488 A2d 299 (1985). A nurse, Corrine Warthen, was fired from a hospital when she refused to dialyze a terminally ill double amputee patient whose dialysis was causing certain complications. Warthen cited in her defense a provision of the *ANA Code for Nurses* which permits conscientious refusal. Generally, employers can fire "at-will" employees for any reason. One exception to this, however, would be if it violates public policy. The New Jersey court declared that protecting the conscience of the nurse in this case did not raise a public policy issue of sufficient importance to qualify as a public policy exemption to the right of the hospital to fire this nurse.
3. For example, see the 1986 information report "Enhancing Quality of Care Through Understanding Nurses' Responsibilities and Rights" submitted to the ANA House of Delegates by the Committee on Ethics.

Nurses' Rights

Claire M. Fagin

The notion that nurses have rights has emerged strongly, and, if anything, is gaining momentum. Years ago, when I was a master's student in psychiatric nursing, my instructor, Hildegard Peplau, introduced us to the notion that nurses had a right to follow their beliefs in participating in patient's treatment. Specifically, we discussed the participation of nurses in electroshock therapy. It was incomprehensible to most of us we could opt for nonparticipation with physicians in this or any other therapy when we were the employees of a hospital or other health agency. Nevertheless, some brave souls did act on their convictions with varying degrees of success. Within that context, nurses' rights could be defined as a refusal to participate in situations in conflict with their preparation, competencies, and beliefs. This is the right *not* to do rather than the right to do.

Recent statements or resolutions on rights in nursing practice have grown out of concerns of nurses regarding the abortion issue and their rights in this matter. Again, this involves a right *not* to do rather than a right to do. Many of the current resolutions regarding the rights of nurses are entitled, "Rights and Responsibilities of Nurses." Few rights are stated that do not have a concomitant responsibility, with the single exception of the refusal to participate. The statements of rights issued by the International Council of Nurses and various state nurses' organizations seem to confuse rights with responsibilities, with that single exception. Nurses' rights, as defined by our organizations, seem to me a kind of double talk on nurses' duties and responsibilities.

The resolution on nurses' rights issued by the Michigan State Nurses' Association has become the model in present usage throughout the United States. The listing of rights in resolution form are as follows:

> RESOLVED, That the nurse practitioner has the responsibility to inform employers, present and prospective, of her educational preparation, experience, clinical competencies and those ethical beliefs which would affect her practice, and be it,
>
> RESOLVED, That the nurse practitioner has the responsibility to alter, adjust to or withdraw from situations which are in conflict with her preparation, competencies and beliefs, and be it,
>
> RESOLVED, That the employer shall provide the resources through which health services are made available to the recipient, and be it,
>
> RESOLVED, That the nurse practitioner has the right and responsibility to collaborate with her/his employer to create an environment which promotes and assures the delivery of optimal health services, and be it further,
>
> RESOLVED, That the nurse has the right to expect that her/his employer will respect her/his competencies, values, and individual differences as they relate to her/his practice(1).

Only the last two statements deal with what I understand as "rights."

RIGHTS VERSUS RESPONSIBILITY

As usually stated, so-called "rights of nurses" make me wonder whether my conception of rights is somewhat off the mark. However, the dictionary, thesaurus, and a handbook of synonyms validate my right to confusion since the actual definitions of rights and responsibilities do not support the blurring nurses' writings would suggest.

The word "right" is defined as a just claim to anything to which one is entitled such as power or privilege. A "right" is that which one may properly demand or claim as just, moral, or legal. A close synonym to right is prerogative.

The word "responsible," on the other hand, means to be accountable, to be answerable for something, to be liable, to be able to satisfy any reasonable claim involving important work or trust; a duty; a charge. It has also been defined as trustworthy, dependable, reliable, expected or obliged. The relationship between these two words, at least from the standpoint of their definitions, seems obscure but I do believe there is an interrelationship. It seems to me that nurses' groups reach the relationship more rapidly than others but, in the process of reaching it too rapidly, tend to lose the focus on rights and increase the focus on responsibilities.

Why does anyone or any group have rights? Are rights given to us at birth? Do we obtain them by virtue of what we do or what we are? Are rights inherited? The answers to these questions would have to be a qualified "yes." It would be difficult, however, to say that everyone in our society is born with rights other than a culturally defined minimum of rights for shelter, food, and education. Clearly, society grants special rights to some individuals or groups in exchange for something society sees of value to it. Individuals endowed with special rights by virtue of fortunate birth must also develop self-systems which enable them to keep these rights. On the other hand, those born with the culturally defined minimum must develop self-systems that enable them to perform those behaviors which permit definition of the rights wanted and the methods of obtaining them.

It is clear that nursing history has mitigated against nursing's awareness and use of rights. Originally, nursing was identified as a religious vocation. This connotation of "service" and "calling" continued in secular nursing and combined with the role of women in society to create an almost impossible barrier of socialization which inhibited a striving for personal or professional rights. In recent years we have begun to give lip-service to the rights and prerogatives that we, as human beings and workers, possess. While we have finally allowed the words to pass our lips, our view of ourselves, from early patterning on, focuses on our responsibilities, duties, charges, and obligations to others.

Until recent years, persons in any of the helping fields, be it nursing, teaching, or ministering, were not seen by society at large as having rights. It is exceedingly difficult for groups, products of their own society, to see themselves any differently from their cultural image. I believe this explains somewhat simplistically our confusion in this area as we attempt to delineate rights and then present papers filled with statements about responsibilities.

HUMAN RIGHTS

Before defining nurses' rights let's focus first on human rights. Philosophically, the rights of a *human* being have to do with permitting humanness—feelings, inclinations, compassions, sympathies, intelligence, and thoughts. One's rights ought to involve the creation of situations to enhance humanness. Clearly, this would include the right to exercise one's abilities, the right to express oneself freely, the right to grow *up* as well as old, the right for fair compensation for one's work, and the right to obtain satisfaction in living. Furthermore, if to humanize is to help someone become kind, merciful, considerate, civilized, and refined, some reciprocal self-enhancement is required to meet this description in relation to others. Thus, rights of humans.

This approach is not original. Many groups are recognizing their lack of rights in the area of humanness and are making conscious efforts to obtain the human rights that they believe have been denied them. The women's rights movement is a case in point.

WOMEN'S RIGHTS

The National Organization for Women, the largest feminist organization in the country, has a statement on rights which interestingly seems to close the circle between rights and responsibilities. According to NOW, the women's rights movements strives for equality and dignity for people through complete freedom of choice in pursuit of their life style and life goals, for access to leadership positions, equality of opportunity, equal pay, and self-determination. They strive to expose and change inequities in the law, in discriminatory policy and practices, in prejudicial myths, and outdated attitudes. They consider equality a birthright and believe women have the right to be in the mainstream of American society, exercising privileges and responsibilities in a truly equal partnership with men. They are dedicated to the proposition that women are human beings, who, like all others in our society, have the right and the opportunity to develop their fullest human potential(2).

In explaining why women have not been more active in securing human rights, NOW points out that women have been conditioned to accept limited and damaging self-concepts accompanied by low aspiration levels and lack of self-identity. One reason for their emphasis on consciousness-raising groups and publicity for their cause is that it is important to share the data regarding the extent of sex bias in everyday life and to help women, together, develop programs for change. In discussing why women ignore opportunities to improve their own lot they point out that women isolate themselves from one another, mistakenly assuming that their problems are personal rather than societal problems. They also point out that women fear losing male approval in our male dominated society. NOW believes that women can achieve equality only by accepting fully the responsibilities they share with all other persons in our society. In order to be part of the decision-making mainstream of American political, economic, and social life, women must create a new image of themselves by acting on their own and speaking out in behalf of their own equality, freedom and human dignity. This is not to be interpreted as seeking special privileges nor as ". . . enmity toward men who are also victims of the current, half-equality between the sexes . . . but rather in the direction of an active, self-respecting partnership. . . . By so doing, women will develop confidence in their own ability to determine actively, in partnership with men, the conditions of their life, their choices, their future, and their society"(3).

In the statements of civil rights groups, consumer groups, and others seeking rights today, the similarities seem more important than the differences. The right to equal and full participation, the right to information and sharing of information, the right to personal growth, and the right to access to power, emerge in all of them. Except for some fortunate groups to whom society grants special rights by virtue of personal or professional inheritance, people seem to obtain rights by having an image of themselves as worthy of rights, through sharing positive information and publicity about themselves, through pressure, and through doing something for society which society values.

How then do nurses' rights differ from human rights or women's rights and where do our particular notions of responsibilities fit? It is interesting to substitute the word "nurses" for "women" in some of the rights statements of the women's movement. To paraphrase them, nurses will do most to create a new image of themselves by acting now and by speaking out in behalf of their own equality, freedom, and human dignity. This acting and speaking will not be in a plea for special privilege nor in enmity towards physicians and others who are also victims of the current inequality between the professionals, but rather in a direction of an active self-respecting partnership with them. In so doing, nurses will develop self-confidence in their own ability to determine actively, in partnership with other health professionals, the conditions of their life, choices, future, and society.

NURSES' RIGHTS

What then does the fact that all human beings have the right to self expression, to full participation, and to enactment of their special abilities, mean to us as nurses? What are our special rights as professionals? I would list the following rights:

1. The right to find dignity in self-expression and self-enhancement through the use of our special abilities and educational background.
2. The right to recognition for our contribution through the provision of an environment for its practice, and proper, professional economic rewards.
3. The right to a work environment which will minimize physical and emotional stress and health risks.
4. The right to control what is professional practice within the limits of the law.
5. The right to set standards for excellence in nursing.
6. The right to participate in policy making affecting nursing.
7. The right to social and political action in behalf of nursing and health care.

I believe there is a direct relationship between human rights and these nurses' rights. Human refers to whatever is descriptive of man and the word "humane" is often used to describe an expectation about the nurse. If we consider the nurse's human rights in terms of professional rights, we could list the right to be heard, the right to participate freely and effectively, the right to satisfaction, and the right to question or doubt. It is when these rights are not fulfilled, that we feel we are not being treated as human beings.

We nurses have made one clear statement of rights—the refusal to participate. To me, the *not* to do, of our rights expression is significant. It's all too close to the level of learning expressed in developmental tasks where children learn who they are by saying they *don't* wish to do. This is an early step in self-development and in the differentiation aspects of who one is. I hope we can move through this step very rapidly and delineate what we have the right *to* do as well as *not* to do.

As June Rothberg has identified, our legal rights to practice and to exercise our professional rights are described in nurse practice acts and in a wealth of common law and tradition(4). In every state of this nation, nurses are legally responsible for their actions and inactions. A key differentiation between nurses and other legally sanctioned health professionals has to do with the public's direct access to service.

One could easily state that there is a strong relationship between such direct access and power, privilege, and rights among the health professions. Society appears to grant rights for valued service directly given rather than service delivered through an intermediary. Without this direct relationship it is difficult for the public to become aware of what a group has to offer. The public is for the most part unaware of what nursing has to offer in the improvement of health care. The public sees nursing as a sub-branch of medicine, ordered and controlled by physicians. If they have received good nursing care in a hospital, for example, they frequently believe that this is the result of physician's orders or some other control outside the realm of nursing practice and decision making.

The law in many instances tends to support this delusion, if indeed it always is a delusion. For example, in order for nurses to be paid by Medicare for their services to patients at home they must have physician's orders for any or all nursing services rendered. Although states may legalize and sanction nurses making judgments about what nursing services patients require, nurses have not been given the right to make this judgment practicable.

The New York State Nurse Practice Act, for example, states that nursing is diagnosing and treating human responses to actual or potential health problems, through such services as case finding, health teaching, health counseling, and initiation of health care. There is power and leverage within this definition. Yet few nurses have so far shown evidence of grasping this inherent power and using it effectively. Nurses, for the most part, play the role described earlier of all women—submissive, dependent, indirect, and frightened. Failure to act on behalf of our rights increases our guilt and low self-esteem and compounds our problems by discouraging the development of enabling behaviors to achieve rights. In seeking security, rather than satisfaction, we are, more often than not, unaware of our lack of achievements. Many of our constituents view their jobs as eight hours of drudgery leading, hopefully, to satisfactions in other areas of life separated from work. In this process we lose the benefits of years of education, our original motivation in becoming nurses, and the potential value of most of our awake lives.

Rather than face this misery openly and honestly we have found it much easier to focus on the responsibilities we ought to have and not have. We are more likely to blame others for the fact that we are not able to carry out the responsibilities we describe in our own nursing literature or in the resolutions quoted earlier. Unfortunately, in this blaming of others we contribute to the alienation of professionals from each other and towards an ever expanding gulf of hostility and non-communication. This is not living, no less professional practice. The highest order of *responsibility* in our priority system should be the responsibility of seeing, through unified action, that our rights are obtained. Leadership in our educational and work situations is required in order to revise the socialization process of nurses and others towards active participation and self-realization. Rigid bureaucratic settings do not encourage active participation. Nor, however, do educational settings which claim to have eliminated the trappings of bureaucracy but through covert and overt messages encourage adjustment and adaptation rather than growth and learning. It behooves us all to examine the conditions of our professional lives in order to ferret out those which inhibit self-enhancement and capitalize on aspects which will encourage our goal of advancing nurses' rights. The climate is now conducive to this goal, providing society sees itself as gaining something in return.

HOW TO KEEP RIGHTS

Nurses' rights and nurses' responsibilities come together, I believe, in the sense that frequently the carrying out of responsibilities on behalf of others will enhance our power base by increasing our support. This broadened power base helps us obtain and keep the rights nurses ought to have in health care systems. For example, new federal guidelines for nursing homes have been issued which even further relax the not-so-high requirements for nursing. No meaningful publicity accompanied this event. How many of the affected individuals and their relatives are aware that the federal government has reduced the standards for nursing in nursing homes? How many nurses are aware that this relaxation not only affects the elderly but has enormous implications for their own livelihoods? Using our rights to act politically would involve a wide range of activities calculated to affect law-making groups on behalf of direct professional interests as well as our responsibilities to the people we are serving. This kind of demand for rights, pertaining to patient care, done noisily and publicly, will help to obtain and keep the power and leverage suggested in the new definitions of nursing practice. We cannot claim what is rightfully ours unless we demonstrate some answerability for our actions. To be responsible and accountable for the delivery of nursing, we must have the authority to act and to do what is necessary to deliver this essential service. We must, through direct action, convince the public that we have a service of great value to deliver. Presently, the public's dissatisfaction with medical and hospital services harbors the threat that some long held rights of power groups may be taken away. It therefore becomes vital, in obtaining and keeping nurses' rights as professionals, to set the highest possible standards for delivering quality nursing care. Consumer validation of our view of quality nursing will clearly have an effect on our rights and legitimacy.

REFERENCES

1. 1973 convention issues: proposed resolution #1 on rights and responsibilities in nursing practice. (News) *Mich. Nurse Newsletter* 46:26, Sept. 1973.
2. National Organization for Women, New York Chapter. *What We're All About.* New York, The Organization, 1973.
3. National Organization for Women. *Statement of Purpose.* Chicago, The Organization.
4. Rothberg, J. S. *Choosing to Use Your Professional Prerogatives.* Paper presented at the Tennessee Nurses' Association Biennial Convention, held in Memphis, Tenn., Oct. 4, 1973.

Do Nurses Have Rights? No

Bertram Bandman

Nurses along with all other health workers, including physicians, have no rights whatsoever in their professional roles. Rather, they have the *privilege* of helping in the care of patients.

Rights are attributable only to *persons*. Insofar as nurses and physicians are persons they have rights, but as persons they only and always have rights equally with all other persons.

A professional role does not confer a right on the practitioner, be that practitioner a government official, a business executive, a policeman, fireman, ambulance driver, or a medical worker. A professional role confers a privilege, not a right. The difference between a right and a privilege is this: A right is a just basis for making a claim while a privilege is "an exceptional or extraordinary power or exemption, one that is revokable"(1). According to Feinberg, a privilege is "carved out" of a right at the pleasure of a right holder(2). A person with a privilege has *authority* but that *authority* is conferred by the right holder; it is "on loan," so to speak.

Applying this notion to the relationship between nurse and patient, I would say that the nurse in respect to the patient has privileges, not rights. These privileges are carved out of the patient's rights by consent of the patient.

Thus, a physician has the privilege of operating on a patient, but it is a patient's right to decide to undergo or to refuse surgery, which is expressed in a patient giving consent or withholding it.

However, a privilege, unlike a right, lacks "guarantee . . . and can be withheld or withdrawn" at one's "pleasure"(2). A physician's privilege, unlike a right, implies no correlative duty on the part of the patient, and the patient may withhold or withdraw the privilege any time he or she wishes(3).

An important part of the difference is this. A patient's right imposes correlative duties on physicians, nurses, other health professionals, the family, and on society to recognize and protect the claims that such a right implies.

But why does a patient and not a nurse or physician have rights? Because the role of patient is an unavoidable and dispositional part of being a person.

The professional role is alterable. Another way of putting this is that a patient is helpless and rights belong to the helpless (persons), not to the powerful.

A nurse or doctor can walk away from being a health worker and, difficult as it may be for some to consider, a nurse or doctor can leave the professional role without ceasing to be persons. A patient during the time she or he is a patient cannot leave that role.

Patients have things done to them as persons that can help or harm them in ways that nurses and physicians, exercising their roles, normally and presumably do not. A patient's role involves his or her being as a person; her or his body "is on the line," so to speak. Life and death, pain, fear, and suffering are at stake for the patient as a person. No similar immediate concern affects a nurse or doctor as a person, unless that nurse or doctor becomes a patient.

A nurse as a nurse and a doctor as a physician therefore have no rights. They have only the *privilege* of treating patients who consent to the regimen of care.

However, within this restriction, a nurse can easily carve out the privilege, for example, of not participating in medical practices, that in the nurse's professional judgment are contraindicated. Nurses could, assuming the law permitted, also have the privileges of diagnosing and treating(4).

Fagin suggests that nurses act "to achieve rights"(5). This is to misconstrue rights, which are reserved for persons. It is better to sharpen our recognition and awareness of the expansion of the rights of persons than to identify rights with the proliferation of social roles, which depend on the dynamics of power.

It is true that workers, slaves, children, blacks, women, and teachers have achieved rights by fighting for them. What they achieved, however, is recognition of their rights as *persons* worthy of dignity and respect. And so it should be for nurses. Their rights as persons should be recognized.

Power is certainly relevant, but rights are not powers. Nor are all rights earned or gained or lost.

The logical correlativity thesis holds that for any right that is accorded to any right holder, (A), there is implied an obligation on the part of someone else, (B), to provide for the exercise of A's right. The logical correlativity thesis states that there is no right for A without a corresponding duty for someone else or for a class of people at large (B) to provide for A's right.

If nurses and doctors have rights, then presumably patients have duties, an odd consequence in attributing rights to nurses and doctors. This raises the issue of conflict of rights among all three groups with no moral priority for any one group. Rights single out the most important values, needs, and desires of a society. Rights hold others accountable for carrying out the duties thus implied. Clearly, rights belong to patients and the duties and privileges thus created belong to professional workers.

Rights are not valid or just or enforceable claims. Rights imply claims by imposing duties on others. Thus, A's right imposes a correlative duty on B, which puts A in a position to impose a duty on B by claiming the right. A also has the appropriate social or legal machinery or procedure to "cash in"
on his right, so to speak, by making an appropriate claim, if necessary, to assure the exercise, enjoyment, and protection of his or her right.

A right accordingly is not a claim, but, rather, a justifiable or warrantable basis for claiming. A right includes the right to make *a strong claim* for one's right.

The right to vote, for example, is a right to vote not just once but whenever there is an appropriate occasion.

Rights are not privileges nor powers; rights are conferred on the powerless among us and are designed to place checks on those who have privileges. Rights, thus, are neither claims, privileges, nor powers. They provide a just basis for claiming one's due.

A person as a patient extends privileges as well as the power to fulfill duties upon medical workers; but rights belong exclusively to persons.

Rights bestow privileges and provide a moral basis for conferring power and authority and title upon the all too often powerless.

REFERENCES

1. Feinberg, Joel. *Social Philosophy*. Englewood Cliffs, N.J., Prentice-Hall, 1973, p. 56.
2. *Ibid.*, p. 57.
3. Bandman, Bertram, and Bandman, Elsie. Rights, justice, and euthanasia. In *Beneficient Euthanasia*, ed. by Marvin Kohl. Buffalo, N.Y., Prometheus Books, 1975, pp. 81–99.
4. Fagin, C. M. Nurses' rights. *Am. J. Nurs.* 75:85, Jan. 1975.
5. Fagin, *op. cit.*, p. 82.

Do Nurses Have Rights? Yes

Elsie Bandman

In the traditional nursing role, as defined by Henderson, the professional goal is to "substitute for what the patient lacks in physical strength, will or knowledge to make him complete, whole or independent"(1). Parsons is said to describe a sick person's appropriate behavior as (a) relinquishing some social responsibility, (b) permitting others to care for him, (c) desiring recovery, and (d) seeking medical advice(2). Although differences in degree of illness require differing amounts of help, all too many persons, such as the mentally disabled, children, the aged, and the economically disadvantaged do not seek help for an actual or potentially unmanageable problem. The notion of the nurse as one providing "physical strength, will or knowledge" in instances of deficiency is a continuous motif in nursing history, dramatized particularly by Nightingale's successful struggle for more nurses and improved conditions during the Crimean War.

In the best tradition of nursing, the imperative has been to safeguard or restore the rights of persons by providing the condition necessary for recovery, "to make him complete, whole or independent"(1). This is possible only when the nurse as a professional practitioner demands conditions necessary to discharge role obligations and responsibilities.

Therefore, I do not agree with the view that rights are attributable only to persons and that insofar as nurses and doctors are persons they have rights, but they only and always have rights equally with all other persons, and that a professional role confers not a right but a privilege.

Legal constraints on professional activity impose both responsibilities and the exercise of rights in support of these responsibilities. As Fagin points out, nurses may exercise their right to refuse to participate in "situations in conflict with their preparation, competencies and beliefs"(3). The right to refuse to participate in abortions, electroconvulsive therapy, research, or experimentation are examples of this right of negation. This right rests on a professional's correlative legal responsibility for his or her own acts.

What about the reverse situation in which the nurse wishes to engage in behavior consistent with preparation, competencies, and beliefs contrary to institutional policy, such as teaching of family planning through the use of contraceptives or the recommendation of early abortion in the case of an unwanted pregnancy from rape? Is this a violation, perhaps, or the nurse's right to practice the profession according to widely accepted standards, or is it a violation of a citizen's right to free speech guaranteed under the Constitution, or is it simply another condition of employment, such as sick leave and vacation, consistent with the institution's objectives and policies?

Even less clear and perhaps the source of most ethical dilemmas are those issues confronting nurses that involve the rights and responsibilities of others. The institutionally employed nurse is faced with three distinctly different, often competing and sometimes contradictory, systems of care demanding response. The first set of expectations is derived from the hospital's provision of safe care, food, shelter, and competent professional services to patients. The nurse occupies the strategic space and time nexus and is thus the coordinating arm of hospital administration. Simultaneously, the nurse is responsible to the physician or medical team as a therapeutic agent responsible for carrying out written, legally sanctioned, medical directives.

The nurse who sees herself or himself as an advocate of a patient's rights perceives considerations which at times may override both these sets of expectations. A position of advocacy may place the nurse in the precarious position of exerting professional rights which may well conflict or compete with the rights of other professionals and the employing institution itself. Dilemmas such as the following are not rare in my experience:

Does the nurse have the right to inform a patient that the recommended treatment is still experimental and that serious side effects are frequent, when the medical staff has failed to do so? Does a nurse have the right to inform families of a seriously ill patient that the institution is dangerously understaffed on weekends, holidays, and night shifts and that some additional coverage for this patient is necessary to safeguard life?

Does a nurse have the right to support striking nonprofessional health workers by refusing to cross picket lines?

Does a nurse have the right to assume advocacy positions on behalf of children, the aged, and the mentally ill or incompetent persons when faced with an indifferent or resistant delivery system providing insufficiently for the patient's care, rights, safety, and welfare?

Does the professional role confer a privilege, a power that is revokable, carved out of a patient's own right to decide, as B. Bandman maintains? Or does the nursing practice act in New York State, for instance, which permits a nurse to diagnose and to treat human responses to actual or potential health problems through case findings, health teaching, and health counseling impose heavy responsibilities on the nurse which require correlative professional rights?

How can a nurse participate in changing social, political, and economic conditions which are major determinants of health without asserting her or his professional right and competence to do so? Or,

as a third option, is the position of retaining some ambiguity of rights as a way of reducing undesirable adversarial relations between systems—as suggested by Willard Gaylin in his remarks on the Quinlan case at the Academy of Science in June 1976—a viable one?

Professional responsibilities must have special professional correlative rights. As nursing emerges from the shadow of medicine, it must, if it is to survive, find its own voice and make its own case for its rights.

The position of advocacy calls for the nurse "to substitute for what the patient lacks in physical strength, will or knowledge to make him complete, whole or independent." Advocacy calls for intervention in systems on behalf of an individual or a class of individuals such as the mentally ill and incompetent persons deprived of their just rights. Nurses can accomplish this only if recognition is awarded to their special rights, based on the professional credentials necessary and sufficient to meet correlative responsibilities and expectations of the profession by the public.

REFERENCES

1. Roy, Sister Callista. *Introduction to Nursing: An Adaptation Model*, Englewood Cliffs, N.J., Prentice-Hall, 1976, p. 7.
2. Schofield, A. Problems of role function. In *Introduction to Nursing: An Adaptation Model*, by Sister Callista Roy. Englewood Cliffs, N.J., Prentice-Hall, 1976, p. 267.
3. Fagin, C. M. Nurses' rights. *Am. J. Nurs.* 75:82, Jan. 1975.

The Human Rights of Patients, Nurses, and Other Health Professionals

Bertram Bandman

If a physician prescribes a drug that is contraindicated in the nurse's judgment and if she finds support for her position from other health professionals and in the New York State Nurse Practice Act, what should she do? In a conflict between a nurse and a physician, who if either of them has the right to decide? Or if a patient refuses a blood transfusion, such as is evident in cases of Jehovah's Witnesses, or if a patient refuses a procedure or medication, which both the physician and the nurse consider essential to life, who if anyone has a right to decide? Does a nurse researcher have a right to determine the limits of a subject's right to refuse? Do nurses and patients have rights? Human rights? What kinds of rights?

In this paper, I shall try to examine what it means to say that patients and nurses and related health professionals have human rights and legal and institutional rights. First, I shall indicate some things that have been said about the meaning of rights and especially about human rights. Second, I shall try to show why patients and nurses have human rights and that in addition nurses and other health professionals have a further role that is best characterized in terms other than rights.

WHAT ARE RIGHTS? WHAT ARE HUMAN RIGHTS?

What Are Rights?

Rights have variously been defined as powers, needs [21], interests, claims, valid or justified claims [15], and entitlements [22,32]. Each of these definitions has strengths and difficulties. Following H. J. McCloskey [22] and Elsie Bandman, in part, I shall refer to rights as *just entitlements* for making effective claims and demands.

What Are Human Rights?

Following in part the work of some recent philosophers [11,15,17,38], I think we may identify a human right as a right that is a moral right of fundamental or "paramount importance" [11], essential to "a decent and fulfilling human life" [30], one that is more important than any other right and is shared equally by all human beings [15, pp. 84–85; 25].

Human rights are important because they are "independent of legal or institutional norms" [25], and I would add, accordingly transcend all other rights. Human rights are so important that they annul, cancel, and override all other rights that conflict with them. Huckleberry Finn has a right to free his friend Jim, no matter what the legal norms of the South are at that time. According to one writer, "human rights serve as an independent standard of political criticism and justification" [25].

There are, I suggest, three conditions for a right of importance, namely, a human right.

Freedom

H. L. A. Hart has well stated that if there are any rights at all, there is at least the equal right to be free [17]. The right to be free is the right to one's *domain*, whether it be one's body, one's life, one's property, or one's privacy. Jeanne Berthold calls this "the right to self-determination" [8, pp. 516–517]. It is the area of one's life over which, as Joel Feinberg aptly puts it, one is "the boss" [14].

John Holt brings out this feature of a right with an example, which applies to any human right: "When the law gives me the right to vote, it is not saying I must vote. It only says that if I choose to vote, it will act against anyone who tries to prevent me." In saying I have a right to vote, the law does not, however, say, "what I must or shall do" [19]. To have a right means you do not have to do what you have a right to do. And "if I have a right to do X," according to Joel Feinberg, "I cannot also have a duty to refrain from doing X" [15, p. 58].

To have a right is also to be free not to use it and also to be immune to a charge of wrongdoing for using or not using it. To exercise one's right may be unwise or foolish, but one is never wrong to exercise one's rights.

The right to be free for nurses, physicians, and patients alike includes the right not to be brainwashed, lied to, kept ignorant, deceived, tricked, involuntarily or unknowingly given drugs or medication, put to sleep, or otherwise unjustifiably coerced, where harm to one's self or others is not involved. The right to be free and autonomous is a necessary condition of a human right and is absolute in the sense that one cannot have these things done and still be free to live a "decent and fulfilling life" as a human being [30].

Rights Imply Duties

A second condition is that rights imply achievable obligations on others [7,11,12,33], obligations that are of the utmost importance [11] to everyone's equal right "to a decent and fulfilling human life" [25]. As Feinberg points out, "rights are necessarily the grounds of other people's duties [15, p. 58].

Rights Presuppose Justice

Freedom and duties are not sufficient to characterize and orient a human right. A right of "paramount importance," like a human right, "is something of which no one may be deprived without a grave affront to justice" [11]. According to St. Augustine, rights flow from justice. There are no rights without justice [29].

Considerations of impartiality and equality are requirements of justice, which includes everyone's equal right to "a decent and fulfilling life" and to the means for achieving such a life. Justice as equality means that everyone is treated in a similar way in similar situations [25]. Justice as equality applied to health care practice means that everyone is justly entitled or has a right to a similar quality of health care.

Justice in connection with human rights means not only that the older political rights, sometimes called freedom or "option rights," are necessary, such as the right to vote, worship freely, and not to be tortured, but also the newer social and economic rights. These rights are known as the rights to well-being, sometimes called rights of assistance or recipience or welfare rights [3,16]. I prefer to call them need fulfillment rights.* These rights include the right to social security, education, and health care. A just conception of rights provides both for option rights and for need fulfillment rights.

Difficulties with Option and Need Fulfillment Rights

One difficulty with the older option rights has been that they were too narrow and exclusive and of benefit to only a few. Large estates and "the high fences" Robert Frost once wrote about no longer "make good neighbors."

A difficulty, however, with the newer rights of recipience or need fulfillment is the *thinning out of rights*. One finds claims for the rights of physicians, nurses, patients, mental patients, cardiac patients, in addition to the rights of policemen, the poor, the aged, Italians, blacks, women, garment workers, the comatose, the gay, prisoners, fetuses, unborn future generations, animals, and trees. The declaration and demand for more and more social, economic, educational, ecological, and health care rights of all kinds can only mean a declining possibility of imposing correlative obligations.

In order to have a right, people have to accept comparable duties implied by the rights they claim. The expansion of claims to rights can have the danger of trivializing and making less valuable each

---

*Joel Feinberg uses this term but in a different connection in Rights, Duties and Claims, *American Philosophical Quarterly* 3:139, 1966.

right, since all rights cannot possibly be fulfilled. The thinning out of rights of need fulfillment is also notable in the role of rights in nursing care. The American Hospital Association's Patient's Bill of Rights promises more than anyone can deliver. For example, the right to complete current diagnostic information along with most other rights cited makes promises that exceed the possibility of implementation.

A solution to both difficulties (of rights being too exclusive and too numerous) is to extend the older rights to include all human beings, recognize basic need fulfillment rights, divide rights into equally small shares as Jesus did with the loaves, but not promise rights that go beyond what human beings can achieve. On this view, human rights are limited to the most essential necessities of life that constitute an equal "floor" of support below which no one falls [25].

There are no rights of importance, no human rights, without freedom, however small the domain has to be cut to make room for everyone's equal right to it, including the freedom to eat and freedom from avoidable pain and disease. Nor are there any rights of value unless others pay the price of that freedom by providing for that freedom in the form of duties [3]. Without correlative duties imposed on and accepted by others, rights are empty. Third, without justice to orient and regulate the relation and distribution between freedom and duties on a rational basis, rights are blind.

HUMAN RIGHTS OF PATIENTS AND CORRESPONDING DUTIES OF HEALTH PROFESSIONALS

The Human Rights of Patients as Option Rights and Need Fulfillment Rights

A human right to life includes not only the option right to be left alone, but as Virginia Held eloquently puts it, "it also includes being able to acquire what one needs to live" [18]. To have any rights of importance is to have not only the equal right to be free, but also the right to "an equally decent and fulfilling human life" and to whatever means are necessary to achieve such a life, including appropriate health care.

The human right to live this sort of life makes the deprivation of one's health care rights "a grave affront to justice" [11]. The Tuskegee syphilis experiment [9], the involuntary Willowbrook Hepatitis program, the use of 600 United States Army servicemen for an LSD experiment without their knowledge [4], and Nurse Ratchet in *One Flew over the Cuckoo's Nest* telling Murphy to take his pills because they are good for him and refusing to tell him why—these are all grave affronts to justice [11]. They violate patients' human rights in health care [4].

The Human Rights of Health Professionals and Patients

Health professionals, including nurses and physicians, have the equal human right to a "decent and fulfilling human life" along with patients.

Claire Fagin cites the human rights of nurses, which include the right to be heard, the right to participate freely, the right to satisfaction, and the right to question or doubt [13]. These rights also include nurses' rights to their beliefs, to advocate patients' health care rights, to refuse to give treatments they believe are contraindicated, the right to challenge, and the right to fulfill oneself professionally and as persons.

Patients' Interests and Rights Paramount

Elizabeth Carnegie ties the nurse's role to the protection of patients' rights. She says, "Nurses have always known that the patient is the chief consideration" [9]. And Carnegie quotes Minnie Goodnow, who said in the early part of this century that "the patient is the main thing—the reason for it all—the unit—the one chief consideration, the one [to] whose welfare all else must be subordinated" [9]. Carnegie concludes, "Patients' rights have always come first with nurses" [9].

If patients' rights are uppermost, nurses may advocate patients' rights quite effectively, it seems, without having to have special rights [6], rights that would imply others' obligations, presumably patients' obligations and, on occasion at least, be in direct collision with patients' rights. If nurses and physicians serve the human rights of patients, there is no reason to accord nurses and physicians special rights, at least when these rights conflict with patients' rights. One of the functions of rights oriented by justice is to protect the powerless, not the powerful, and in the relationship of the patient to the health professional, the patient is relatively powerless.

Attributing rights to nurses and physicians also adds to the population explosion of rights and a resulting *thinning out* of everyone's rights. Such a thinning out generates needless conflicts between patients' and nurses' rights, with a resulting loss to patients' rights, where it even becomes possible for the investigator to "usurp the individual's right to freedom of choice" [8, p. 518]. If the patients' interests are paramount, the role of health professionals would seem to be to serve those interests and not be in a position to usurp them.

Nurses and Other Health Professionals Have Duties But No Special Rights Against Patients

To have a right is to have the right to be free to do or not do what the right provides. To have a right is also to have a right not to. The odd thing about nurses' rights is that if nurses are free, nurses can choose not to exercise their rights. For example, if a health professional has a right to stop a patient from bleeding to death could not the health professional also say, "I have a right to stop this bleeding, but as with my right to vote or to play golf, which I'm also free not to do, I'll exercise my right and not stop the patient from bleeding to death"?

The statement that "if I have a right to do X, then I cannot also have a duty" either to do or "to refrain from doing X" [15] also spotlights a difficulty for those who champion nurses' and physicians' (special) rights. This difficulty is that, first, the so-called right is *to* prescribe and apply appropriate treatment, and second, it is not to permit medications and drugs that are contraindicated in place of X. In the first case this right is a duty *to do*, to prescribe, and to treat, and in the second case it is a duty to refrain, cancel, or refuse. If X is believed to be contraindicated, a health professional has a duty, not a right, to refrain from administering or prescribing it.

The absence of a duty or the absence of a duty to refrain from doing something is not applicable to the so-called special rights of health professionals. If they fail to do or omit to do what they say they have a special right to do or not to do, but which it is their duty to do or refrain from doing, then they are liable, culpable, and open to the charge of wrongdoing and malpractice. Hence their duty is hardly a "right" that one is free to exercise with immunity to the charge of wrongdoing.*

If patients have a right and thus a choice, others then have a duty and no choice. If health professionals refuse to carry out their duties, they become liable to malpractice. For example, if a nurse is in a conflict with a physician, believing that a medication is contraindicated, is it the nurse's right or her duty to refuse to give the medicine to the patient? If, as I think, the nurse has a duty to refuse, she cannot have a right to decide whether to refuse; but neither does the physician have a right to decide; he, too, clearly has a duty not to do what is contraindicated.

I turn next to the correlation between rights and duties. The right to refuse to be a research subject implies the duties others have to forebear from research. Yet one finds that "the nurse has . . . the right to conduct research" [1, p. 105; 8; 26]. Even Jeanne Berthold weakens her protection of patients' and subjects' rights by asking, "When is it the responsibility of the investigator to usurp the individual's right to freedom of choice?" [8, p. 521]. Recalling Cranston's remark, "a human right is something the deprivation of which is a grave affront to justice" [11], we can interpret an investigator's responsibility to mean that it can never be to usurp an individual's right to freedom of choice, for this usurpation would be a gross violation of a human right.

If nurses have a right to "usurp the individual's right" for purposes of research, this right means that others, presumably subjects, have a corresponding duty to submit to such research. This assumption would seem to be a patently absurd consequence of patients' or subjects' rights to refuse to participate in research projects.

Ernest Nagel similarly suggested a difficulty in ascribing to presently living geneticists the right to plan future generations [24]; for presumably the

---

* For those who like logical symbolism, by a familiar *modus tollens* argument, one can derive the following conclusion:
1. If I have a right to prescribe X_1 (or refuse X_2), then I cannot also have a duty to prescribe X_1 (or refuse X_2, whichever the case may be).
2. *But I have a duty to prescribe X_1 (or refuse X_2).*
3. Therefore, I cannot have a right to prescribe X_1 (or refuse X_2, whichever the case may be).

right to plan future generations would imply correlative obligations on future generations not yet born to provide for and accept the geneticists' right to plan.

If it is a nurse's right to administer blood or give a medication or participate in sterilizing a patient or do research, it is then a patient's corresponding duty not to interfere or refuse and to submit and be a willing recipient to the experiment or transfusion or medication or sterilization. If nurses and physicians have rights, presumably patients have duties, an absurd consequence in attributing special rights to nurses and physicians that conflict with patients' rights.

If, however, a patient has a right to refuse X (medication, sterilization, or blood transfusion), but the health professional also has a right to administer X, in a conflict of rights, one right or the other gives way. Either the patient receives X or not. But we cannot have two rights simultaneously, at least not two conflicting rights that generate contradictory obligations, a patient's right to refuse and the right of health professionals to administer X. But if rights imply duties, including patients' rights to refuse X, then health professionals have a duty to protect the patients' rights of refusal. Otherwise, there are no real rights to refuse.

However, if patients have rights, others have duties toward right-holders: and with respect to the rights of patients, health professionals cannot have rights that coincide with patients' rights without colliding with patients' rights.

If rights collide and some rights are to be satisfied, some rights will need to be set aside or vacated in favor of others. In a conflict, patients' human rights, being the fundamentally important rights, override, cancel, and annul the special rights of nurses and physicians. Accordingly, it appears to be an anomaly to ascribe specialized role-derived rights to health professionals that conflict or may conflict with patients' fundamentally important human rights, rights that are important enough to override or cancel all other rights.

NURSES AND PHYSICIANS HAVE DUTIES AND PRIVILEGES

Rights, Duties, and Privileges

What is the special role of nurses in relation to patients? I believe nurses and physicians have no special rights, only privileges [2]. Privileges are "carved out" of rights, as Feinberg points out [15]. To have a privilege, to cite a second metaphor Feinberg adopts from more imaginative writers, is to have a key to a lock that belongs to a right-holder. If the right-holder is unable to unlock the gate, he or she may extend the privilege of using the key to another person—an advocate, one might say.

If patients' interests and rights are of "paramount importance" to nursing, as Carnegie [19], Porter [27], Berthold [8], and others contend [10,20,23,28], and if nurses regard themselves as protecting patients' rights as advocates, then nurses have the duty and also the privilege of acting on behalf of patients, but not the right to do so. However, having the duty does not give nurses the right or freedom to decide whether or not to act on patients' behalf. Nurses have no choice in the matter, and hence they could not possibly have a right in the matter.

For a patient to have general and special human rights in his or her role as patient is to have rights that are fundamentally important, and they are more important than any other legal or institutional, role-derived rights that may be regarded as privileges instead. At the top of the scale of importance, we refer to patients' human rights. In marked contrast and at a subordinate level of the scale, we may refer to an instrumental privilege, a means of doing something for someone.

In this juxtaposition of rights and privileges, we move away from the rights of nurses and physicians and relocate their roles as clearly subordinate and instrumental to that of patients—akin to Hume's dethroning of reason and relocating it as "the slave of the passions." The role of health professionals, being responsible and having duties to patients, is to serve the health needs, interests, and human rights of patients.

What is a privilege? According to Feinberg's citation in *Black's Law Dictionary*, a privilege is "an exceptional or extraordinary power or exemption," and one that is revokable [15, p. 56].

Nurses and physicians are privileged. They are "permitted to carry keys to the lock on the gate" of a patient's domain of freedom, when this domain includes a patient's body. To shift to a woodcutting metaphor: Privileges are "carved out" of rights at the right-holder's request and at the right-holder's pleasure, assuming the right-holder is informed and the consent is voluntary. The physician and the nurse do not "carve out" a privilege without the consent and pleasure of the right-holder. The hand may be the nurse's or physician's, but the decision is the patient's.

A physician's privilege of operating on a patient depends on a patient signing a consent form. The physician operates only with the *consent* of the patient (except in an emergency). This privilege is recognized in law as a patient's right to decide what happens in and to his or her body [2; 5, pp. 95–96]. However, a privilege, unlike a right, "lacks guarantee . . . and can be withheld or withdrawn at one's pleasure" [15, p. 57]. A license gives a person a privilege, not a right. A physician's privilege, unlike a right, implies no correlative duty on the part of the patient, and the patient may withhold or withdraw the privilege at any time, just as a subject or patient may terminate an experiment at any time.

If a right invests a right-holder with the authority to hold others responsible [2], in a patient-physician or patient-nurse relation, the physicians and nurses are responsible to their patients. If, moreover, those who are held responsible are accorded privileges, which by definition are revokable, physicians and nurses have the privilege of serving their patients. Consequently, in a rights-privilege relationship, patients have the right to treatment, and physicians and nurses have the privilege rather than the right to treat patients.

The Subordination of Health Professionals' Privileges to Patients' Human Rights

However, within this restriction, one can easily "carve out" the privilege in place of the special right which Fagin, Peplau, Elsie Bandman, Catherine Murphy, and others understandably wish to confer on nurses, the privilege,* for example, of not participating in a medical practice, such as electroshock therapy, that, in a nurse's professional judgment, is contraindicated. In addition, the sort of positive right Fagin wishes to confer on nurses can also be expressed as a privilege, such as the privilege of "diagnosing and treating human responses" in accordance with the New York State Nurse Practice Act, for example.

Rights single out the most important values, needs, and desires of a society. Rights hold others accountable for carrying out the duties thus implied. On this basis, rights are clearly attributable to patients, and duties, responsibilities, and privileges thus created from such rights belong to health professionals.

Since human rights, being fundamentally important, are independent of and transcend other legal and institutional rights, they are of greater importance than other rights, including the so-called special role-derived rights of health professionals. One way to mark off this distinction is to refer to patients as having rights and health professionals as having corresponding duties and privileges.

A Limited Case for Special Rights Against Other Health Professionals

There may, nevertheless, be a small but vital area in which nurses have special rights. The role of involved advocacy may sometimes make some rights voluntarily transferable. In the law, a will manifests the transferability of rights. Transferability may also occur in common law, for example, when a foster parent becomes deeply and beneficially involved with a child. The foster parent may gain the esteem and confidence of that child to the point where the child develops a deep sense of trust in the foster parent. This relationship may be due to the fact that the foster parent has made evident that he or she is disposed to protect or provide for the child's *vital rational interests*. In such relationships, a foster parent may, in the eyes of the child, act on the child's behalf. What may have begun as a privilege may end up as a special right, somewhat as a relationship between friends or lovers may eventuate in marriage.

The relationship in the nurse-patient relation is analogous. Deep involvement with each other may render rights transferable. In this sense, nurses have special rights to help and sustain their patients. It is in this sense, too, that nurses may have special rights *against* other health professionals. Nurses have such rights whenever they are demonstrably in the *right* and others are in the *wrong*. (The etymological connection between *having a right* and being *right* or between *rights* and what is morally or legally right is not—nor was it ever—unintended [9, p. 442].) Nurses gain or earn special rights through training, competence, and experience along with their natural sympathy and understanding, and often their judgments and beliefs

---

* Insofar as a nurse's role does not conflict with a patient's, but rather with the role of a physican or another nurse, a nurse's special human rights of challenging and doubting may also come into play.

coincide with rationally justified beliefs about what serves the vital interests of their patients.

Although, according to this account, nurses do not have special rights against patients, they may very well have special rights against other health professionals. The converse, too, is true, that is, other health professionals may have special role-derived rights against nurses. But no health professionals have special role-derived rights against patients' *human rights,* and the determination as to who in a given situation has special rights depends on the extent to which a given health professional is serving the *vital rational interests* of patients. That is why, to return to the case cited at the outset, a nurse does have a right against a physician whenever a physician's order is contraindicated. But it could be the other way; that is, the physician could be right and the nurse wrong.

For a nurse correctly to claim that a physician's order is contraindicated, however, is the *exception* rather than the *rule.* As Dorothy Nayer has pointed out to me, quite correctly I believe, the paradigm of physician-nurse-patient relationships is that the physician is ordinarily recognized to "give the orders" for the patient. The physician is acknowledged legally, historically, and traditionally, and on sound grounds, to *know* more than other health professionals; and he or she is consequently considered the most essential link in the restoration of health.

The physician is primarily and ordinarily responsible for the patient, and the physician ordinarily gives the orders, *unless* they are contraindicated, either because the physician does not really know the patient's condition or medication, or is negligent or overworked, or demonstrably has an interest other than the patient uppermost in mind. In such cases—but it would seem to apply only in such cases—the nurse not only has the legal right to refuse to do what the physician orders, but also a moral basis for exercising a role as an advocate for the patient.[*]

Thus the nurse ordinarily respects the contractual relation between the physician and the patient *unless* there is a clear-cut case of the physician not putting the patient's interest first. A physician gives the orders *unless* these orders are contraindicated.

If the physician makes an error, who best safeguards the patient's health interests? The family is not always present. The patient may be too sick. The persons who are naturally most suitable to safeguard the patient's interests are those who give continuous care, namely, nurses. Thus a defeasible clause provides protection of the patients' rights and interests if physicians fail to provide for their patients' rights and interests in health care. The special rights nurses would have against physicians would be provided by the defeasible provisions of contracts that physicians have with their patients.

The principle governing the attribution of special rights is the consistency of role-derived rights with the general human rights from which such special rights are logically derivable. And the test of consistency between special role-derived rights and general human rights is, it seems, quite effectively put by Carnegie, Minnie Goodnow, and others, namely, that the patient comes first [10].

Since, unlike Claire Fagin, I see no real difference between a right *against* and a right *to,* I also see a case for a nurse's special role-derived right *to* do things on behalf of the rational vital interests of her patients, providing, however, that such rights never collide with the patients' human interests and rights and have been knowingly and voluntarily transferred by the patients to the nurse.

CONCLUSION

Patients and health professionals share equally in having fundamentally important human rights. But to distinguish and subordinate the specialized role of health professionals from patients, patients have special health care rights and health professionals have the privilege and the duty of correcting each other's mistakes whenever indicted. Finally, if there are instances in which rights are transferable, such as when deep attachments develop, nurses may gain special rights to provide for and protect their patients' rational vital interests and even exercise these rights against other health professionals.

The reason I think it is nevertheless rare that nurses have special rights is that to have such rights is to know and to be in a position systematically to care for the rational vital interests of patients. But who is ever really in a position to know or care that much for someone else?

In any event, the test of the privileges and special role-derived rights of health professionals is the

---

[*] The notion of "unless" clauses in contractual relations is known in law and morality as "defeasibility"; it consists in the elucidation of those conditions that would "defeat" a contract. It was first given philosophical prominence by H. L. A. Hart in "The Ascription of Responsibility and Rights," in A. Flew (ed.), *Logic and Language* (Oxford: Blackwell, 1952).

consistency of privileges and rights with the fundamentally and overridingly important human rights of patients. For without human rights, which imply freedom, duties, and justice, there are no rights at all.

REFERENCES

1. American Nurses Association. The Nurse in Research: ANA Guidelines on Ethical Values. New York: American Nurses Association, 1968. (Also in *Nurs. Res.* 17:104, 1968.)
2. Bandman, B. Nurses have no rights. *Am.J.Nurs.* 78:1, 1978.
3. Bandman, B. Some legal, moral and intellectual rights of children. *Educational Theory* 27:169, 1977.
4. Bandman, E. L., and Bandman, B. Rights are not automatic. *Am.J.Nurs.* 77:5, 1977.
5. Bandman, B., and Bandman, E. L. Rights, Justice and Euthanasia. In M. Kohl (ed.), *Beneficent Euthanasia.* Buffalo, N.Y.: Prometheus, 1975. Pp. 96–98.
6. Bandman, E. L. The Rights of Nurses and Patients: A Case for Advocacy. This volume, Chap. 48.
7. Benn, S., and Peters, R. S. *The Principles of Political Thought.* New York: Collier Books, 1959. Pp. 102–103.
8. Berthold, J. S. Advancement of science and technology while maintaining human rights and values. *Nurs. Res.* 18:514, 1969.
9. Brandt, R. B. *Ethical Theory.* Englewood Cliffs, N.J.: Prentice-Hall, 1959. Pp. 436–442.
10. Carnegie, M. E. The patient's bill of rights and the nurse. *Nurs. Clin. North Am.* 9:557, 1974.
11. Cranston, M. Human Rights, Real and Supposed. In D. Raphael (ed.), *Political Theory and the Rights of Man.* Bloomington: Indiana University Press, 1967. Pp. 49–52.
12. Cranston, M. *What Are Human Rights?* New York: Basic Books, 1962. P. 41.
13. Fagin, C. Nurse's rights. *Am.J.Nurs.* 75:82, 1975.
14. Feinberg, J. Voluntary Euthanasia and the "Inalienable Right to Life." Paper presented at Bioethics and Human Rights Conference at Long Island University, Brooklyn, N.Y., April 9, 1976, and forthcoming in *Philosophy and Public Affairs,* winter 1978.
15. Feinberg, J. *Social Philosophy.* Englewood Cliffs, N.J.: Prentice-Hall, 1973.
16. Golding, M. Towards a theory of human rights. *Monist* 52:4, 1968.
17. Hart, H. L. A. Are There Any Natural Rights? In A. I. Melden (ed.), *Human Rights.* Belmont, Calif.: Wadsworth, 1970.
18. Held, V. Abortion and Rights to Life. This volume, Chap. 11.
19. Holt, J. Why Not a Bill of Rights for Children? In B. and G. Gross (eds.), *The Childrens' Rights' Movement.* Garden City, N.Y.: Anchor Books, 1977. P. 321.
20. Kelly, L. The patient's right to know. *Nurs. Outlook* 24:26, 1976.
21. McBride, A. Can family life survive? *Am.J.Nurs.* 75:1651, 1975.
22. McCloskey, H. J. Rights. *Phil. Quart.* 15:118, 1965.
23. Murphy, C. P. The Moral Situation in Nursing. This volume, Chap. 46.
24. Nagel, E. Comments on the Presentations of Drs. Ehrman and Lappé. This volume, Chap. 9.
25. Nickel, J. Are Social and Economic Rights Real Human Rights? Paper presented at Society for Philosophy and Public Affairs, City University of New York, Graduate Center, New York City, March 1977.
26. Notter, L. Protecting the rights of research subjects. *Nurs. Res.* 18:483, 1969.
27. Porter, K. Patient's rights and nurse's responsibilities. *Hospitals* 17:102, 1973.
28. Quinn, N., and Somers, A. The patient's bill of rights: A significant aspect of the consumer revolution. *Nurs. Outlook* 22:240, 1974.
29. St. Augustine. *The City of God* (translated by G. Walsh et al.). Garden City, N.Y.: Image Books, 1958. Pp. 468–472.
30. Scheffler, S. Natural rights, equality and the minimal state. *Can. J. Phil.* 6:64, 1976.
31. Schlotfeldt, R. Can we bring order out of the chaos of nursing education? *Am.J.Nurs.* 76:105, 1976.
32. Wasserstrom, R. Rights, Human Rights and Racial Discrimination. In A. I. Melden (ed.), *Human Rights.* Belmont, Calif.: Wadsworth, 1970. Pp. 96–110.
33. Williams, P. Rights and the Alleged Right of Innocents to Be Killed. This volume, Chap. 18.

A Bill of Rights for Nurses

H. Michael Bennett

1. The nurse has the right to be treated considerately and respectfully by the patient. In the event the patient becomes combative, the nurse may take reasonable steps to defend himself/herself. Likewise, if the patient's behavior is such that it threatens his own safety or that of others, the nurse may, without prior authorization, restrain the patient provided immediate notice is given to the attending physician.

2. The nurse has the right and obligation to maintain a careful vigil over the patient, and this right takes precedence over the patient's right of privacy when, under the circumstances, a failure to oversee the patient's activities may be reasonably expected to result in physical harm to the patient.

3. The nurse has not only the right, but the obligation, to question any order of a physician which is believed to be unreasonable. In the event the physician demands compliance with the order, after it is duly questioned, the nurse has both the right and obligation to refuse to carry out any order which is patently erroneous. Marginal orders, on the other hand, after they have been questioned, should either be carried out or refused in accordance with standard hospital policy.

4. The nurse has the right to expect a duly licensed physician to impart to the patient the necessary information regarding the risks and consequences of and alternatives to the prescribed treatment whereby the patient may give an informed consent. If the patient expresses reservations or doubts concerning this consent, after the aforementioned explanation, the nurse has the further right to expect the physician to answer these additional questions and resolve any misunderstandings prior to the treatment being undertaken. Absent legislation to the contrary, the nurse's only right and obligation regarding patient education is to inform the patient and his family regarding basic self care.

5. The nurse has the right to expect the hospital to provide adequate nursing personnel to assure prompt recognition of an untoward change in a patient's condition and to facilitate appropriate intervention by the nursing, medical, or hospital staffs. At a minimum, the hospital should provide such staffing as is necessary to comply with the local rules and regulations of the Department of Public Health.

6. The nurse has the right to expect that within its capacity a hospital will provide adequate and efficient support staff to enable nursing personnel to provide quality patient care.

7. The nurse is entitled to receive a written job description setting forth the duties and responsibilities required. Said description should likewise include a description of fringe benefits including meals and breaks. Though the nurse is entitled to certain time for meals and breaks, these privileges do not take priority over quality patient care. Nevertheless, when the demands of the patient preclude the nurse from receiving such breaks, the nurse should be duly compensated for such time by the employer.

8. The nurse has the right and obligation to refuse any patient assignment for which he/she does not possess the necessary technical skills required by the assignment. This right, however, does not give the nurse an absolute right to refuse to float or to accept additional patients when understaffing occurs. As an employee, the nurse agrees to carry

Bennett, H. B. (1982, November–December). A bill of rights for nurses. *Critical Care Nurse*, 2, 88. Reprinted with permission of © *Critical Care Nurse*. All rights reserved.

out a coordinated plan of care for the patient and must assume any assignment for which he/she possesses the necessary expertise.

9. The nurse has the right to be informed regarding mechanisms within the hospital for the initiation, review, and resolution of complaints concerning fellow nurses, the medical staff, or hospital policy in general. The nurse likewise has the right of input into the hospital's quality assurance program. Whether the nurse files a formal complaint or offers suggestions for improvement of patient care, he/she has the right to know and expect that complaints and/or recommendations will be given due consideration by the appropriate authorities and will not serve as a basis for disciplinary action. Finally, the nurse has the right to be advised of any complaints or grievances filed against him/her by fellow staff members or patients and to offer a written explanation in response thereto.

10. The nurse shall be afforded impartial treatment regardless of race, sex, religion, or national origin.

STUDY AND DISCUSSION QUESTIONS
NURSES' RIGHTS

1. Do you agree with Fagin's assertion that the history of nursing has "mitigated against nursing's awareness and use of rights?"

2. Fagin wrote in 1975 that the public is for the most part unaware of what nursing has to offer? Is this still the case?

3. What is your assessment of Fagin's analysis of why nurses have not obtained the power and authority to carry out their role?

4. Should nurses have the right to refuse to participate in certain treatments or refuse to care for certain clients? Compare the ANA Code for Nurses statement and interpretive statements. Consider the following: abortion, sterilization, psychosurgery, electro-convulsive therapy, application or withdrawal of life, prolonging technology to the terminally ill, AIDS clients, suctioning, and other unpleasant care.

5. Bertram Bandman asserts that only persons (not professions or anything else) can be rights holders. Do you think something other than a person can have rights?

6. Bertram Bandman argues that nurses have revocable privileges and not rights. Can you think of any "rights" that impose obligations on clients that are exclusive to nurses and that the client cannot revoke?

7. Bertram Bandman maintains that it is a feature of true rights that the rights holder can fail to exercise the right without failing in a duty. Do the professional rights suggested in the articles by Fagin, Elsie Bandman, and Michael Bennett pass this test?

8. Consider Bertram Bandman's exception to special nursing rights—a nurse may act on the rational vital interests of a patient if knowingly and voluntarily transferred. Does this pass his own tests for being a right—that is, does the nurse also have the right to refuse the transfer and watch the patient's vital interests go unprotected?

9. Is it as difficult to know another person's "rational vital interests" as Bertram Bandman suggests?

10. How many of Bennett's rights in his bill of rights are exclusive to nurses and pass the tests outlined by Bertram Bandman?

11. How would you wish to characterize the special authority that nursing needs (individually and professionally) to carry out its role? Would you wish to call them "rights" even though failure to exercise them can be blameworthy (like a duty) and, in addition to which, they cannot supersede the human rights of a client?

4

The Nurse–Physician Relationship:
I. Sexism and Hierarchy

INTRODUCTION

The nurse–physician relationship is an acknowledged impediment to the realization of the role of the nurse as client advocate. Historically, physicians have
been overwhelmingly male and nurses overwhelmingly female. This statistical
imbalance has in the past, at least, been coupled with male and female stereotypes—physicians idealized the masculine and nurses the feminine. The four
articles included in this chapter explore some of the difficulties that this historical and cultural legacy has created in nursing.

Leonard Stein's classic 1987 article, "The Doctor–Nurse Game," describes
patterns of nurse–physician communication patterns, the origin of the game in
medical and nursing education, and some of the factors that perpetuate the
game.

Virginia Cleland, in her classic 1971 article, "Sex Discrimination: Nursing's
Most Pervasive Problem," argues that sex discrimination is the most fundamental problem in nursing because it is a women's occupation in a male-
dominated culture.

A moral critique of sexism and a discussion of whether the professions of nursing and medicine require sex-linked characteristics is the focus of Richard
Hull's article, "Dealing with Sexism in Nursing and Medicine."

Lastly, Catherine Watson queries the implications of the phenomena of men
acquiring leadership positions in nursing in numbers far exceeding their general representation in nursing.

A more detailed examination of these articles follows.

STEIN

Psychiatrist Leonard Stein's often cited "The Doctor–Nurse Game" describes the way open conflict between nurses and doctors is avoided. Nurses must conceal their recommendations in the guise of questions and hints. Doctors must be savvy enough to pick up on these recommendations and also to subtly ask for recommendations. From the doctor's perspective, the well-played game preserves the doctor's sense of omnipotence and omniscience and cashes in on the valuable contributions of the nurse. Additionally, a successful transaction benefits the nurse who is able to meet the client's need and also avoid the ridicule and humiliation that a more direct communication might provoke.

Why is the game played? It has the obvious positive reinforcements just described as well as penalties for deviation for both parties. Obtuse doctors can be given a hard time by nurses or the nurse who communicates directly may be labeled a "bitch" or as suffering from "penis envy." Additional factors that reinforce the game are medical and nursing education, factors that Stein claims foster attitudes of omnipotence and omniscience in the one and sub-servience in the other; a mind set that views suggestions as insulting and belit-tling; a sense of security engendered by the ideal of one omnipotent leader; and the acting out of stereotypical sex roles—masculine physicians dominant and feminine nurses passive.

According to Stein, this is an inefficient form of communication that is sti-fling and anti-intellectual. It is also rather telling that other professionals will not play this game with physicians and demand a more direct communication.

One may be tempted to defend this game on the grounds that it works and that there is nothing insidious in showing respect and using tact. But as Stein later wrote, nurses contribute to their own oppression and inhibit the au-tonomous development of the profession by playing this game.[1]

CLELAND

Nurse educator Virginia Cleland's thesis is stated in the title of her 1971 arti-cle: "Sex Discrimination: Nursing's Most Pervasive Problem." At first glance, this thesis would seem paradoxical since nursing is primarily female and fe-males hold most positions of power. The actual difficulty emerges when nurs-ing is viewed as a women's occupation in a male-dominated culture. The importance of positions of authority in nursing is diminished when it is noted that they are available only with the approval of male-dominated power struc-tures. Cleland believes that there has been a failure in nursing leadership that, since the 1940s, has produced a generation of acquiescing, submissive, and overly cautious leaders who are acting out professionally the stereotypical sex roles they were taught as little girls. Most tellingly, nursing has difficulty *inter alia* in gaining control over its own budgets, establishing and maintaining its own standards of practice, and failing to use the shortage of nurses to enhance and strengthen the profession.

Cleland proposed a number of ways in which this sexism could be attacked. Included are proposals to revamp the curriculum and make the occupation more attractive to males by emphasizing more decision-making freedom and responsibility. Cleland also envisions distinguishing between the technical and the more autonomous professional nurse with perhaps a new title—nursologist. Cleland, however, thought that women in society would be more successful in obtaining equal rights than nursing would be. This in turn would, she predicted, create problems in recruitment.

HULL

Philosopher Richard Hull examines the underlying thought that informs some of the sexual stereotypic attitudes in nursing and medicine. There is a theory with some etymological and historical support that views nursing as the skilled application of maternal skills and doctoring as the skilled application of paternal or masculine skills. This theory is augmented by other conjectures that declare that these traits are sex linked by nature or culture.

If one takes such a position, it becomes easy to see that it is "natural" or commonsense that males should dominate medicine, females dominate nursing, and combinations like male nurse or female physician appear a bit odd.

Hull does not attack these views head on. Rather, he illustrates how they pervade nursing and medicine and offers a moral critique of it. As in most kinds of stereotyping, sex role stereotyping is unfair to individuals who are not evaluated and utilized on the basis of capacities he or she actually possesses. This wastes individual talent as well as affecting quality health care. (A notorious example of sexism's influence has been the dismissal of many complaints by women as psychosomatic.) A further consequence of sex role stereotyping is that it becomes self-confirming in the sense that many adopt these role expectations or confirm them by struggling against them. For example, a female physician who goes out of her way to show how tough, authoritative, and decisive she is, is confirming that these are positive traits to be associated with physicians.

Hull concludes that society would be better off if we did not view the professions of nursing and medicine as having sex linked characteristics. Unfortunately, he does not foresee any substantial changes in these attitudes soon. Individuals may resist this stereotyping of the profession and our educational systems may try to combat it, but ultimately we may have to wait until the present generation dies off and hope that not too many of our future generations are infected with such older sexist ideas.

WATSON

Catherine Watson, in "These Men Worry Me," is concerned that men are taking over leadership roles in nursing in numbers disproportionate to their numbers generally. In England, for example, although men constitute only 10 percent of all nurses, 50 percent of the candidates for the United Kingdom Central Committee (UKCC), the professional governing body for nurses, is male.[2] Watson believes that this is due to sexism. Males are socialized to be confident leaders and females passive and unassertive. It is expected of men to be leaders. However, it is not expected of men to be kind and compassionate. Watson believes that nurses themselves overvalue this quality in men, but expect it in women. A significant cause for this disparity perhaps can be found in education where males are encouraged in leadership career expectations but females not.

If such trends continue, nursing, in the United Kingdom at least, will have a male-dominated leadership in a largely female profession. That in itself may be a neutral fact, but Watson fears that males may not know or represent the desires of the majority of female nurses.

This point is illustrated by the differing analysis Watson and a male nurse educator gave to a televised portrayal of a nurse who was asked to explain her beliefs and actions concerning a patient. She lapsed into timidity and confusion. The male nurse diagnosed the problem as a lack of command of the nursing process. Watson, however, saw the problem as related to the socialization process in which women are passive and unconfident.

SUMMARY

The lower status of women in society seems intimately related to the fortunes of nursing as a profession where such problems are often magnified. Ironically, however, if Cleland's predictions are correct, improved status of women in society will not necessarily parallel or provoke an improved status of nursing. If nursing is associated with female role-related characteristics, it may not be attractive to men or "liberated" women. Except for perhaps Lisa Newton (chapter 1), no one has extolled the "feminine" side of nursing. Rather, there seems to be agreement that such stereotyping is harmful to the profession and perhaps indirectly to clients.

No author presented here is overly optimistic about sudden changes that would eliminate sexist attitudes from health care fields. Hull and Cleland agree that nursing education should play a role. The influx of men into nursing may help reduce stereotyping but even here Watson is cautious. For her, sexism is not just a matter of waiting for old guard physicians to retire. Many nurses share the role expectations expressed by such physicians as well.

NOTES

1. Leonard I. Stein, "Liberation Movement: Impact on Nursing," *AORN Journal* 15 (April 1972):75–79. This article mostly recapitulates "The Doctor–Nurse Game" with a few more pertinent remarks, including his belief that the doctor–nurse game is responsible for a decline in the number of persons choosing a career in nursing.

2. The UKCC or the United Kingdom Central Council for Nursing, Midwifery, and Health Visiting has the principal functions of establishing and improving standards of training and professional conduct for nurses, midwives, and health visitors in the United Kingdom.

The Doctor–Nurse Game

Leonard I. Stein

The relationship between the doctor and the nurse is a very special one. There are few professions where the degree of mutual respect and cooperation between co-workers is as intense as that between the doctor and nurse. Superficially, the stereotype of this relationship has been dramatized in many novels and television serials. When, however, it is observed carefully in an interactional framework, the relationship takes on a new dimension and has a special quality which fits a game model. The underlying attitudes which demand that this game be played are unfortunate. These attitudes create serious obstacles in the path of meaningful communications between physicians and nonmedical professional groups.

The physician traditionally and appropriately has total responsibility for making the decisions regarding the management of his patients' treatment. To guide his decisions he considers data gleaned from several sources. He acquires a complete medical history, performs a thorough physical examination, interprets laboratory findings, and at times, obtains recommendations from physician-consultants. Another important factor in his decision-making are the recommendations he receives from the nurse. The interaction between doctor and nurse through which these recommendations are communicated and received is unique and interesting.

THE GAME

One rarely hears a nurse say, "Doctor I would recommend that you order a retention enema for Mrs. Brown." A physician, upon hearing a recommendation of that nature, would gape in amazement at the effrontery of the nurse. The nurse, upon hearing the statement, would look over her shoulder to see who said it, hardly believing the words actually came from her own mouth. Nevertheless, if one observes closely, nurses make recommendations of more import every hour and physicians willingly and respectfully consider them. If the nurse is to make a suggestion without appearing insolent and the doctor is to seriously consider that suggestion, their interaction must not violate the rules of the game.

Object of the Game

The object of the game is as follows: the nurse is to be bold, have initiative, and be responsible for making significant recommendations, while at the same time she must appear passive. This must be done in such a manner so as to make her recommendations appear to be initiated by the physician.

Both participants must be acutely sensitive to each other's nonverbal and cryptic verbal communications. A slight lowering of the head, a minor shifting of position in the chair, or a seemingly nonrelevant comment concerning an event which occurred eight months ago must be interpreted as a powerful message. The game requires the nimbleness of a high wire acrobat, and if either participant slips the game can be shattered; the penalties for frequent failure are apt to be severe.

Rules of the Game

The cardinal rule of the game is that open disagreement between the players must be avoided at

Stein, L. I. (1967, June). The doctor–nurse game. *Archives of General Psychiatry, 16*, 699–703. Reprinted with permission of © American Medical Association. All rights reserved.

all costs. Thus, the nurse must communicate her recommendations without appearing to be making a recommendation statement. The physician, in requesting a recommendation from a nurse, must do so without appearing to be asking for it. Utilization of this technique keeps anyone from committing themselves to a position before a sub rosa agreement on that position has already been established. In that way open disagreement is avoided. The greater the significance of the recommendation, the more subtly the game must be played.

To convey a subtle example of the game with all its nuances would require the talents of a literary artist. Lacking these talents, let me give you the following example which is unsubtle, but happens frequently. The medical resident on hospital call is awakened by telephone at 1 AM because a patient on a ward, not his own, has not been able to fall asleep. Dr. Jones answers the telephone and the dialogue goes like this:

This is Dr. Jones.

(An open and direct communication.)

Dr. Jones, this is Miss Smith on 2 W—Mrs. Brown, who learned today of her father's death, is unable to fall asleep.

(This message has two levels. Openly, it describes a set of circumstances, a woman who is unable to sleep and who that morning received word of her father's death. Less openly, but just as directly, it is a diagnostic and recommendation statement; ie, Mrs. Brown is unable to sleep because of her grief, and she should be given a sedative. Dr. Jones, accepting the diagnostic statement and replying to the recommendation statement, answers.)

What sleeping medication has been helpful to Mrs. Brown in the past?

(Dr. Jones, not knowing the patient, is asking for a recommendation from the nurse, who does know the patient, about what sleeping medication should be prescribed. Note, however, his question does not appear to be asking her for a recommendation. Miss Smith replies.)

Pentobarbital mg 100 was quite effective night before last.

(A disguised recommendation statement. Dr. Jones replies with a note of authority in his voice.)

Pentobarbital mg 100 before bedtime as needed for sleep, got it?

(Miss Smith ends the conversation with the tone of a grateful supplicant.)

Yes I have, and thank you very much doctor.

The above is an example of a successfully played doctor–nurse game. The nurse made appropriate recommendations which were accepted by the physician and were helpful to the patient. The game was successful because the cardinal rule was not violated. The nurse was able to make her recommendation without appearing to, and the physician was able to ask for recommendations without conspicuously asking for them.

The Scoring System

Inherent in any game are penalties and rewards for the players. In game theory, the doctor–nurse game fits the nonzero sum game model. It is not like chess, where the players compete with each other and whatever one player loses the other wins. Rather, it is the kind of game in which the rewards and punishments are shared by both players. If they play the game successfully they both win rewards, and if they are unskilled and the game is played badly, they both suffer the penalty.

The most obvious reward from the well-played game is a doctor–nurse team that operates efficiently. The physician is able to utilize the nurse as a valuable consultant, and the nurse gains self-esteem and professional satisfaction from her job. The less obvious rewards are no less important. A successful game creates a doctor–nurse alliance; through this alliance the physician gains the respect and admiration of the nursing service. He can be confident that his nursing staff will smooth the path for getting his work done. His charts will be organized and waiting for him when he arrives, the ruffled feathers of patients and relatives will have been smoothed down, his pet routines will be happily followed, and he will be helped in a thousand and one other ways.

The doctor–nurse alliance sheds its light on the nurse as well. She gains a reputation for being a "damn good nurse." She is respected by everyone and appropriately enjoys her position. When physicians discuss the nursing staff it would not be unusual for her name to be mentioned with respect and admiration. Their esteem for a good nurse is no less than their esteem for a good doctor.

The penalties for a game failure, on the other hand, can be severe. The physician who is an unskilled gamesman and fails to recognize the nurses' subtle recommendation messages is tolerated as a "clod." If, however, he interprets these messages as insolence and strongly indicates he does not wish to tolerate suggestions from nurses, he creates a rocky path for his travels. The old truism "If the nurse is your ally you've got it made, and if she has it in for you, be prepared for misery," takes on life-sized proportions. He receives three times as many phone calls after midnight than his colleagues. Nurses will not accept his telephone orders because "telephone orders are against the rules." Somehow, this rule gets suspended for the skilled players. Soon he becomes like Joe Bfstplk in the "Li'l Abner" comic strip. No matter where he goes, a black cloud constantly hovers over his head.

The unskilled gamesman nurse also pays heavily. The nurse who does not view her role as that of a consultant, and therefore does not attempt to communicate recommendations, is perceived as a dullard and is mercifully allowed to fade into the woodwork.

The nurse who does see herself as a consultant but refuses to follow the rules of the game in making her recommendations, has hell to pay. The outspoken nurse is labeled a "bitch" by the surgeon. The psychiatrist describes her as unconsciously suffering from penis envy and her behavior is the acting out of her hostility towards men. Loosely translated, the psychiatrist is saying she is a bitch. The employment of the unbright outspoken nurse is soon terminated. The outspoken bright nurse whose recommendations are worthwhile remains employed. She is, however, constantly reminded in a hundred ways that she is not loved.

GENESIS OF THE GAME

To understand how the game evolved, we must comprehend the nature of the doctors' and nurses' training which shaped the attitudes necessary for the game.

Medical Student Training

The medical student in his freshman year studies as if possessed. In the anatomy class he learns every groove and prominence on the bones of the skeleton as if life depended on it. As a matter of fact, he literally believes just that. He not infrequently says, "I've got to learn it exactly, a life may depend on me knowing that." A consequence of this attitude, which is carefully nurtured throughout medical school, is the development of a phobia: the overdetermined fear of making a mistake. The

development of this fear is quite understandable. The burden the physician must carry is at times almost unbearable. He feels responsible in a very personal way for the lives of his patients. When a man dies leaving young children and a widow, the doctor carries some of her grief and despair inside himself; and when a child dies, some of him dies too. He sees himself as a warrior against death and disease. When he loses a battle, through no fault of his own, he nevertheless feels pangs of guilt, and he relentlessly searches himself to see if there might have been a way to alter the outcome. For the physician a mistake leading to a serious consequence is intolerable, and any mistake reminds him of his vulnerability. There is little wonder that he becomes phobic. The classical way in which phobias are managed is to avoid the source of the fear. Since it is impossible to avoid making some mistakes in an active practice of medicine, a substitute defensive maneuver is employed. The physician develops the belief that he is omnipotent and omniscient, and therefore incapable of making mistakes. This belief allows the phobic physician to actively engage in his practice rather than avoid it. The fear of committing an error in a critical field like medicine is unavoidable and appropriately realistic. The physician, however, must learn to live with the fear rather than handle it defensively through a posture of omnipotence. This defense markedly interferes with his interpersonal professional relationships.

Physicians, of course, deny feelings of omnipotence. The evidence, however, renders their denials to whispers in the wind. The slightest mistake inflicts a large narcissistic wound. Depending on his underlying personality structure the physician may obsess for days about it, quickly rationalize it away, or deny it. The guilt produced is usually exaggerated and the incident is handled defensively. The ways in which physicians enhance and support each other's defenses when an error is made could be the topic of another paper. The feelings of omnipotence become generalized to other areas of his life. A report of the Federal Aviation Agency (FAA), as quoted in *Time Magazine* (Aug 5, 1966), states that in 1964 and 1965 physicians had a fatal-accident rate four times as high as the average for all other private pilots. Major causes of the high death rate were risk-taking attitudes and judgments. Almost all of the accidents occurred on pleasure trips, and were therefore not necessary risks to get to a patient needing emergency care. The trouble, suggested an FAA official, is that too many doctors fly with "the feeling that they are omnipotent." Thus, the extremes to which the physician may go in preserving his self-concept of omnipotence may threaten his own life. This overdetermined preservation of omnipotence is indicative of its brittleness and its underlying foundation of fear of failure.

The physician finds himself trapped in a paradox. He fervently wants to give his patient the best possible medical care, and being open to the nurses' recommendations helps him accomplish this. On the other hand, accepting advice from nonphysicians is highly threatening to his omnipotence. The solution for the paradox is to receive sub rosa recommendations and make them appear to be initiated by himself. In short, he must learn to play the doctor–nurse game.

Some physicians never learn to play the game. Most learn in their internship, and a perceptive few learn during their clerkships in medical school. Medical students frequently complain that the nursing staff treats them as if they had just completed a junior Red Cross first-aid class instead of two years of intensive medical training. Interviewing nurses in a training hospital sheds considerable light on this phenomenon. In their words they said,

> A few students just seem to be with it, they are able to understand what you are trying to tell them, and they are a pleasure to work with; most, however, pretend to know everything and refuse to listen to anything we have to say and I guess we do give them a rough time.

In essence, they are saying that those students who quickly learn the game are rewarded, and those that do not are punished.

Most physicians learn to play the game after they have weathered a few experiences like the one described below. On the first day of his internship, the physician and nurse were making rounds. They stopped at the bed of a 52-year-old woman who, after complimenting the young doctor on his appearance, complained to him of her problem with constipation. After several minutes of listening to her detailed description of peculiar diets, family home remedies, and special exercises that have helped her constipation in the past, the nurse politely interrupted the patient. She told her the doctor would take care of the problem and that he had to move on because there were other patients waiting to see him. The young doctor gave the nurse a stern look, turned toward the patient, and kindly told her he would order an enema for her that very afternoon. As they left the bedside, the nurse told him the patient has had a normal bowel movement every day for the past week and that in the 23 days the patient has been

in the hospital she had never once passed up an opportunity to complain of her constipation. She quickly added that if the doctor wanted to order an enema, the patient would certainly receive one. After hearing this report the intern's mouth fell open and the wheels began turning in his head. He remembered the nurse's comment to the patient that, "the doctor had to move on," and it occurred to him that perhaps she was really giving him a message. This experience and a few more like it, and the young doctor learns to listen for the subtle recommendations the nurses make.

Nursing Student Training

Unlike the medical student, who usually learns to play the game after he finishes medical school, the nursing student begins to learn it early in her training. Throughout her education she is trained to play the doctor–nurse game.

Student nurses are taught how to relate to physicians. They are told he has infinitely more knowledge than they, and thus he should be shown the utmost respect. In addition, it was not many years ago when nurses were instructed to stand whenever a physician entered a room. When he would come in for a conference the nurse was expected to offer him her chair, and when both entered a room the nurse would open the door for him and allow him to enter first. Although these practices are no longer rigidly adhered to, the premise upon which they were based is still promulgated. One nurse described that premise as, "He's God almighty and your job is to wait on him."

To inculcate subservience and inhibit deviancy, nursing schools, for the most part, are tightly run, disciplined institutions. Certainly there is great variation among nursing schools, and there is little question that the trend is toward giving students more autonomy. However, in too many schools this trend has not gone far enough, and the climate remains restrictive. The student's schedule is firmly controlled and there is very little free time. Classroom hours, study hours, meal time, and bedtime with lights out are rigidly enforced. In some schools meaningless chores are assigned, such as cleaning bed springs with cotton applicators. The relationship between student and instructor continues this military flavor. Often their relationship is more like that between recruit and drill sergeant than between student and teacher. Open dialogue is inhibited by attitudes of strict black and white, with few, if any, shades of gray. Straying from the rigidly outlined path is sure to result in disciplinary action.

The inevitable result of these practices is to instill in the student nurse a fear of independent action. This inhibition of independent action is most marked when relating to physicians. One of the students' greatest fears is making a blunder while assisting a physician and being publicly ridiculed by him. This is really more a reflection of the nature of their training than the prevalence of abusive physicians. The fear of being humiliated for a blunder while assisting in a procedure is generalized to the fear of humiliation for making any independent act in relating to a physician, especially the act of making a direct recommendation. Every nurse interviewed felt that making a suggestion to a physician was equivalent to insulting and belittling him. It was tantamount to questioning his medical knowledge and insinuating he did not know his business. In light of her image of the physician as an omniscient and punitive figure, the questioning of his knowledge would be unthinkable.

The student, however, is also given messages quite contrary to the ones described above. She is continually told that she is an invaluable aid to the physician in the treatment of the patient. She is told that she must help him in every way possible, and she is imbued with a strong sense of responsibility for the care of her patient. Thus she, like the physician, is caught in a paradox. The first set of messages implies that the physician is omniscient and that any recommendation she might make would be insulting to him and leave her open to ridicule. The second set of messages implies that she is an important asset to him, has much to contribute, and is duty-bound to make those contributions. Thus, when her good sense tells her a recommendation would be helpful to him she is not allowed to communicate it directly, nor is she allowed not to communicate it. The way out of the bind is to use the doctor–nurse game and communicate the recommendation without appearing to do so.

FORCES PRESERVING THE GAME

Upon observing the indirect interactional system which is the heart of the doctor–nurse game, one must ask the question, "Why does this inefficient mode of communication continue to exist?" The forces mitigating against change are powerful.

Rewards and Punishments

The doctor–nurse game has a powerful, innate self-perpetuating force—its system of rewards and punishments. One potent method of shaping behavior is to reward one set of behavioral patterns and to punish patterns which deviate from it. As described earlier, the rewards given for a well-played game and the punishments meted out to unskilled players are impressive. This system alone would be sufficient to keep the game flourishing. The game, however, has additional forces.

The Strength of the Set

It is well recognized that sets are hard to break. A powerful attitudinal set is the nurse's perception that making a suggestion to a physician is equivalent to insulting and belittling him. An example of where attempts are regularly made to break this set is seen on psychiatric treatment wards operating on a therapeutic community model. This model requires open and direct communication between members of the team. Psychiatrists working in these settings expend a great deal of energy in urging for and rewarding openness before direct patterns of communication become established. The rigidity of the resistance to break this set is impressive. If the physician himself is a prisoner of the set and therefore does not actively try to destroy it, change is near impossible.

The Need for Leadership

Lack of leadership and structure in any organization produces anxiety in its members. As the importance of the organization's mission increases, the demand by its members for leadership commensurately increases. In our culture human life is near the top of our hierarchy of values, and organizations which deal with human lives, such as law and medicine, are very rigidly structured. Certainly some of this is necessary for the systematic management of the task. The excessive degree of rigidity, however, is demanded by its members for their own psychic comfort rather than for its utility in efficiently carrying out its mission. The game lends support to this thesis. Indirect communication is an inefficient mode of transmitting information. However, it effectively supports and protects a rigid organizational structure with the physician in clear authority. Maintaining an omnipotent leader provides the other members with a great sense of security.

Sexual Roles

Another influence perpetuating the doctor–nurse game is the sexual identity of the players. Doctors are predominately men and nurses are almost exclusively women. There are elements of the game which reinforce the stereotyped roles of male dominance and female passivity. Some nursing instructors explicitly tell their students that their femininity is an important asset to be used when relating to physicians.

COMMENT

The doctor and nurse have a shared history and thus have been able to work out their game so that it operates more efficiently than one would expect in an indirect system. Major difficulty arises, however, when the physician works closely with other disciplines which are not normally considered part of the medical sphere. With expanding medical horizons encompassing cooperation with sociologists, engineers, anthropologists, computer analysts etc, continued expectation of a doctor-nurselike interaction by the physician is disastrous. The sociologist, for example, is not willing to play that kind of game. When his direct communications are rebuffed the relationship breaks down.

The major disadvantage of a doctor-nurselike game is its inhibitory effect on open dialogue which is stifling and anti-intellectual. The game is basically a transactional neurosis, and both professions would enhance themselves by taking steps to change the attitudes which breed the game.

Mrs. Gertrude Hermsmeier, RN, Mrs. Joyce McCollum, RN, Arnold M. Ludwig, MD, and Arnold J. Marx, MD, of Mendota State Hospital, aided in this report.

Sex Discrimination:
Nursing's Most Pervasive Problem

Virginia Cleland

A study I undertook a few years ago was focused upon the perceived inducements and consequences of married nurses reactivating their careers after a period of inactivity. The conclusion of this reactivation study which relates to the career motivation of married nurses was:

> For the male, work dominates the life space regardless of whether he is married or single, rich or poor, educated or uneducated. The male, even when he is widowed or divorced and possessing custody of children, is still expected first of all to provide for his family economically. . . . In contrast, the life space of the employed, married woman has two focuses—employment and family. The female also bears responsibility to an extended family in that she (rather than her brothers) is more often expected to provide a home for elderly parents and other relatives. For nurses this family demand may be increased to include care of the sick. . . .

> . . . One may conclude that the inducements offered by nursing are not sufficient (. . . in terms of the inactive nurse's values and . . . the alternatives open to her), to motivate her to make the contributions demanded if she is to reactivate her career. Employment of married nurses can most often be characterized by the principle of immediate gratification, namely:

> 1. Rapid job turnover and change of work status when family problems arise.
> 2. Acceptance of dead-end jobs which are compatible with family needs and demands.

> 3. Work goals which focus upon maintenance of existing skills rather than advancement or growth.(1)

From that study, I concluded that nurses *could* combine career and marriage, but that careful planning is necessary to avoid sacrifice of one or the other. Two of the premises I then offered upon which change could be built were that employment for married women must be planned as secondary to family responsibility, but satisfying and meaningful within that framework, and the model of male employment need not be the model for the employment of married women.

About one year ago, I became seriously interested in the women's rights movement. Like most nurses, I had not felt discriminated against. My earliest participation ostensibly was for the purpose of lending support to faculty colleagues working in fields where sex discrimination is frankly overt. From Betty Friedan's *Feminine Mystique*, Caroline Bird's *Born Female*, Kate Millett's *Sexual Politics* and innumerable other reports, articles, and news clippings, I began to recognize how closely the entire social issue of equal rights for women actually relates to nursing. Today, there is no doubt in my mind that our most fundamental problem in nursing is that we are members of a woman's occupation in a male dominated culture(2,3,4).

Millett has defined sexual politics as power-structured relationships whereby one group of persons is controlled by another. Control is exerted through either consent or force. In the instance of sexuality, it is by consent through the process of socialization. In the realm of temperament, the male is socialized to display the stereotype of aggression, intelligence, and efficiency; the female, passivity, ignorance, docility, virtue and ineffectuality. Millett shows that the patriarchal system is supported by every social and economic force including the military, industry, technology, universities, science, political office, and finance, each of which is entirely within male hands. The power of patriarchy is probably most pervasive because of its universality and longevity(5).

Marriage and divorce laws also have supported this view and only in recent decades has a woman been permitted an economic existence separate from that of her father or her husband. The wife was entitled to room and board in exchange for housekeeping functions and sexual availability. If you have seen the movie *M.A.S.H.*, you know that nursing is indeed a woman's occupation.

NURSING AUTONOMY A FALSE PREMISE

At one time, I thought nursing had an advantage over other women's occupations since in nursing women held all of the positions throughout the hierarchy, unlike the occupations of teaching, social work, and library science which in numbers are dominated by women but where power positions are held by men. I thought nursing had more autonomy because of this. Now, I believe this was an incorrect assumption. Rather, nursing is weaker because of the almost complete absence of men. Nursing, in its utter isolation from all vestiges of power except within its own group, can be likened to the exploitation of Negroes in our culture. With women, as with Negroes, dominance is most complete when it is not even recognized. Only those who are closest to the goal of freedom are concerned about the lack of freedom. The majority of nurses, like the majority of Southern blacks, have not been vocally or obviously concerned about their lack of power.

Nursing leaders have often displayed marked similarities to black principals in the separate Southern black school systems(6). The dual system of education in the South offered graduates of Negro colleges an opportunity for unlimited advancement within the system. They could become teachers, supervisors, and principals. The black schools provided upward mobility for a group to whom other routes were closed. Nursing, too, has

provided upward mobility to large numbers of women for whom other routes were closed because of sex discrimination.

The Negro principal in the all black school system was a "big" man and the director of nursing or dean of a collegiate school in an all woman system is a "big" woman. The Negro principal, frequently, was the only channel of communication between the black and white communities, for he was the only one with whom the white power structure would deal. He couldn't get the top position without approval of the white community and in exchange for the cloak of authority, he was supposed to speak with authority and finality on all questions relating to the black community. The greatest impact of all of this was in the minds of black children who saw this Uncle Tom in the principal's office, tried to act like him, and dreamed of standing in his shoes one day.

Likewise, administrative positions in nursing generally are available only with the approval of the male systems in medicine, hospital administration, and higher education. The top nurse communicates to the male systems with authority and finality on all questions relating to the nursing community. And worst of all, younger nurses have viewed the position without seeing the acquiescing behavior of Aunt Jane. They ape her and dream of standing in her shoes some day. Unconsciously, in a search for autonomy and self-actualization, we chose as our role models the Aunt Janes, who really have no power except over the hapless and are only female Uncle Toms.

Nursing in the 1940's, 1950's and 1960's did not have the leadership it had at the turn of the century, or even during the first three decades of this century (an impression which the writer cannot document). I believe that these past 30 years of weak and unimaginative leadership parallel the growth of the cult of women as sex symbols. The influence of Freud's writings and his belief that anatomy is destiny cannot be overestimated(7). As his ideas found their way into the popular literature there developed a common belief that women would find happiness through mothering broods of children in suburbia. The route to fulfillment was by way of the uterus.

Betty Friedan, in 1963, described the feminine mystique. She traced its origins, in part, to the work of Farnham and Lundberg who wrote *Modern Women: The Lost Sex* in 1947. Friedan describes the book as holding forth a "warning that careers and higher education were leading to the 'masculinization of women with enormously dangerous consequences to the home, the children dependent on it, and to the ability of the woman, as well as her husband, to obtain sexual gratification'"(8).

The women who never had a chance nor any desire to be anything but housewives could now feel vindicated. The housewife-mother became the model for all women. Friedan writes:

The feminine mystique says that the highest value and the only commitment for women is the fulfillment of their own femininity. It says that the great mistake of Western culture, through most of its history, has been the undervaluation of this femininity. It says this femininity is so mysterious and intuitive and close to the creation and origin of life that man-made science may never be able to understand it. But however special and different, it is in no way inferior to the nature of man; it may even in certain respects be superior. The mistake, says the mystique, the root of women's troubles in the past is that women envied men, women tried to be like men, instead of accepting their own nature, which can find fulfillment only in sexual passivity, male domination, and nurturing maternal love.(9)

Most of nursing's leaders probably have felt less than adequate when comparing themselves against the social standard of the "women-as-sex" symbol (a feeling shared by many other nurses). Simultaneously, they have had to play the game of professional leadership wherein all the rules have been established by males. This double jeopardy with its accompanying risks of double failure has produced a generation of acquiescing, submissive, overly-cautious leaders.

The female can win individual plays but the game itself must be won by the male. The socialization of a little girl dictates that she must learn how to lose. She is supposed to acquiesce and please whomever is the master. If she doesn't learn how to lose, her sex identity has not been "correctly" learned. She learns to fail and she learns to hate herself. The flagellant, self-hatred phenomenon seen so often in women and in nurses is similar socially and psychologically to the self-hatred phenomenon common with Negroes.

LEADERSHIP DOES NOT CONTROL

The general lack of leadership in nursing, I believe, derives directly from the social position of women in our society. It is the occupation's most pervasive problem. The leadership deficiency is most apparent in the areas of decision making, communicating needs and resources, establishing and maintaining professional standards, and functioning consonantly with the economic system of the working world. I am appalled every time I am forced to recognize that the vast majority of directors of nursing do not control their departmental budgets, even though the nursing department frequently spends 80 to 85 percent of the total personnel budget of the institution. I cannot imagine a man accepting a similar title with such absence of corresponding authority.

In educational institutions I see nurse faculty members who fail to assume responsibility for helping to formulate educational policy. In service institutions I see nurse practitioners negating their responsibility to be involved in establishing policies pertaining to nursing practice. Nurse faculty members and professional practitioners must assume more autonomous behavior. The practice, so common within nursing, of turning to administrative authority for direction is, I believe, a result of the socialization process of girls. Marjorie Batey has written discerningly about the difference in the normative expectations of the two types of institutions(10).

For 30 years, the occupation of nursing has been faced with inadequate numbers of personnel to meet the increasing demand. It is a frank indictment of nursing's leadership that during this period the supply-demand principle has not been used to create a more financially rewarding and attractive occupation. In situation after situation, we see directors of nursing fighting collective bargaining, written contracts, grievance procedures, et cetera, most often at the request of male administrators. These leaders have risked the lives of patients rather than take forceful, public stands to insist on the closing of improperly staffed areas. I personally have known of only one director of nursing who has had sufficient courage and conviction to use her power to close units.

Instead of offering money for professional services, we see directors who confuse the sex role and the professional role in job recruitment. For example, a recent advertisement from the *Journal* reads:

Face to face
with one another,
telling secrets,
killing lies.
Sharing love's own

silent language,
speaking only
with our eyes.
Come to me
across the space
of love's own
private sky.
Fly to me on
wings of truth,
unmasked and pure as I.(11)

Who would have guessed the sponsors wanted a nurse for an infirmary! In other advertisements in the *Journal* another institution, which makes no mention of its nursing staff, pointedly relates that it employs 200 staff doctors, 250 residents, 30 interns and has a medical school affiliation(12). Still another shows an attractive young lady sitting with her son by the fireplace with a dog at her feet(13). The entire advertisement is written in the past tense with the clear implication that this woman's hunting days are over and she achieved matrimonial success while working at X institution!

When directors of nursing permit the use of such outrageously sexually motivated advertisements, I can only conclude that they would rather entice nurses by cheap sexual inducement than pay an honest salary. Could this common practice be called "procuring"?

The acquiescing behavior of nurse directors and deans is often "wife-like" toward the male hospital or university administrator like housewives asking for grocery money. Yet, some can intelligently and effectively defend their departments' needs in the face of growing demands or impending budget cuts. Nursing desperately needs leaders who will insist on being involved in decision making related to program priorities of their institutions.

professionally whether a nurse lives alone, lives with another female, lives with a male, or is married. These are personal decisions each woman makes for herself. It is sexism at its worst to use marital status as a symbol of success or failure.

A married woman may wish to work part-time. And, nursing can certainly experiment with ways to provide alternatives to the usual full-time, 40-hour-week employment. Part-time work is an important way to prevent career discontinuity, a way to avoid retreading later, a way to keep, not lose, nurses. However, employing nurses part-time must be balanced economically so that full-time staff are not penalized.

Marriage for those who make that choice need not be a male dominated state. When I attended several sessions of the Women's Teach-in on the campus last fall, I was excited to learn that the number of men who want equality in marriage is certainly growing.

When there is equality within the family, a sharing of all rights and responsibilities, men will also find a new freedom. For freedom built upon dominance and oppression is not freedom; it is license. When sex is accepted as a biologically given rather than as an attained role, men will be free to be themselves and so will the children. With a fusion of the social manifestations of the sex roles, there will be less exploitation. As smaller families become commonplace, the youngest child will usually be of school age when the mother is about 32. She will then have 25 to 30 years in which to establish her own identity apart from that of Henry's wife or Tommy's mother. But, the opportunities will be hers only if she starts by removing the social constraints within the family. The alternative is to be a "functionless" woman at 45.

DISCRIMINATION CAN BE ATTACKED

If sex discrimination is acknowledged as a problem within nursing, it can be attacked within both spheres of a woman's life space simultaneously; the family structure and the professional structure.

I believe we could start by ignoring the marital status of women. Let us strike out marriage as a distinguishing symbol. Just think of all the paper work the profession could eliminate! Marriage is a personal relationship that should have no professional significance. It should not make any difference

RECRUITMENT PROBLEMS LIE AHEAD

Within the profession itself equal employment opportunity may not be a significant issue. However, when attending meetings on women's rights, I have heard nursing used time and time again as *the* illustration of discrimination. The assumption always is that if a nurse is intelligent, educated, and capable, she is a nurse instead of a physician only because of sex discrimination. I predict that nursing is going to have an increasingly difficult time in trying to recruit intelligent young women.

Equal pay for equal work is a very relevant issue. Title VII of the 1964 Federal Civil Rights Act prohibits discrimination because of race, color, religion, sex, or national origin in hiring, upgrading, and all other conditions of employment among private employers of more than 25 persons(14). Executive Order No. 11246, as amended, extended the law to include employment by federal contractors and subcontractors and employment under federally assisted construction contracts regardless of race, creed, color, sex, or national origin. The vast majority of all U.S. colleges are subject to this order because of their acceptance of federal teaching and research grants. Similarly, hospitals usually receive funds from federal agencies.

I am currently a member of the group at Wayne State University which has filed a complaint with the Department of Health, Education, and Welfare for noncontract compliance by Wayne with regard to sex discrimination. Although it is not true at Wayne, many universities, rank for rank, pay nurse faculty less than they pay faculty members in other colleges of the university. It is also becoming public knowledge that within the same discipline men may be paid 10 to 30 percent more than women of the same rank in the same department(15,16).

Graduate school admissions is another important area of discrimination. Nursing suffers greatly because its members face sex discrimination when trying to get admitted to graduate school and then when trying to get the types of financial support available to male students. The University of Michigan has appealed to the Secretary of Health, Education and Welfare to have graduate school admissions excluded from the jurisdiction of the contract compliance regulations because graduate students "are not employees." Others of us have been writing to Secretary Richardson to urge that he rule to include graduate and professional school admissions under the regulations. We maintain that these schools are the gateway to the professions and to employment as faculty members. The situation is comparable to the need to integrate apprenticeship programs in order to make employment in the building and machine trades available to blacks. The nurse scientist programs which prepare nurses at the Ph.D. level would most likely be unnecessary if sex discrimination within graduate schools were prohibited.

Fringe benefits is still another area where women need to impose their thinking. The monthly retirement payment under the Teachers Insurance and Annuity Association, the retirement plan used in so many universities, reflects the actuarial fact that women live longer than men. Thus, the monthly payment women receive is less than the monthly payment men receive. But is it reasonable to expect women to live on less than men? Rather, women faculty members should be advocating a change so that there is no sex discrimination in the monthly payment, as is true of Social Security benefits. (There are other sex inequities with Social Security which I will not go into.)

REVAMPING IS NEEDED

I expect and hope that the 1970's will bring important social and economic changes for women. Nursing has much to gain by establishing new employment styles which will include discrimination *for* women where pregnancy and young children are involved. The employment picture for women will improve, but I am very pessimistic about nursing. I do not believe nursing leaders see the need for the drastic change in nursing I believe is necessary.

We can only grow as a profession by becoming less isolated. This means joining the mainstream of society. It means revamping the profession in rather drastic ways to make nursing acceptable to males.

Society needs first rate nurse clinicians to fill the gap between the technical nurse and the specialist physician. Patients need the services of a nurse prepared in the behavioral sciences as the physician is now prepared in the natural sciences. But we cannot prepare such a nurse by taking her through the steps of a traditional curriculum. With traditional preparation, we prepare a trained dependency characterized by high predictability of behavior. Instead, we need professional nurses who are perceptive, who possess great social sensitivity, and who will take calculated risks in making decisions. This is in contrast to the nurse who strives to never make a mistake and who fails to realize that decisions which were never made can be just as wrong.

Many women do not want this type of freedom and responsibility. For them, technical nursing has much to offer. We must make clear distinctions between the roles of these nurses, distinctions which physicians and patients alike will appreciate. Perhaps we could call the newer types of nurse practitioner a nursologist. The nursologist would be to the nurse what the pharmacologist is to the pharmacist or what the anesthesiologist is to the anesthetist. Nursing's long insistence that a nurse is a nurse is a nurse is patently untrue and is illustrative of the indecisiveness of the occupation. We cannot recruit or retain the type of people needed to fill the health care gap until we put our house in order, until we design a new career in nursing which will be attractive to both men and women.

It means the development of nurses who will not only accept but also seek freedom and responsibility. Just as the black school system in the South had to go because it wasn't good enough to meet societal needs, so must the all female system of nursing go. Closed systems have no future, even though they offer protection to the incumbents. Promotions are probably easier when you don't face open competition. My fear is that a desire for protection will win over a bolder plan involving more calculated risks. If that happens, nursing will continue to be consumed by more aggressive groups.

REFERENCES

1. Cleland, Virginia, and others. Decision to reactivate nursing career. *Nurs.Res.* 19:446–452, Sept.–Oct. 1970.
2. Friedan, Betty. *Feminine Mystique.* New York, Dell Publishing Co., 1965 (Originally published by W. W. Norton, 1963)
3. Bird, Caroline, and Briller, S. W. *Born Female.* New York, David McKay Co., 1968.
4. Millett, Kate. *Sexual Politics.* Garden City, N.Y., Doubleday and Co., 1970.
5. *Ibid.,* p. 25.
6. James, J. C. Black principal. *New Repub.*
7. Shainess, Natalie. In Robin Morgan (ed.) *Sisterhood is Powerful.* New York, Random House, 1970.
8. Friedan, *op. cit.,* p. 37.
9. *Ibid.*
10. Batey, Marjorie V. Two normative worlds of the university nursing faculty. *Nurs. Forum* 8(1):4–16, 1969.
11. Advertisement. *Am.J.Nurs.* 70:2456. Nov. 1970.
12. *Ibid.,* p. 2443.
13. *Ibid.,* p. 2445.
14. U.S. Women's Bureau. *Laws on Sex Discrimination in Employment.* Washington, D.C., U.S. Government Printing Office, 1970.
15. *Research on the Status of Faculty Women, University of Minnesota.* Minneapolis, Minn., Planning and Counseling Center for Women, 1970.
16. *Study of the Status of Women Faculty at Indiana University.* Indiana Chapter, Committee on the Status of Women, American Association of University Professors, 1971.

Dealing With Sexism in
Nursing and Medicine

Richard T. Hull

Assessing the extent and character of sexism in nursing and medicine is made difficult by virtue of subtle complexities involved in the question. Let me point out three such complexities.

Traditionally, nursing has been regarded as a field in which skilled nurturing has been the chief mode of interaction between the nurse and the patient. Indeed, from its early history, the shared view of nursing has been based on an analogy between nurse and mother.[1] A similar analogy has been made between physician and father.[2] Therefore, the first part of the question is theoretical: Is the view that the nurse performs skilled applications of maternal functions and that the physician performs skilled applications of paternal or masculine functions essentially correct theory or theory that is sexist?

Second, women have been regarded culturally as naturally possessing personality traits that lead to superior performance of nurturing tasks and as lacking the natural traits of decisiveness and leadership required for the tasks of physicians. Nightingale and other "originators of nursing saw nursing as a natural vocation for women second only to motherhood. Nightingale viewed women as instinctive nurses, not physicians."[3] Thus the view arose that nursing as a vocation was more suited to women than men, since women naturally perform such actions as nurturing, caring, and education. Inherent in this view is that men lack natural aptitude in these skills and must struggle to acquire them in an imperfect and artificial manner that runs counter to their more aggressive natural traits.

Third, some will grant that the natural propensities of the good nurse may be sufficiently plastic to be acquired by both women and men. Nonetheless, there is a strong cultural bias in our society as well as most others toward cultivating nurturing traits in women and not in men. (Proponents of this view are thus able to dismiss the different sex distributions in nursing and medicine in other countries, such as Russia and China, as irrelevant to an assessment of the distribution patterns in the United States—quite possibly a subtle appeal to Americanism.)[4,5] Moreover, the role of caring for the sick has been viewed as a natural extension of the woman's "responsibility to an extended family . . . to provide a home for elderly parents and other relatives."[6] Hence, the strong statistical skew indicating women as the better source for personnel in the nursing profession and men in the medical profession is justified as being a product of our culture.

These three positions can be tendered in defense of the preponderance of women in nursing and men in medicine, and even in defense of certain attitudes towards men and women who individually seek to move against that preponderance. At the same time, opponents of these distribution patterns may elect to disagree with any one or a combination of these positions. For example, one might agree that nursing is properly characterized by modes of behavior that are primarily nurturing, but deny that women naturally manifest nurturing character traits any more than do men. Or, one may hold that while there is a cultural bias toward producing certain clusters of traits in women and others in men, such a bias is unjustly discriminatory against both men and women and requires positive redress. Or, one may hold that, however nature and culture distribute nurturing character traits among women and men, nursing is wrongly viewed as a profession requiring just that particular set of characteristics.

Answering such questions definitively within the scope of a journal article is impossible. But it may be possible to trace some of the subtle connections between these three positions and the more obvious instances of blatant sexism encountered by nurses, in order to suggest directions for further thought and action by practitioners of this "profession in transition," and ways of understanding and dealing with the more onerous types of sexism encountered in that profession.[7]

One final, prefatory comment. Men have been criticized for engaging in efforts to contribute to the growing body of feminist literature and theory because they have not experienced the forms and types of sexist discrimination encountered by women. But I think such criticism is not valid for two reasons.

First, much of human evaluative and critical thought rests on one person's ability to empathetically assess the experiences of another. Any ethical theory that requires one engaged in moral deliberation to project consequences of various alternatives for the happiness of others (act utilitarianism) or to discriminate between competent and incompetent decisions (legitimate paternalism) or to balance competing needs within a context of limited resources (theories of justice) also requires that such deliberation be conditioned by empathy. Even the fundamental element in virtually all ethical theories, personified in the Golden Rule, would be empty of any concrete content if it did not implicitly make reference to the perceptions and needs of others. Otherwise, one like John Hinckley, Jr. could claim a moral justification for attempting the assassination of the president on the grounds that he wishes his own destruction and is simply doing unto others as he would have them do unto him. Moreover, the ability to change one's undesirable attitudes through education and "consciousness-raising" depends on one's ability to transcend the gaps in one's own experience by participating imaginatively and vicariously in others' lives and to recognize analogies between one's own experience and that of others. Since humans have these abilities, it is false that a man cannot understand the discrimination suffered by a woman, a white person that by a black, a Protestant or Catholic that by a Jew.

Second, sexism is a two-edged sword; it hurts both women and men alike by excluding each from certain spheres of experience that are thought reserved for the other. Sexism in nursing and medicine is not just the problem of women nurses, women doctors,

and women patients; men suffer from it as well, although in different ways.[8]

INSTANCES OF SEXISM IN NURSING AND MEDICINE

The following illustrations of sexism in nursing and medicine are drawn from the writings of nurses about their profession.

1. "I recall a conversation with an extremely well-respected hospital administrator regarding the clinical placement of nursing students. He assured me that there would be ample opportunity for students to rotate through all of the services provided by the hospital, particularly for the male nurses to experience emergency room care and for the female students to affiliate in labor, delivery, and postpartum care. When questioned about his placement concepts, he responded that any male in nursing is a frustrated physician, and thus would enjoy the decisive atmosphere of emergency nursing, whereas women were drawn to nursing because of their innate motherly qualities. Furthermore, he stated his belief that all male nurses were homosexuals."[9]

2. "The gynecological clinic is extremely busy this morning. There are 35 clients enrolled for clinic appointments. The three physicians are kept busy with a variety of pressing complaints. One of the physicians comes out and picks up Mary's chart. She is 13 years old and her chief complaint is 'cramps.' The physician throws her chart on the desk and tells you to give her the standing prescription and send her back to school. He adds, 'We don't have time to see hysterical women today.'"[10]

3. "It is not uncommon to hear the complaints of nurses that female physicians are more demanding and degrading than their male colleagues. It is permissible for a male physician to excuse the female nurse for her shortcomings, to try to protect and lead her through the maze of medical miracles. Such protective, paternalistic behavior on the part of a female physician would be inappropriate and might even be misread as symbolic of masculinization, with lesbian overtones. . . .

"Once graduated and licensed, she must choose between the role of authoritarian medical doctor with no option for paternalistic relationships with subordinate staff, or she may attempt to establish collegial relationships with female health professionals—with the attendant risk of perception as a weak sister, probably better suited to nursing, in the eyes of her male peers."[11]

4. "Men who do succeed in challenging and surmounting the sexist barriers confronting them when entering the career of nursing are rewarded for their gender in one way in which their female colleagues are not. A man in nursing is much more likely to be perceived as a leader or teacher, or in other authoritarian roles, than is a woman. Although men comprise less than seven percent of all registered nurses, it is estimated that they comprise fifteen percent of registered nurse administrators. When gaining entrance to the profession, they are advanced along assumptions of maleness even in the female world! Their colleagues are more likely to tolerate assertive behavior and the attributes of leadership from a male than from a female; thus, men in nursing are able to move up the supervisory ladder more rapidly than their female peers of equal education and competence."[12]

ANALYSIS OF THE ILLUSTRATIONS

These illustrations are but four of an increasing number of examples in the literature testifying to the belief that sexism is a major source of bias in both nursing and medicine:

The first illustration suggests that female nurses are perceived as naturally inclined toward nurturing and caring functions, understood on the basis of the motherhood model. Thus, nursing experience with labor, delivery, and postpartum care is perceived by the administrator as the ideal clinical experience for the female nursing student. There, he believes, she will achieve the integration of training and personal characteristics that will move her toward being an effective practitioner. The corollary view is that female nurses would be least happy in the emergency room where decisiveness and other masculine characteristics are required, traits antithetical to the female nurse's natural inclinations. She would have to apply not only nursing knowledge and skills in that unit, but also practice characteristics that she does not naturally possess. By contrast, the male nurse, because of his being male, is perceived as having the qualities of decisiveness and emotional control that would permit a natural integration of training and personal characteristics to

move him toward becoming an effective practitioner in emergency or trauma practice. Maternity services call for characteristics that are thought to be natural for the female and foreign to the male nurse. In addition, based on the unfounded assumptions that all male nurses are homosexuals and that homosexuality is rooted in a deep hostility toward women, the administrator no doubt thinks that the presence of a male in the maternity unity poses an actual threat to the patients. Childbirth is a period of great psychological vulnerability that would, by its quintessential female character, exacerbate the male homosexual's hostility.

Analysis of this illustration uncovers several important features of sexism as it is operant in nursing. First, there is an implicit theory about personality traits that are coordinated with sex, in which traits are identified as either masculine or feminine. Second, this coordination of traits and gender is the result of natural, rather than cultural determination. Third, various nursing services can be classified as more or less feminine and more or less masculine to the extent that practice in them involves a greater preponderance of feminine or masculine traits. Thus, nursing services seem to be arrayed in the administrator's mind along a continuum. At one end are characteristics perceived as wholly feminine, at the other end those wholly masculine. In between are mixtures of masculine and feminine characteristics, ordered according to how much utility is attached to decisiveness, empathy, diagnostic or mathematical reasoning, nurturing, or education.

The second illustration embodies an even narrower conception of feminine characteristics. Here, the physician's reaction to menstrual problems is that they are usually psychosomatic and involve hysterical conversions of physical signs and symptoms of menstruation by neurotic women. Menstrual tension is thought to be psychogenic in origin because the physical disorder categories familiar to the physician contain no element that would account for it. The fact that this might be due to a deficiency in the physician's knowledge or command of diagnostic categories, as opposed to a complex set of personality traits of women, would strike the physician as implausible. Both his training and his perceptions of women preclude drawing such a belief into question.

But the roots of this physician's response go deeper. Not only is it conditioned by a set of beliefs instilled through training and other cultural influences, it is an expression of a much more common physician response: loss of perspective that the patient is a whole person and not just a set of complaints and causes. The tendency of interns and residents to convert "the patient in room C-7 with cirrhosis of the liver" to "the liver in C-7" is notorious, rooted in medicine's preoccupation with diagnosis and treatment of organic pathologies and the fledgling physician's sense of the power of the knowledge he or she is struggling to master. Most physicians come through this stage showing respect to patients whose complaints are based on identifiable organic lesions; the physician is never so civil and supportive as when he can exercise his powers to the patient's benefit and appreciation. But the patient whose complaints defy the diagnostic powers of the medical model, or whose organic complaint defies treatment, tends to challenge the limits of the physician's knowledge. Because physicians do not learn to deal with the finitude of their powers but instead learn to practice with the heady sense of omnipotence, such patients are dismissed in some way. When viewed from the perspective of medical education and the sexist account of the female character, the behavior of the physician who dismisses menstrual cramps by saying that the patient is not really sick is not so surprising.

The third illustration gives another insight into the dynamics of sexism. Because of the dichotomies of masculine and feminine traits and identification of nursing chiefly as a feminine occupation and medicine as a masculine one, the female physician becomes enmeshed in a Catch-22 situation. Unfortunately, part of the bind is created by the perceptions and attitudes of nurses themselves. That is, just as a male nurse was perceived by the hospital administrator as a frustrated physician, so a female physician is frequently perceived by male physicians and nurses as a frustrated male. It is rather shocking to read, for instance, Florence Nightingale's description of the few female physicians of her day, "They have only tried to be men, and they have succeeded only in being third-rate men."[13]

Having adopted a profession that is perceived as essentially a masculine one, a female physician (like a male nurse) is perceived as a walking contradiction, as unnatural, involved in a complex denial of her natural propensities. Unfortunately, these attitudes can be easily acquired by the female physician herself. To prove that she is as good a physician as her male colleagues, she will become (1) uncompromisingly authoritarian with respect to subordinate

nursing staff, (2) possessed by the discipline and intellect of the male physician, and (3) increasingly devoid of the more feminine characteristics, whose mixture in her personality and behavior might be perceived as indicating a confusion of sex identity. It is difficult enough for a woman to enter a man's profession; but it is perceived as inappropriate, with homosexual overtones to act like a man in that practice, just as it is for a male nurse to display maternal characteristics while practicing a woman's profession. Women who enter the medical profession receive less subtle cues about their sexual identity in those specialities that cast them in quasi-maternal support roles. Therefore, a significant number of female physicians specialize in pediatrics, family practice, and psychiatry, and not in surgery and emergency medicine.

Finally, the fourth illustration shows that the nursing profession's internal system of advancement and rewards is perhaps marred by discriminatory attitudes and practices. One must again postulate the belief that either inherent or culturally ingrained differences between male and female nurses justifies the disproportionate advancement of male nurses to positions of administrative power. The illustration suggests how this may happen. A female nurse's behavior that would be perceived in a man as signifying qualities of leadership and administrative skill is viewed as inappropriate in a woman. There is a kind of pejorative conjugation at work: he is persistent, aggressive, ambitious; she is stubborn, pushy, overreaching. He is on good terms with the administrator; she plays up to the administrator. He has his favorites among the subordinate staff; she is cliquish.* As a result, it becomes far more difficult for a female to achieve advancement in competition with similarly qualified males; a much narrower range of behaviors is deemed appropriate and tolerated. Like Caesar's wife, the female nurse who aspires to advancement must be above and beyond reproach.

ETHICAL ANALYSIS OF SEXISM IN THE HEALTH PROFESSIONS

Establishing that sexism is a major ethical problem for nursing is yet a further task. Fenner sees the chief objection to sex stereotyping in nursing

---

*These are characterizations that I heard while working as an employment counselor in a personnel agency, when checking applicants' references or interviewing personnel directors to determine why positions were vacant.

and medicine to be its cost. "The assumption of appropriate behavior and attributes on the basis of gender prevents health consumers and health professionals alike from realizing their true roles and contributions to and benefits from the health care system. . . . The limitation of a person by pigeon holing according to characteristics other than capabilities and capacities is not only unfair; it's wasteful."[14] Of course, the health care industry in a society of plenty has not been moved by accusations of waste. Nadelson and Norman come closer to the mark in saying, "As a result, the wide range of talents and abilities of many providers is not utilized."[15] But such waste is perceived as tolerable, since a reasonably high standard of care is maintained. Ashley argues that the systematic injustice against women in the health sciences has resulted in adverse effects on the quality of health care that is delivered.[16] This observation provides a major ground for ethical criticism of sexist patterns of inclusion and exclusion.

Fenner's point that sexism is unfair is perhaps the other most important wrong in an external critique of the situation. Sexism has robbed the public of the best possible health care by pitting professionals against one another in the "doctor–nurse game," with the patient usually suffering the effects.[17] Sexism has delayed advances in our medical understanding of problems identified wrongly as psychosomatic. Sexism violates the fundamental guarantees of a society that prides itself on its commitment to equality of opportunity. Such opportunity extends to those hardy women who survive entry into the professions, but who all too frequently become disillusioned and leave them in droves.[18] The terrible impact in discovering that one's abilities and acquired skills are devalued solely on the basis of sex, and that one possesses a kind of second-class citizenship in the world of power, despite all one's efforts at professionalization is responsible in the eyes of one psychologist for the "well established fact that women are two to three times more prone to depression and hysteria than men."[19]

The last observation suggests the major ethical wrong of sexism in terms of the values within medicine and nursing. Sexism tends to be self-confirming—that is, it is a normal tendency for people to behave as they are expected by others around them. When the dominant perceptions of women—whether patients or nurses or physicians—are sexist, a climate of expectations and interpretations is created in which the so-called feminine characteristics are rewarded and the so-called masculine characteristics are discouraged

in women—the reverse being true for men. Hence, even the male nurse who knows he is heterosexual struggles with the subtle challenges to his masculinity and tends to traverse the paths where he encounters the least resistance—paths leading into those levels and divisions of nursing that are perceived as more appropriate for men. Women, who possess the drive and qualities of decisiveness and leadership to become administrators or emergency or trauma nurses, either become discouraged in those efforts by the lack of sympathetic support mechanisms or find that they must suppress the more affectionate, nurturant parts of their personalities and learn to play at "being men." Nightingale's unfortunate observation missed the central facts underlying her perception of women physicians. It is "inappropriate" for women to become physicians but acceptable for them to become nurses because of the way those professions are biased, not because of any inherent link between the qualities of a good physician or a good nurse and sex-dependent features of character. The tragedy of sexism in health care is that it is ultimately an iatrogenic phenomenon, self-confirming, not based on a realistic assessment of the potentials and possibilities for human growth and development that still remain unexplored promises of the free society.

The terrible irony is that medicine and nursing, with the historically persistent commitment to the Hippocratic maxim, *primum non nocere*—above all, do no harm—are structured in practice so as to preserve a set of assumptions that may well produce as much harm as any pathogenic agent.

DEALING WITH SEXISM IN NURSING AND MEDICINE

There are no easy prescriptions for dealing with sexism in a profession. Nevertheless, one may gain some perspective on it if one thinks about how sexism manifests itself in one's own life, works constructively on those aspects that are amenable to change, and adopts an understanding, indirect intolerance for the rest.

One's personal sexist attitudes and practices may be the most difficult things to perceive, and, having perceived, to change effectively. The illustrations suggest places in one's professional practice in which sexist attitudes intrude. For instance, one might deal with one's reactions to male nurses and female physicians by using more sensitivity and circumspection. Empathy for such individuals may provide them with deeply needed encouragement and support. A similar attitude can be taken with patients—that is, by seeking to maintain the same standards of professionalism in one's behavior toward male and female clients, one may clarify the degree to which one's personal attitudes have been influenced by sexist thinking. Finally, one can establish a bulkhead against sexist undermining of one's own enlightenment by good-spirited but firm resistance to being subjected to sexist patterns of discrimination by both physicians, other nurses, and even patients.

One caveat: Focusing most of one's efforts against sexism at the personal level may invite extreme frustration, for sexism, like other forms of prejudiced thought, tends not to yield to direct confrontation. A digression into the history of science can clarify the point.

Even in so supposedly rational an enterprise as scientific theory construction, validation, and replacement, the history of science shows that theoretical revolutions occur not through conversion of the proponents of one theory by those of another but rather through their replacement. Adherents to theories such as geocentrism or phlogiston tended to maintain their adherence to those theories despite mounting contrary evidence and the availability of promising alternatives. Theoretical change occurred mainly by the emergence of generations of younger scientists who did not accept the old views; instead, they were excited by the promise and prospects of developing alternatives that contained fewer of the old anomalies and presented a fresh set of new problems.[20,21]

Like some scientists, sexists generally do not change when challenged with evidence that runs contrary to their views. This occurs in part because they insulate themselves from criticism by employing tactics such as creating *ad hoc* criteria for the admissibility of contrary evidence. Firmness and diplomatic resistance can sometimes limit their power to enforce their sexism, but the real change comes when new generations, who have acquired views that are less oriented toward preservation of the status quo, move into positions of leadership.

It becomes important, then, to make an impact on the problems of sexism at the educational level. Actions to be taken can range from encouraging the admission of individuals into professional study who are not predisposed toward the older sexist views of the professions to restructuring educational faculties, course materials, and content so that unquestioned assumptions of previous generations can be subjected to critical scrutiny. This process gradually creates role models in both professional education and practice who have successfully resisted the biasing influences of their education, and who, by precept and example, serve as living refutations of the powerful assumptions of sexist psychology. As Stromberg observes, "Nursing educators need to become aware that the prevalent conforming orientation of the female precludes the acquisition of those traits which are valued by the profession . . . the resolution of this disharmony can be facilitated by providing time within the curriculum to explore with the students the inherent conflicts of the two roles (sex role and professional role) and to provide opportunity for the students to verbalize how they can most effectively deal with this conflicted area."[22] Similar counsel, of course, can be extended beyond basic preparatory programs to administrators of continuing nurse education and inservice programs.

The nurse who perceives her or his role as independent of sex-determined qualities, who openly encourages that view in others, and who supports those who run counter to the prevailing gender distributions in the professions may not see the day when sexism in nursing becomes a thing of the past. But that nurse will nonetheless have contributed to the eventual liberation of the health professions from this wasteful, harmful, and unfair bias.

REFERENCES

1. Nadelson, C. C., and Notman, M. T. Women as health professionals. In *Encyclopedia Of Bioethics*, ed. by W. T. Reich. New York, The Free Press, 1978. Vol. 4, pp. 1713–1720.
2. Hull, R. T. Defining nursing ethics apart from medical ethics. *Kans.Nurse* 55:5, 8, 20–24, Sept. 1980.
3. Nadelson and Notman, *op.cit.*, p. 1716.
4. *Ibid.*, p. 1717.
5. Sidel, V. W. The right to health care: an international perspective. In *Bioethics and Human Rights*, ed. by E. L. Bandman and Bertram Bandman. Boston, Little, Brown & Co., 1978, pp. 341–350.
6. Cleland, V., and others. Decisions to reactivate nursing career. *Nurs.Res.* 19:446–452, Sept.–Oct. 1970.
7. Churchill, L. Ethical issues of a profession in transition. *Am.J.Nurs.* 77:873–875, May 1977.

8. Fenner, K. M. *Ethics and Law in Nursing*. New York, D. Van Nostrand Reinhold Co., 1980. pp. 182–183.

9. *Ibid.*, p. 183.

10. Steele, S. M., and Harmon, V. M. *Values Clarification in Nursing*. New York, Appleton-Century-Crofts, 1979, p. 144.

11. Fenner, *op.cit.*, pp. 181–182.

12. *Ibid.*, p. 183.

13. Ehrenreich, B., and English, D. *Witches Midwives and Nurses: A History of Women Healers*. 2nd ed. Old Westbury, N.Y., Feminist Press, 1973.

14. Fenner, *op.cit.*, p. 184.

15. Nadelson and Notman, *op.cit.*, p. 1718.

16. Ashley, J. A. *Hospitals, Paternalism, and the Role of the Nurse*. New York, Teachers College Press, Columbia University, 1976.

17. Stein, L. I. The doctor–nurse game. *Arch.Gen. Psychiatry* 16:699–703, June 1967.

18. Wolf, G. Nursing turnover: some causes and solutions. *Nurs.Outlook* 29:233–236, Apr. 1981.

19. Lewis, H. B. Sex differences in adaptation to exploitative society. In *Bioethics and Human Rights*, ed. by E. L. Bandman and Bertram Bandman. Boston, Little, Brown & Co., 1978, pp. 299–304.

20. Kuhn, T. S. *The Structure of Scientific Revolutions*. 2d ed. Chicago, University of Chicago Press, 1970.

21. Lakatos, I., and Musgrave, A., eds. *Criticism and the Growth of Knowledge*. Cambridge, England, The University Press, 1970.

22. Stromberg, M. F. Relationship of sex role identity to occupational image of female nursing students. *Nurs. Res.* 25:363–369, Sept.–Oct. 1976.

These Men Worry Me

Catherine Watson

I LIKE working with male nurses—generally, they are kind and straight-forward. Usually they are competent nurses, and usually they are relaxing company. They don't sulk in the sluice, go off in a huff or moan under their breath in the canteen about other nurses.

But I am worried by them. I am worried about what they are doing *in* nursing and I am worried about what they are doing *to* nursing.

Events of the past week have done nothing to allay my worries. First, there are the nominations for the UKCC. The figures will have changed slightly by the time this column appears, but it appears that 50 per cent of the nurses standing for the UKCC are men—a percentage much larger than the number of men in nursing (only 10 per cent of nurses are men, and most of them are psychiatric nurses; in general nursing it is about 3 per cent).

Second, there was the business of George Castledine. George, as I am sure most of you know, is a lecturer in nursing at Manchester University, the co-author of a book on the nursing process and a writer for *Nursing Mirror*. For those of you who have not seen him in person, he is also a big, beefy, handsome and incredibly nice fellow.

I recently heard him give a lecture on the nursing process in which he said in essence that the nursing process will give nurses a voice. With a logical approach to their work, nurses will gain self-respect and the respect of others.

To illustrate this he described a scene from the television series *Doctor's Dilemmas* in which a nurse was asked to explain her actions and beliefs about a patient. Apparently she could not and lapsed into confusion. As George told this anecdote, he became the nurse. His shoulders rose up to his ears in shyness. His head tilted to one side in timidity and hesitancy. His voice faltered. And his face broadcast the message: "What I think is not important. My opinions have no value."

Now his diagnosis was that here was a nurse who badly needed the nursing process. Had she had it, she would have confidently stated her case. She would have known why she did what she did and she would have said so.

My diagnosis, on the other hand, was that the nurse was a woman and that, nursing process or no nursing process, she would not have ever confidently stated her point of view in front of the cameras.

But what worries me about this incident is that George and I saw two different scenes when we looked at the same incident. He came away thinking "We need the nursing process." While I, empathising with that poor nurse facing the television cameras, came away thinking: "We need to help women to believe in themselves."

He concluded from this scene that the nursing profession must implement the nursing process correctly. While I concluded that the nursing profession must be sensitive to, fight against and *not contribute to* the socialisation of women into passive unconfident people.

If he, a male nurse, and I, a female nurse, interpreted so differently the same incident, what is going to happen to nursing when an increasingly male leadership interprets what it is that the bulk of nurses (women) want? I predict a leadership more and more out of touch with the needs of nurses.

But given that men are socialised from birth to have high self-esteem and high expectations of themselves, is it the nursing profession's fault if male nurses surge up through the ranks and into positions of authority?

Watson, C. (1983, March). These men worry me. *Nursing Mirror, 156,* 32. Reprinted with permission of © *Nursing Times.*

Well, this is where the "student's view" comes in. I cannot prove it, it is only an educated guess on my part. And I would love corroboration or contradiction from other nurses. But I think male student nurses are treated differently from female students.

Male student nurses are regarded as exceptional. They are treated as more mature and more authoritative than their female counterparts. They come under less criticism because, unlike female nurses, there is no stereotype to which they must conform, and in fact, their eccentricities are often viewed with tolerance or even enjoyment by senior nurses.

This difference in treatment helps male student nurses to trust in their abilities and to envisage themselves in jobs of responsibility.

Since nursing incorporates many attributes that are traditionally female—such as empathy—a male nurse *is* exceptional when he shows those attributes. This leads us to praise in male student nurses what we expect from female student nurses.

I remember being moved when I saw a male student nurse sit down with a confused and upset patient and quietly stroke the patient's head until he had calmed down. What a compassionate man, what a good nurse, I thought. And he was.

But I realise now that much of the impact of that scene lay in the fact that it was a man being gentle and kind. I would have been less moved if the nurse had been a woman—I would have expected compassion.

So what needs to change to ensure that nursing does not acquire a leadership unrepresentative of most nurses? I do not think that the confidence of male student nurses ought to be undermined, but I do think nursing needs to be aware of the sexism that leads us to overvalue the work of men and to take for granted the creativity, energy and competence of women.

Sisters and tutors should encourage female student nurses to believe in their ability and to pursue jobs of leadership. They should also ask themselves whether, in fact, they are more lenient with male student nurses and have different career expectations of them.

Finally, I think male nurses at all levels should ask themselves whether they understand the experience of their female co-workers and whether it really is in the best interests of nursing that they speak for them.

STUDY AND DISCUSSION QUESTIONS
THE NURSE–PHYSICIAN RELATIONSHIP: I. SEXISM AND HIERARCHY

1. Stein's article on the doctor–nurse game was published in 1967. Do you think this game is still being played?

2. Do you think there is something distinctive about the educational and historical backgrounds of these professions that accounts for the doctor–nurse game or is it inherent in any power hierarchy such as employer–employee?

3. If Stein is correct and other professions will not play the doctor–nurse game with physicians, how can we account for that?

4. Is the doctor–nurse game merely a sign of respect for physicians and tact or is it inherently demeaning?

5. Should nurse's play the game if that's what it takes to meet the client's needs with certain doctors? That is, does the end of client care justify the means?

6. Can the doctor–nurse game be called sexist even if male nurses play it?

7. Cleland's 1971 article claimed that the sex discrimination that goes along with being a female occupation in a male-dominated culture is nursing's most fundamental problem. Is this still a problem today?

8. Why has nursing attracted so many women and so few men?

9. What would make nursing attractive to men?

10. Cleland suggested two kinds of classifications: one for nurses who do not want the freedom and responsibility that goes with it and another for professionally autonomous nurses who will take risks and make decisions and who might be called "nursologist." Do you agree?

11. Do you think it is true that males typically exhibit qualities good physicians need and that females typically exhibit qualities good nurses need?

12. Cleland predicted in 1971 that unless nursing altered its image it would have recruitment problems. Was she correct?

13. Do you agree with Hull's pessimism regarding the changing of sexist attitudes?

14. Should schools of nursing attempt to change the views of students if they see the nursing role as having certain sex-linked qualities?

15. Do female nurses overvalue the contributions of their male colleagues?

16. Why is it that men assume positions of power and leadership in nursing disproportionate to their numbers?

17. Can men accurately represent the desires of the majority of nurses?

18. How would you assess the situation of the nurse described by Watson? Is her timidity due to socialization as a woman, as Watson believes, or lack of command of the nursing process as George Castledine claims?

19. Is the title "nurse" appropriate today or would another title enhance or alter some stereotypical mind sets?

5

The Nurse–Physician Relationship:
II. Somera and Tuma

INTRODUCTION

As particularly noted in the Winslow article (Chapter 1), two cases have been significant in the evolving role conception of the nurse. The first is the case of Filipino nurse Lorenza Somera who was sentenced to a year in prison for the death of a 13-year-old girl undergoing a tonsillectomy. Somera had merely carried out a confirmed order for cocaine when the doctor had apparently wanted procaine. Somera had acted precisely as she had been trained and nursing textbooks of the time had prescribed. Somera was not to question the orders of a physician except to verify it. This she did but was nevertheless held criminally liable for her action.

The frequently cited case of Jolene Tuma is more recent. Tuma was acting according to the prescriptions of the ANA Code for Nurses and attempting to meet the informational needs of a cancer patient. She thought she was acting within the scope of professional practice. However, the Idaho Board of Nursing agreed with a complaining physician that Tuma had unprofessionally interfered with the doctor–patient relationship and suspended her license for six months.

Sensing the importance of this case, Tuma brought it to public attention through a letter to the editor of *Nursing Outlook*. That letter and the related editorial, "The Right to Inform," by Edith Lewis sparked a prolonged debate in that journal. Those letters are anthologized here. Also included is Sister Teresa Stanley's analysis of the case.

THE SOMERA CASE

The 1929 case of Lorenza Somera was brought to the attention of nurses through articles by Elizabeth Grennan in *I.C.N.* (reprinted here) and a briefer notice in the *American Journal of Nursing*.[1] Somera was the only person convicted in the death of the 13-year-old patient. The International Council of Nurses, however, with the help of others was able to effect a conditional pardon for Somera. Grennan views the Somera case as an apparent tragedy that has worked out for the good of the profession. In convicting Somera, the courts made it clear that following orders was not a defense available to nurses. In doing so, Grennan asserts, "these decisions . . . lift nursing from a subservient place to one of equality in responsibility and dignity with that of the doctor."

THE TUMA CASE

At the beginning, the Jolene Tuma case focused on "the right to inform" and the meaning of unprofessional conduct, but as reaction to the case grew and new information emerged the issues became more complex. We have set out here the historical record of the reaction to the Tuma case as it appeared in the pages of *Nursing Outlook* from September 1977 to July 1979. A digest and analysis of the entire case is contained in Teresa Stanley's "Ethical Reflections on the Tuma Case: Is it Part of the Nurse's Role to Advise on Alternative Forms of Therapy or Treatment?"

The letters to the editor can be *roughly* described as falling into three categories: (1) informative, (2) supportive of the issues raised, and (3) critical.

Among the informative letters are Bullough (who mentions the content of the Idaho Nurse Practice Act), Bejsovec (who explains why the Idaho Nurses' Association supported the decision to suspend Tuma's license), and Vahey (who comments on the Idaho Supreme Court's ruling that reversed the decision of the Idaho Board of Nursing).

The majority of letters were supportive of Tuma or the issues raised by the case.[2] These letters saw the Tuma case as emblematic of the grave difficulties besetting the profession.[3] Among the issues raised are concern about professional autonomy, the rights of patients, the control of nursing, nursing practice acts, the failure of the board to recognize the ANA Code for Nurses, the failure of professional organizations to support Tuma's actions, the disagreement among nurses about professional role responsibilities, and concern that the ideals expressed in the code and taught by nursing faculty may lead to the suspension of the license of any nurse who practices accordingly.

Some letters, however, were critical of Tuma—Baldini, Wilson, Hohle, and Ferguson and Fletcher. A common theme of these letters is the breakdown of communication, collegiality, and teamwork. Underlying much of this criticism is the view that nursing is a subordinate profession. Baldini writes, "Our duty is to follow the physician's orders, not compete with him in the treatment of a patient. . . . True, the patient has the right to know, and the nurse has the right to inform, but only if she has the physician's consent." Ferguson and Fletcher believe that meeting with the patient and family, disclosing the side effect of a drug, or mentioning alternative treatments in the absence of the physician or without the physician's consent is to assume the "medical management" of the patient and thus interfere with the physician–patient relationship.

A full presentation of the facts of the case is made in Stanley's article, but it is worthwhile to clarify a point of dispute in the letters. According to the Bejsovec letter, one of the reasons the Idaho Nurses' Association supported the decision of the Board of Nursing was that ". . . the physician's course of treatment . . . was interrupted." This leaves the impression that the interruption was Tuma's doing. The facts as stated in the Idaho Supreme Courts' opinion[4] make it clear that it was the doctor who stopped the chemotherapy without discussing it with either Tuma or the patient. He cancelled the treatment when he was informed by the patient's daughter-in-law that the patient had some questions about the therapy and that the family was going to meet with a nurse to talk about it. The treatment and the meeting were scheduled for 8:00 PM. The doctor resumed treatment after the meeting at 9:15 PM. The patient had never refused the treatment.

A related issue that deserves some mention is the criticism of the Idaho Board of Nursing, the Idaho Nurses' Association, and the American Nurses' Association Committee on Ethics for their actions or lack thereof. In this vein are the letters of Partridge, Storlie, and Summers as well as Stanley's article. Storlie writes, "The Idaho Board of Nursing has in my opinion, made an error that will go down in history to the shame of nursing."

NOTES

1. Elizabeth M. Grennan, "The Ultimate Problem of Ethics: A Brief Review of the Somera Case," *American Journal of Nursing* 30 (June 1930):733–734.
2. Nurses in general may have been more supportive of Tuma than the actions of the Idaho Board of Nursing and the INA would suggest. In 1981, *RN* published a survey of 12,500 nurses that, among other things, asked a question loosely modeled on the Tuma case. The question was stated as follows:

   > A 54-year-old cancer patient is scheduled for surgery tomorrow morning. Extremely agitated, he tells his nurse, "I'm really scared about this operation. There *must* be other treatments, but the doctor refuses to tell me about them. Can't you help me?" The nurse fully explains the various alternatives but avoids making any recommendations. Afterwards, the patient clearly seems relieved and remarks to the nurse on the way out, "Well that certainly gives me a lot to think about!" Do you think the nurse was right in answering the patient's question?

   Eighty-three percent said the nurse did the right thing (while 17 percent thought the nurse violated the doctor–patient relationship. See Ronni Sandroff, "Protect the MD . . . or the Patient?: Nursing's Unequivocal Answer," *RN* 43 (February 1981)), p. 30.
3. Among letters in this category are Peplau, Phaneuf, Kohnke, S. Adasczik, Opie, Greene, King, Talento, Grissum, Summers, D. Adasczik, Mauksch, Partridge, Brose et al., and Storlie.
4. *Tuma v. Board of Nursing* 593 P.2d 711 (1979).

The Somera Case

Elizabeth M. Grennan

The case of the Filipino nurse, Lorenza Somera, who was condemned in May, 1929, at Manila to one year's imprisonment, in connection with the death of a young girl in the operating theatre, caused much concern and deep-felt sympathy in a large section of the nursing world during the latter half of last year. Miss Somera had been accused, together with Drs. Gregorio Favis and Armando Bartolome, of "homicide through reckless imprudence." The following is a summarized statement of this important case, and describes the course of events from the time of the operation down to the movement which ultimately secured Miss Somera's pardon, granted by the Governor-General of the Philippines.

FACTS AS STATED IN THE TESTIMONY

Several days previous to May 26th, 1928, Pedro Clemente took his daughter Anastacia Clemente, not yet fourteen years of age, to Dr. Gregorio Favis at Manila. After examination Dr. Favis decided to perform a tonsillectomy. He instructed the father and daughter to go to St. Paul's Hospital where he would perform the operation at 7 A.M. on May 26th.

Dr. Favis then called up Sister Mercedes at St. Paul's Hospital and had the operation fixed for the date and hour agreed. He said he would follow the same orders given in previous tonsillectomy cases done there.

The head nurse in the operating room on the morning in question was Lorenza Somera. Valentina Andaya and Consolacion Montinola were student nurses working in the operating room under Miss Somera. Consolacion Montinola was the sterile nurse, Dr. Bartolome was the assistant surgeon.

Dr. Favis arrived a little before 7 A.M., scrubbed his hands and examined the patient, who was already present. He then asked for 10 per cent cocaine with adrenalin and swabbed the throat of the patient. Before this was done, as the clock was striking 7, Dr. Bartolome arrived. He scrubbed and came to assist Dr. Favis. The sterile table was prepared with the solutions and other needed articles. Dr. Favis asked Dr. Bartolome for the novocaine solutions. Miss Montinola handed Dr. Bartolome a syringe of solution, which Dr. Favis received from him and injected into the patient. After a few minutes Dr. Favis asked for and injected more solution.

Dr. Bartolome noticed that the patient became pale and acted as if dizzy, and called Dr. Favis's attention to this. Dr. Favis said this was not unusual. Dr. Favis then asked for, received and injected a third syringe of solution. A few minutes later the patient showed symptoms of convulsions. Dr. Bartolome again called Dr. Favis's attention to the condition of the patient. Dr. Favis ordered adrenalin, which was injected. A second injection was also administered. The patient again showed symptoms of convulsions and died in a few moments.

Dr. Favis then asked if the novocaine was fresh. Miss Somera replied: "It was not novocaine but 10 per cent cocaine." Upon direct examination Miss Consolacion Montinola when questioned by the prosecution affirmed firstly that she did not know who prepared the drugs, and secondly that she heard Dr. Favis order cocaine with adrenalin for injection and also heard Miss Somera verify the order. When questioned by the defence she again testified

Grennan, E. (1930). The Somera case. *International Council of Nurses Congress, 5,* 325–333. Reprinted with permission of © International Council of Nurses Congress. All rights reserved.

that she heard the order given and verified. This point is important—even the prosecution brought out that Dr. Favis ordered 10 per cent. cocaine for injection and that Miss Somera verified the order.

The autopsy report and the testimony of Dr. Anzures showed that the patient was suffering from *status lymphaticus*. He also testified that such patients have been known to die with even so slight an injury as the prick of a needle; also that the organs of a person dying from this disease (after a very slight injury as the prick of a needle) which he had examined, were in practically the same condition as those of the deceased.

Facts not brought out in the trial are: that Miss Somera had only finished her training on May 20th, 1928; that she had not yet received her registration certificate and was not an experienced graduate, as stated in the prosecution; that Dr. Favis had operated for tonsillitis but once previously in St. Paul's Hospital and that Miss Somera had not been on duty in the operating room at the time; and that no order from Dr. Favis was given her before his arrival.

DEFENCE IN THE LOWER COURT

The defence was conducted by Mr. Courtney Whitney, who has been practising law in Manila for a number of years and previous to that time was a member of the Legal Department of the United States Army.

He brought out the following points:

1. That there was no competent evidence to clothe Lorenza Somera with the crime.
2. That if the testimony of Consolacion Montinola that Miss Somera prepared the drug is accepted, it must also be accepted that she did it upon the order of Dr. Favis. Her testimony must be either accepted *in toto* or rejected *in toto*.

Dr. W. H. Waterous and Dr. Rufino Abriol, both of whom had operated for many years in St. Paul's Hospital, testified that both in that institution and elsewhere nurses are under a semi-military training and are required to carry out the orders of the doctors for drugs. That when a doctor orders a solution for injection the nurse does not know how much he intends to use of the amount prepared. That furthermore a doctor learns the actions of drugs by administering them and that, therefore, the nurse's training and experience are not adequate to this knowledge and that this responsibility belongs to the doctor. They also testified that

cocaine both was and had been used for injection by many doctors.

A resolution approved by the Educational Section and by the Executive Board of the Filipino Nurses' Association was presented. This resolution affirmed that nurses are taught that they must not question the order of a doctor for drugs except to verify it. The Chairman of the Curriculum Committee of the Educational Section and Principal of a School of Nursing testified to the same, and nursing textbooks were presented to support the testimony.

3. That the prosecution had failed to establish whether the cause of death was due to cocaine poisoning or *thymus lymphaticus*. The testimony of Dr. Anzures, as given in the facts above, and that of Dr. Waterous indicate that the patient could have died irrespective of the solution used. "The fact that Anastacia Clemente died subsequent to surgical procedure does not in itself make any of those in professional attendance upon her *prima facie* responsible."

DECISION OF THE LOWER COURT

The case dragged along from May 26th, 1928, to May 7th, 1929, when the following decision was rendered:

Wherefore the Court absolves the two said accused, Gregorio Favis and Armando Bartolome, of the crime of which they are accused in this case, ... and declares Lorenza Somera guilty of the crime imputed in the complaint and in conformity with the provisions of Article 568, Section I, of the Penal Code, *without finding any modifying responsibility as none has been shown*, condemns her to suffer one year and one day imprisonment, to indemnify the heirs of the deceased Anastacia Clemente in the sum of One Thousand (1,000) Pesos with subsidiary imprisonment in case of insolvency and to suffer further the accessories provided in Article 61 of said Code and to pay one-third of the costs.

EXTRA LEGAL ASSISTANCE

On May 10th the Legislative Committee met, appointed Mrs. Diaz (President of the Nurses' Association) and Miss Macaraig (Chairman of the

Educational Section) to serve with the Chairman, Miss Grennan, as a Special Committee. The Special Committee was to take the following course: prepare articles for the newspapers; send the facts of the case to nursing journals throughout the world; present the whole case with request for advice to the International Council of Nurses; consult the medical advisers to the Governor-General.

A few days later materials for publication, setting forth the professional and humanitarian aspects of the case, were presented to Attorney Whitney for approval. As he had already filed the case with the Supreme Court and believed they would reverse the decision, and as the Committee might be liable for contempt of court if they discussed too freely a case pending before the Supreme Court, he advised the Committee to drop its programme. Dr. Waterous when consulted was of the opinion that the safer course would be to wait quietly and depend on the Supreme Court for justice. The Committee considered this advice carefully. (A high government official had just received a sentence for contempt of court.) However, after careful thought the three members of the Committee decided that this case was legitimate nursing business and must go before the International Council of Nurses; and also that the Medical Advisers to the Governor-General were sympathetic friends of nursing and that a confidential report to them could not do any harm. Furthermore, they judged that if any untoward results came from this course of action they would come to them personally.

Consequently a detailed report was prepared and one copy sent with Miss Macaraig to Montreal and another copy (with verbal explanation) filed with Colonel M. A. Delaney and Major George Lull at Malacañang.

THE DEFENCE BEFORE THE SUPREME COURT

Mr. Whitney based his plea before the Supreme Court on six points. In these he showed that the conclusions of the Court of First Instance were not supported either by the evidence or by the actual facts of the situation, all of which had not been brought out. He pleaded the case upon professional and humanitarian as well as legal grounds, bringing in and using those facts which had escaped the Lower Court.

THE SUPREME COURT DECISION

On December 20th, 1929, Justice Villareal with Justices Street, Ostrand and Johns, handed down the following decision:

Wherefore, finding the decision of the Lower Court to be in accordance with the facts and law, it is confirmed in all respects with costs against the appellant.

Ten days from the promulgation of this sentence, let sentence be entered accordingly, and five days later return the record to the Lower Court.

MOTION FOR RECONSIDERATION

As soon as this decision was announced Attorney Whitney filed a very carefully prepared Motion for Reconsideration.

PARDON

As a Motion for Reconsideration is only granted in very rare instances the Committee of Nurses began working for the pardon. A radio was sent immediately to the International Council of Nurses, asking their co-operation in securing a pardon. The Council had previously written the Governor-General drawing his attention to the professional aspects of the case, and asking his interest.

A petition to the Governor-General was prepared setting forth the professional and humanitarian aspects of the case. The Committee took the stand from the beginning and refused to withdraw from it: That this young nurse had merely followed the rules which she had been taught. That these rules had been formulated for the good of the general public and had been practised in every country where nursing has been known. That the Committee, representing the group which determined what a Filipino nurse should be taught, had seen to it that Filipino nurses were so taught. That this programme had been followed in the full faith and credit that it was in entire accordance with the law of the land; if it was not, we the leaders of the profession were guilty and culpable and not this young nurse. That the punishment should be ours and that making her a substitutionary sacrifice for us was a gross injustice that before God ought not to be.

This petition was presented to all the women's clubs in Manila and received unanimous approval. A copy was sent to each hospital and was signed by hundreds of nurses and scores of doctors.

Attorney Whitney secured the signature of two members of the Supreme Court who sat on the case (Justices Street and Ostrand) and presented the matter to the Legal Advisers to the Governor-General. The Committee visited the members of the Pardon Board[1] and the Legal Advisers and Medical Advisers to the Governor-General. All of these were in entire sympathy with the plea of the nurses and each did his part in bringing about the pardon.

It is reported that at midnight on January 30th, 1930, His Excellency Dwight L. Davis, Governor-General of the Philippine Islands, after a long conference with his Legal Adviser, Colonel Blanton Winship, signed a conditional pardon absolving Lorenza Somera from her sentence. The length of the conference is not to be interpreted as any reluctance on the part of the Governor-General to release this girl from a prison sentence. His Excellency was faced with two perplexing problems. One of the fundamental principles of American Government is that the Executive shall not interfere with the Judiciary. Also, pardons are granted upon good behaviour after part of a sentence has been served, and to pardon someone condemned by the Courts without his even entering the prison would establish a dangerous precedent. So to frame the pardon as to obviate these difficulties was a task requiring careful consideration.

On the morning of January 31st, 1930, Miss Somera, accompanied by the Committee, appeared before Judge Diaz and heard the pardon read.

Counsel for the defence inserted the following statement in the Court record:

Upon the confirmation of the sentence of this Court by the Supreme Court, on behalf of Lorenza Somera I sought from the Governor-General a full, unconditional pardon. This the Governor-General refused to consider on the ground that it was contrary to the policy of the Chief Executive to thus set aside the mandates of the Courts, but in view of the recommendation of two of the Justices of the Supreme Court who reviewed the case upon appeal, the unanimous recommendation of the Board of Pardons, and the petition of the Philippine Nurses' Association for executive clemency in some degree, as well as because of certain exceptional extenuating circumstances apparent to him in this case, the Governor-General remitted that part of the sentence as called for prison confinement, upon the condition that Lorenza Somera should not in the future violate any of the penal laws of the Philippine Islands.

Although disappointed in not being granted the full and unconditional pardon from the Governor-General which she had through her counsel sought, Lorenza Somera has formally accepted the conditional pardon His Excellency has extended.

I therefore hand the Court a signed copy of the conditional pardon of the Chief Executive and a signed copy of Lorenza Somera's acceptance thereof, and move the Court to order the release of the young nurse convicted, and the exoneration of her bond.

In reviewing this case we are casting no aspersion whatever on the Courts. We believe they were discharging their sworn duty in the application of the law. While we do not know the working of their minds in relation to the case, we would say that if their decisions were influenced by the thought that human life is precious and must be guarded at any cost, and that it can better be guarded by two responsible persons, a doctor and a nurse, rather than by one, a doctor and a less responsible person, we agree with them entirely. We not only agree with them but thank them for these decisions which lift nursing from a subservient place to one of equality in responsibility and dignity with that of the doctor.

But while we are grateful to these we want to pay a special tribute to those men, including His Excellency the Governor-General, the Legal Advisers, the Medical Advisers, the Pardon Board and the two members of the Supreme Court, who have hearts and minds big enough to admit that the most carefully and perfectly made human law sometimes fails, but that the law of God, which is true justice, never fails and must be put above human law. We wish also to express our appreciation of Dr. W. H. Waterous and Attorney Courtney Whitney who were our constant and unfailing friends

---

[1]The Pardon Board consists of Under-Secretary of Justice Torres, Colonel Sweet, of the Constabulary, and Dr. Jose Fabella, Welfare Commissioner.

during the darkest hours. These men were our professional, financial and legal backing. They defended the case for the sake of justice and the nursing profession and that without remuneration. The International Council of Nurses also sent a letter of appreciation to the Governor-General. All of these were thanked by the Legislative Committee both personally and by letter.

What at times looked like a tragedy has worked together for the good of our profession. We not only feel that the Philippine Islands are safe for nursing, but that we are sure of the sympathy and co-operation of our Government in effecting advances in nursing education which will not only greatly benefit the public here, but establish precedences of help to nurses everywhere. These plans have not yet been perfected and presented, but we have assurances of support.

One of the finest results of the Somera Case is the strengthening of professional consciousness in our group. The humblest nurse in the farthest place in the Philippine Islands is no longer an isolated, forlorn worker, but a part of a great organism that not only suffers when she suffers and rejoices when she is made glad, but is ready with advice and help—the International Council of Nurses.

The Right to Inform

Edith P. Lewis

First, read the letter that appears on page 546. It is ironic that it should appear in the same issue as an article about credentialing which discusses, among other things, nurse practice acts. "Licensure is presumed to prevent or eliminate poor practice," the author says, "because the process of licensure is controlled by the professionals concerned." Later, she points out that each profession holds this internal control to be essential, on the basis that ". . . only one's professional peers can judge competent practice."

Well, in the situation described in the letter, the nurse *was* judged by her peers—the board of nursing in her state—and found guilty. The decision was to suspend her license for six months because, in the words of the hearing officer (not a nurse), the nurse had violated the state's nurse practice act ". . . by interfering with the physician–patient relationship and thereby constituting [sic] unprofessional conduct." This ruling is now being appealed.

We bring this matter to the attention of our readers because we believe that, regardless of the specifics of this particular controversy—who was right and who was wrong—it represents a set of circumstances that, in today's health care climate, could arise again. If this is true, then the situation raises some urgent and realistic issues to which the profession must address itself. For a beginning, it forces us to think seriously about the meaning of "professional," since we are now confronted with a ruling which suggests that a major component of professionalism may be *not* to interfere with the physician–patient relationship.

This, then, leads us to the doctor–patient relationship itself and what the nurse did that interfered with it. Here, one can only speculate, but her alleged misconduct seems to have consisted of giving the patient information that the physician had not given her, did not believe should be given her, believed it not in his patient's best interest to have, or ran counter to his recommended treatment. The alternatives mentioned by the nurse (this all took place in March 1976, remember) are unconventional ones, but a careful reading of the hearing officer's report does not indicate that the *nature* of the information given the patient and her family was the point at issue. Rather, it seems to be that the nurse intervened in the situation at all.

And this brings us smack up against some values that nurses hold high these days: the nurse as the patient's advocate, her accountability to that patient, her responsibility in ensuring that the patient's consent to treatment is truly "informed"—that is, that he is aware of all the options. Another concept that nurses value—one that is frequently mentioned in the literature, emphasized in the education of students, and, as a matter of fact, spelled out in the Idaho nurse practice act—is to "make judgments and decisions regarding patient status and take appropriate nursing interventions."

In this situation, however, the judgment of one professional—the nurse—ran ahead on into the judgment of another professional—the physician. Which brings us to the old "captain of the team" question. We have gotten around this delicate issue by talking about "interdependent functions" and a collegial relationship. The latter, however, is a two-way street. The nurse may assert that she is the physician's colleague, but if the physician does not see her in those terms, what restrictions does this, or should this, place upon the nurse's functioning?

Among the "findings of fact" of the hearing officer is that the nurse presented the information to the patient and family ". . . without the knowledge and consent of the attending physician . . ." While the hearing officer did not directly link this observation with his finding of interference with the physician–patient relationship, the fact that it is mentioned at all raises one final question: Is there an implication here that, unless the nurse first secures the physician's consent, she must not discuss treatment alternatives with the patient? Or anything else, for that matter?

I do not raise these questions lightly, nor am I trying to prejudge the case. As I have thought about it, I have tried to put myself in the position of the patient, her family, the physician, and the nurse, and I have found myself troubled from all vantage points. Like most other nurses, I value the concept of the nurse as a self-directing professional, responsible for and capable of making independent judgments in the patient's behalf. But I also acknowledge that the law, as represented in the nurse practice acts and interpreted by the legally constituted authorities, determines the scope and limits of nursing practice. This situation suggests—to me, at least—that these two views of the professional practice of nursing are at variance.

The implications of the issues raised here—for our practice, our teaching, our responsibility to the public, and our claims for our profession—are far-reaching. Comments from readers would be most welcome.

Professional Misconduct?

Jolene L. Tuma

The patient's right to know has been well established by the publication of the Patients' Bill of Rights, but how about the nurse's right to inform?

The Idaho State Board of Nursing has given an order to suspend my license to practice nursing because I informed a terminally ill patient and her family, at their request, about alternate methods of treatment for cancer: namely, the natural approach such as nutrition, herbs, touch therapy, and Laetrile.

The board affirmed the hearing officer's conclusions that I was "unprofessional" because my actions disrupted the physician–patient relationship. The nurse practice act does not specify this type of action as being unprofessional. In fact, what I did was truly professional. It takes a true professional nurse to assess the needs, physical, emotional, and spiritual, of a dying patient and intervene accordingly. Both Kubler-Ross and Hans Maukksch express how poorly doctors do this and generally how poorly nurses react. I felt I was fully within the scope of nursing practice set forth in ANA's *Code for Nurses*. At my hearing, however, the ANA *Code* could not be entered as an exhibit because I was told it was not recognized by the board. "Professional shock" has overcome me at times lately.

Here was a 59-year-old woman, fully coherent, who had been told the night before by her doctor that she was going to die. He offered chemotherapy as a last resort. I approached this patient with the drug, accompanied by a student. The patient had been crying and, while I disclosed the side effects of this drug, she began to relate to me her own beliefs about God and herself. She had controlled her leukemia for 12 years with natural foods and she felt God would perform a miracle on her behalf. She was apprehensive about the drug, but gave consent because her son wanted her to take it. We discussed other forms of treatment for cancer and I told her they were not sanctioned by the medical profession. She asked me to return in the evening to talk with her son and daughter-in-law. I consented to do this. Her son, angry with the impending death of his mother, told her doctor. He brought charges against me.

Does the nurse have the right to assist the patient toward full and informed consent? Litigation against nurses already shows us we have the responsibility when we do not properly inform the patient. But do we have the authority to go along with this responsibility as the patient's advocate? Please consider "The Patient's Right to Know," published in the January 1976 issue of *Nursing Outlook*. Also "Therapeutic Touch: The Imprimatur of Nursing," in the May 1975 *American Journal of Nursing*.

Presently my case is being appealed to the state supreme court on the ground that the nurse practice act is void because of vagueness and was applied ex post facto.

This has been a long hard struggle, and I feel the general masses of nurses across the country should be participating, at least intellectually, in this perhaps precedent-setting event for nursing. I would appreciate your making this event public by giving it space in your journal.

Tuma, J.L. (1977, September). Professional misconduct. *Nursing Outlook, 25,* 546. Reprinted with permission of © American Journal of Nursing Company. All rights reserved.

Letters to the Editor of *Nursing Outlook:* The Tuma Case

The September editorial was informative and provocative and clearly outlined some ominous dimensions of a serious issue to which the strength of ANA and NLN should be brought to bear.

I'd like to raise a few other related questions. Is it really in the best interests of patients for a single one of the several health care professions to have unilateral control over the information given to patients? Do patients have autonomy and choice? Or, to put it another way, are the wishes of patients—for information from many sources, for example—to be respected and honored?

To put it more bluntly, who owns the patient? Who should control the choices and life of a patient? How should professionals view patients: as fragile china cups that break easily and must be protected, or as persons who have already survived stresses and strains and who are capable of using information to choose their own directions for living?

In the Tuma case it seems that the central issue—the patient's rights—is being overlooked, and the nurse practice act instead is put on the defensive. In such circumstances Illich (*Medical Nemesis*) sounds ever more convincing!—Hildegard E. Peplau, R.N., Madison, N.J.

While I would not have selected the same alternatives as Ms. Tuma did—and apparently the physician on the case holds the same misgivings about her choices as I do—that is beside the point. She has the right and the responsibility to listen to her patient, assess that patient's needs, and give the emotional support and information which she feels are called for.

I question the legality of the Idaho Board of Nursing's suspension of Ms. Tuma's license on the grounds that she interfered with the physician-patient relationship. I have the 1971 version of the Idaho Nurse Practice Act before me and I cannot find anything in it about not interfering with the physician–patient relationship. The Idaho statute differs from most state nurse practice acts in that it does not spell out the specific grounds for suspension or revocation of a license. It does indicate that in so far as possible these policies should conform to policies and practices of the American Nurses' Association, the National League for Nursing, and the National Federation of Licensed Practical Nurse State Associations, Inc. The pronouncements I have heard from these bodies in recent years have supported the right and obligation of nurses to assess their patients' needs for support and teaching and to give that support and do that teaching. Moreover, the Idaho definition of the practice of professional nursing includes "observation, care and counsel of the ill" (Section 54-1413). That is what Ms. Tuma did. It seems to me that the Idaho Board of Nursing has made an error.

I would like to see us unite to support this nurse. If we do not, all our recent talk about the patient's right to information and our right to professional status will be hollow rhetoric.—Bonnie Bullough, R.N., Long Beach, Calif.

The editorial clearly identifies critical issues in professional practice which relate to possible "interference" in the physician–patient relationship, while Ms. Tuma's letter centers on the nurse's right to inform and a confrontation which resulted from "informing" a patient.

I do not believe the facts as presented in the letter permit a judgment in the case. However, the situation raises the interesting question of whether "the right to know" and "the right to inform" are not far more complex than is generally recognized.

Letters to the editor of *Nursing Outlook:* The Tuma case. (1977, December), *Nursing Outlook, 25,* 737, 740, 742–743.

The focus on a "disrupted" physician–patient relationship suggests a simplistic view of rights. As a result, courts will center on physician–nurse conflict and territorial professional grounds. This raises a risk of precedent-setting decisions that will not be in the public interest, or in the legitimate interest of either profession.

The right to inform entails accountability, which requires sound clinical judgment about both content and timing of information, as well as concern for the patient and his well-being as the primary focus. The first admonition for physicians and nurses is that they shall do no harm to patients. This, alone, suggests the complexities involved in the who, what, when, how, and why of exercising the right to inform. These complexities are compounded because the patient's right to know is basic to his right to make informed decisions about his course of action in the face of various options.

In following through on the issues raised in the editorial, I urge highly disciplined thinking that goes to the root of values and value formation and then clearly establishes a moral ground on which nursing can stand as it increases, refines, and intensifies its professional interventions.

The Tuma case is an example of the need for such thinking.—Maria C. Phaneuf, R.N., San Diego, Calif.

The Tuma case seems to be one in which the goals of a nurse were in conflict with the rights of a nurse. Because the patient is our primary concern, we professional nurses tend to concentrate solely on what is best for the patient, sometimes overlooking the fact that the patient also has a physician.

We must never forget that there is a difference between the privileges of a physician and the privileges of a nurse. As nurses, our rights do not include suggesting treatments or drugs to a patient without the physician's consent, nor do they give us the authority to interfere with the treatment that a doctor has ordered for his patient. We do have the right to consult the physician in regard to his treatment for a patient, question his treatment, or suggest an alternate treatment to him; we do not have the right to suggest an alternate treatment to the patient.

Our duty is to follow the physician's orders, not to compete with him in the treatment of a patient. The nurse and physician must work together, not against each other, for the welfare of the patient.

True, the patient has the right to know and the nurse has the right to inform, but only if she has the physician's consent. We do not have the right to interfere with the physician–patient relationship,

only the right to be part of that relationship by working with the physician for the benefit of the patient. This case should remind us that there are boundaries and limits in the practice of nursing.— June Baldini, R.N., Nashville, Tenn.

The editorial is right. This situation does indeed raise some serious questions, not only for the professional who believes she must act as the patient's advocate, but also for me, a professor who teaches a graduate course in advocacy. Am I, for instance, teaching students to act in a manner that may well result in suspension of their licenses? If so, where does culpability lie?

Are we so divided and estranged from one another in nursing that what we teach in our professional schools can then be labeled as unprofessional by our nursing practice boards? Are these boards so estranged from their professional organization that they can ignore the code of ethics for nurses? Is the code we teach our students not recognized by a state nursing board? The answer seems to be "yes." If so, what a sad day this is for nursing in a year we call "The Year of the Nurse."

We have often said that if we don't get our act together, someone else will. In the same issue of *Outlook*, Lucie Kelly said that that time has already come, and someone else is.

Despite all the warnings we have had, and continue to hear (and ignore), one must raise the serious question of care. The word is a hallmark of nursing, but whom do we care for? Or should we ask, do we care at all for anyone? Do we care for students if we teach them to practice in a way that will get their licenses suspended? Do we care for nurses when we penalize them for practicing as professionals? And do we care for patients when we abandon them to states of unknowing because of our fear for ourselves?

These are serious questions which demand thoughtful consideration. Or have we become so indoctrinated by the hospitals and the medical profession that we are indeed even afraid to think? Where are our courage, our convictions, our principles? Have we compromised them all away in efforts to appease, to be loyal members of the team? Have we become so brainwashed in what some call the "interdependent" nature of the system that we are willing to sell out the authority over nursing practice and its autonomy?

Perhaps we should have a moratorium on admitting students to schools of nursing until we figure out what is safe to teach, a moratorium on nursing practice until it is safe to practice, or, perhaps, a moratorium on ourselves until we figure out what our principles are. Until we can straighten our profession out we can only advise each student and practicing nurse to seek within herself the principles of a caring practice; to act in a thoughtful manner that will bring honor on herself and her practice; to continue to care, no matter what the risk.

I believe that nursing today is beset by forces that it has never before seen, both from within and without, and it will take individual courage, thoughtfulness, and even prayer for it to survive. I suggest all three in equal doses.—Mary F. Kohnke, R.N., New York, N.Y.

It would seem that Ms. Tuma has been made a scapegoat by her fellow health care professionals. She made the tactical error of attempting to "captain her own ship" under a banner of accountability to her client, rather than sail a smoother course under orders from a more traditional physician-captain. Since I firmly believe that all health care professionals must be accountable in their own right for their own actions, the old view that nurses intervene only under a physician's orders is untenable to me.

And since I also hold to be both true and necessary the idea that clients are consumers with both the right and need to participate in decisions affecting their own health wellness outcomes, I find it difficult to understand the state board's action; in effect, it ordered Ms. Tuma's license suspended for intervening in a manner that served to protect her client's right to be given information influencing a health-related decision.

That the content of the information was not questioned, but rather the fact that she intervened at all in the situation, causes me profound concern for the future of professional nursing.

It frightens me to think that the Idaho Board of Nursing may be setting a precedent that will contribute in the future to downgrading nursing practice, in terms of nurses fearing reprisal in the event that they choose to practice as sentient, knowledgeable, caring, and accountable professionals.—J. Patricia Adasczik, R.N., Clark, N.J.

I believe that Ms. Tuma did nothing wrong and was punished unfairly—and by a committee of her peers!

The basic problem lies in the evolution of present day nursing, the socialization of women to subservience, and the control of nursing practice by

physicians. I find it interesting that doctors will allow us to do many things on their say-so, but resist all efforts to legalize those practices for nursing. Qualifications, patients' rights, demands from the public, and logic seem to have little bearing.

This incident reinforces my thinking that we very much need nurse practice acts that protect nurses and help to clarify nursing roles and responsibilities. Teaching patients is not a medical regime, it is a part of the health care regime.

This case also points to the responsibility of nurses not only to assess patient needs and develop therapeutic plans of care, but also to share the information with other team members and try to arrive at more mutual goal setting. The patient/client needs to be a part of the decision-making process.

This is not and will not be easy to accomplish, but I think we nurses must take the bull by the horns and become the responsible members of the team. We are stepping on what many other professionals consider their "turf" these days, and we will continue to experience retaliation. We will be more successful in our efforts and we will find more cooperation when we seek more cooperation. The patients' best interests will also be better served.—Nancy Opie, R.N., Cincinnati, Ohio.

Poor communications caused the entire incident, I believe. The patient had not communicated to her son what she actually wanted (and thus her consent was not really a consent); she also didn't communicate to her doctor what she actually wanted: an alternate form of cancer treatment.

Good communication between a patient and her physician—in the form of consent for treatment—establishes a team through which a goal is reached. If the ultimate goal of the physician–patient team is to arrest a disease process, the nurse functions as the link between the team and the goal. Actually, she serves as a member of the team; she "carries the ball." Without the nurse, the goal is not attained.

What happens if one member of the team decides to rescind her side of the contract? In this case, the patient began to question whether or not she really wanted chemotherapy. It was therefore the patient, not the nurse, who interfered with the physician-patient relationship. She should have informed the other team members (physician and family) of her new wishes.

This is where the responsibility of the professional nurse comes into play. If she is functioning as the link between the team and the goal, does she not also serve as the messenger from one end to the other? If the terms of the contract have changed, the doctor should be notified by either patient or nurse. Then the doctor will be able to respect the wishes of the patient. Ideally, he should welcome this information from the other team member, the nurse.

The fact that the nurse gave the patient information about cancer treatments is not an issue; the patient could just as easily have read about it. Does it make a difference that the patient asked the nurse and not the physician? Would he not have had to give her the same information? It was unfortunate that this was seen as a "disruption of the physician–patient relationship," when the nurse was merely fulfilling her role as the messenger of the patient to her family and doctor. The family, learning of the patient's reconsideration, should have communicated this to the doctor. Then the basic right of the patient to choose a particular treatment method would not have been violated, while the nurse could have been praised for identifying the true needs of her patient and ultimately drawing the team members together in respecting the patient's new status.—Paula Galandak, R.N., Middletown, Conn.

From where I sit it looks as though Ms. Tuma needed to go ahead with the medical order prescribed *with* the patient's consent *by* her physician —and *then* discuss the patient's misgivings with her physician at the earliest chance possible.

Collaborative nursing performed by nurse practitioners in many community health nursing settings requires varying degrees of physician input. But where prescription medication is concerned, and until laws are changed, we cannot act as independently as we would like.

Our influence with physicians can create an impact, however, with a "stop-and-think" approach to such dilemmas as the one so painfully described by Ms. Tuma.—Patience Wilson Cameron, R.N., Cleveland, Ohio.

I find it incomprehensible that a professional nurse has had her license suspended because she was acting as a patient advocate. We declare that the nurse's responsibility is to meet the patient's defined need for help. Clearly, Ms. Tuma identified and met the patient's need by informing her of alternative methods of treatment for cancer. The fact that the doctor brought charges against her and won the case proves to me that "R.N. is subservient to M.D."; we cannot move without doctor approval.

Obviously, if this case is defeated in the state supreme court we are still "playing games" with the doctor and are independent practitioners in name only. I feel that we as nurses have a professional responsibility to rally to the aid of this nurse. There is much more at stake than the license of a fellow colleague—namely, the role of the nurse in today's health care system.—Marie Greene, R.N., Boston, Mass.

The key issue, I believe, is the "physician–patient relationship"—whatever that is. The days of the old country doctor administering care to the grateful and ignorant patient, who gazed up with eyes of childlike trust and innocence, are long gone!

It seems to me that the burden should be on the physician to prove that Ms. Tuma had interfered with his "relationship." I'd be willing to bet that no scientific data can be found to support the belief that a "relationship" adds to or subtracts from a patient's chance for recovery.

Furthermore, if all Ms. Tuma told the patient was what was mentioned in her letter, it was only information that the patient could easily have found in any consumer magazine.

I'm certain there are many aspects of this case of which I am unaware. However, I can't help but feel that this nurse has been unjustifiably abused.— (Name Withheld), Alabama.

The editorial was far too benign concerning a question that is so vital to the basic concepts of individualized nursing care, proper nursing assessment, and informed consent. This nurse simply made the patient aware of all the options, in accordance with the patient's request.

Have we forgotten that our primary commitment should be to the individual patient—not the family, not the physician, but the patient? In this instance the nurse, very properly, put the interests of the patient first, answered her questions, and permitted her to express her fears. This, in my opinion, was proper nursing intervention and must have served to allay some of the patient's anxiety. This case raises issues that are vital to the nursing profession. We must not stand by, abdicating our responsibility to make our voices heard concerning this issue.—Walter King, R.N., Campton, Calif.

I support Jolene Tuma's right to practice professional nursing to its fullest measure. To this end, I am sending a copy of her letter and the September editorial to the political action committee of my professional organization.

In my roles as both practitioner of nursing and teacher, I hold dear the patient's right to know and the nurse's right to inform. To me, anything less would not be professional nursing.—Barbara Talento, R.N., Brea, Calif.

Surely, the doctor–patient relationship is not a part of Idaho's nurse practice act! And, surely, the doctor–patient relationship is no more sacred than the nurse–patient relationship. The implication from the information available is that it will jeopardize the physician's "claims" on the patient. If that is in fact the crux of the matter, our profession is in grave difficulty.

For a panel of so-called professional peers to affirm that a nurse is "unprofessional" because she disrupted the physician–patient relationship is beyond the scope of my imagination! To have that same panel refuse to recognize such an innocuous statement as the ANA *Code for Nurses* seems incomprehensible.

In my opinion, the professional nurses in this country should support any nurse who is being accountable to her patients and who is willing to risk the wrath that will likely befall her when she challenges others in more powerful positions. Especially when, through her actions, she demonstrates where they have failed to meet the total needs of the patient.—Marlene Grissum, R.N., Fayette, Mo.

More is involved in the Tuma case than "informed consent." The following statement from Pat Jory, president of the Idaho Nurses Association, explains why the INA board supported the state board of nursing's decision to suspend Ms. Tuma's license.

. . . The original complaint by the physician to the clinic administration and by them to the board of nursing was that the physician's course of treatment had been interrupted—which, in fact, it was. On that basis she was suspended.

Mrs. Tuma did what a lot of us do; she attempted to meet a dying patient's need to discuss her situation. As I understand it, during the discussion of the chemotherapy treatment she was about to begin, what some would consider as alternatives to that treatment were discussed. However, at the patient's request, Mrs. Tuma came back on her own to discuss those alternatives with the family without first talking with

the physician about the situation. She even asked them not to tell the physician they were discussing it. If she was a colleague of the physician, as she claimed, he should have been consulted.

Nowhere was there any indication that the nurse does not have the right to do patient teaching. The Patient's Bill of Rights indicates the patient has the right to knowledge about his treatment from any and all members of the health team. But it should be a team approach.

Laetrile (or vitamin B-17, as some refer to it) was only one of the alternatives discussed. Whether you favor its use or not, if she asked, the patient had the right to know something about it. The problem arose with Mrs. Tuma's indicating to the patient that this illegal drug could be made available to her. Whether we agree or disagree with the FDA's opinions, we, as professionals, should not promote therapy which is illegal.

Mrs. Tuma never discussed the alternatives as cures. But she did ask her student not to discuss the conversation. She did request that the family not discuss the conversation with the physician. And the physician's course of treatment—which is the present accepted medical treatment for the patient's diagnosis—was interrupted. On that basis, the Idaho Nurses Association board felt obligated to support the board of nursing's decision. . . .

The above appeared in the October issue of INA's newsletter. When the INA board decided to support the board of nursing's ruling, the following statement was released:

We recognize that the state board of nursing protects the consumer and that INA protects the professional nurse. However, the common goal is high quality patient care. Therefore, having considered the facts presented in the recorded testimony of the hearings of the Tuma case, INA supports the decision of the board of nursing.

—Joseph L. Bejsovec, executive director, Idaho Nurses Association, Boise.

Having been in circumstances similar to Ms. Tuma's, I can truly empathize. The whole situation is appalling, but the most disturbing part is that the state board, in effect, nullified (by failure to recognize) the standards of care adopted by the representative body of the nursing profession, the ANA. What are the priorities for nursing and who establishes them, if not nursing's representative? What is the point of teaching students to guide their care of patients according to the carefully developed guidelines agreed upon by the experts in the area, when the students can then pick up a magazine and read that someone was punished by the regulatory branch of nursing for using the guidelines?

Even sadder, unless the Tuma ruling is overturned, is that the stigma of suspension will follow her for the remainder of her career, even though it may have been undeserved. What a commentary on the state of the profession that we cannot even support our own. There are many nurses who through their own fault remain oblivious to the beliefs and practices of contemporary nursing. Why should someone so informed and courageous be punished?

I feel as though the profession has really been undercut from within. When are we going to have the power to become a truly objective, intelligent, self-regulating profession? If nurses cannot practice without feeling intimidated by the other disciplines caring for the patient—and, indeed, by members of the profession itself—some of us may choose not to practice at all, but rather to go into health fields other than nursing. At times we seem to be our own worst enemies.—Ann Summers, Hornell, N.Y.

Jolene Tuma defends her actions by citing patients' rights and the nurse's right to inform. But she does not mention the "colleague" relationship between the physician and nurse. The conclusion that one could draw, based on the information she gives, is that Ms. Tuma assumed that *she alone* was the patient's advocate.

Did Ms. Tuma relate to the physician as a colleague? Did she discuss with the physician the patient's apprehensiveness and invite him to participate in her discussion with the patient and family? Did she advise the physician that the patient and family had requested an appointment with her to discuss alternative cancer treatments so that he could be present if he wished? Did Ms. Tuma give the physician the opportunity to object or did she assume the physician would object?

I wonder if Ms. Tuma would have taken the action she did if the health provider had been another nurse instead of a physician.—Beth M. Hohle, R.N., Glendale, Calif.

One of the issues in the Tuma case is that of control. Who indeed is in charge? Is it the physician? Or is it the patient, who is crying out for some hope, however slight? Are nurses the patients' advocates or the physicians' handmaidens? Just what do our nurse practice acts say? Apparently they can be interpreted and misinterpreted arbitrarily.

As Lucie Young Kelly stated in "The Patient's Right to Know" (*Outlook*, January, 1976), the patient needs a nurse who cares and dares, who will stand up and be counted, and be punished, and fight back. Well, Ms. Tuma has taken a stand. I for one am impressed by her courage and by her concern for her patient.—Doris C. Adasczik, R.N., Toms River, N.J.

The issue has relevance not only for nursing but also for other professional groups in our society and for the general public. The basic issue is inherent in the question raised in the September editorial: "Is there an implication here that unless the nurse first secures the physician's consent, she must not discuss treatment alternatives with the patient? Or anything else for that matter?"

The same question might be asked about other professionals—for instance, a social worker, a psychologist, and a nutritionist, or a teacher and a psychologist—who work jointly in the delivery of services to the consumer. In other words, there are many instances where services are rendered collaboratively by two or more members of different professions. Under these circumstances one must ask: Is there always a rigidly defined captain of the team? And, if so, does this preclude professional autonomy and the exercise of those prerogatives to which each profession is committed? I believe that nursing as a profession needs to address itself to this issue, in a different way, perhaps, from the way in which the court in Idaho will adjudicate this matter.—Ingeborg G. Mauksch, Velere Potter Distinguished Professor of Nursing, Vanderbilt University, Nashville, Tenn.

This tragic event embodies so many of nursing's problems: nebulous, untested autonomy as a profession; divided, ineffective responses to attacks on professional boundaries (where were the ANA and INA in all of this?); disagreement among nurses as to what our real rights and prerogatives are and should be; and nursing's unwillingness (or inability) to recognize the precariousness of our "professional" status and to deal with it.

I'm afraid we prefer to perpetuate myths that beguile us. If this incident doesn't mobilize significant numbers of nurses to demand a full investigation and proper redress, nothing will, I fear. How much more significant this issue is than salary.—Kay Partridge, R.N., Baltimore, Md.

We are responding to the September editorial regarding the Tuma situation because there are important ethical and professional issues to be addressed.

Nurses and women are most sensitive to being excluded from the policy-making arena and to being considered less than professionals. In the profession's zeal for inclusion, as well as in advocating on behalf of the patient, nurses must not lose sight of the right of the physician to prescribe the medical therapeutic regimen. Concomitantly, as the health care team grows in size and complexity, the right of many to advocate for the patient must be recognized. The need for continuous dialogue and collaboration is crucial as all of us strive to provide the best, most humane, and responsive care for patients.

On the basis of the facts presented in Ms. Tuma's letter, which also appeared in the September *Outlook*, we must conclude that she acted unilaterally in three instances of the therapeutic management of the patient's care. Each instance considered alone constituted a compromise of the physician–patient relationship, but when all three are taken together, the suggestion is very strong that Ms. Tuma's decisions resulted in her assuming the authority of the physician in the patient's medical management.

(1) "I disclosed the side effect of this drug," she said. If the physician had not already disclosed the side effects in the context of offering chemotherapy, it was her responsibility to point out this omission to him and see that the proper information was given.

(2) "We discussed other forms of treatment for cancer and I told her they were not sanctioned by the medical profession." Discussion of alternate medical treatments is a necessity for informed consent, but the physician should be the one to review the alternatives. Again, if this important element was missing from the original discussion of chemotherapy, it was the nurse's duty to call attention to it and see that alternatives be explored.

(3) "She asked me to return in the evening to talk to her son and daughter-in-law. I consented to do this." The nurse allowed herself to be "triangled" between a patient and her physician, to the extent that she was perceived by the patient's son as a rival to the physician.

Ms. Tuma had other options, but she did not use them. She could have insisted that the issues of risk and alternative treatment had not been thoroughly explained and called for a meeting between her and the physician or the physician, nurse, patient, and family. If the physician had refused to meet, she could have justifiably refused to participate until these wrongs had been righted. An option of last resort was to report the facts to the person in administrative authority over the physician and withdraw from the patient's care. The *Code for Nurses* of the American Nurses' Association supports all of these alternatives.

We believe that Ms. Tuma's observations were sound. Here was a patient who had not been well informed and had not discussed her religious beliefs with her physician. She chose to tell the nurse instead of her second thoughts about chemotherapy. It happens frequently that the patient will reveal his true thoughts to someone other than the physician. Ms. Tuma made, in our view, the wrong decision by keeping the information to herself and proceeding to assume the responsibility that should have been the physician's. The original communication from the patient regarding her fears about the drug belonged to the physician as well as the nurse. Because Ms. Tuma deprived the physician of this knowledge she did him an injustice and, it could be said, even showed contempt for his real authority for the patient's medical management. It is ironic that a nurse so dedicated to being an "advocate" for the patient should exclude the physician from the knowledge of important information.

The outcome of having charges brought against her was inevitable when Ms. Tuma accepted the patient's suggestion for a family conference. The priority here was for skillful intervention by the nurse in the patient's behalf, not an assumption of responsibility for medical management. The skills of confrontation and negotiation are needed and must be learned and applied skillfully in today's complex care scene, with due regard for their effect on the patient.

The lesson from this case is that nurses (and physicians) should not restrict their options when in ethically charged situations. Possibly Ms. Tuma was afraid for herself and the patient and fear played a role in restricting her alternatives. Good communication, especially about strong feelings and fears, is a prerequisite for the maintenance of high ethical standards. Ms. Tuma, unfortunately, allowed herself to be cut off from others during the most important decisions she made.—Vernice Ferguson, R.N., Chief, Nursing Department, and John Fletcher, Assistant for Bioethics to the Director, The Clinical Center, National Institutes of Health, DHEW, Bethesda, Md.

We strongly support Jolene Tuma's nursing action and recognize those actions as falling within legal and moral functions of the professional nurse. The action taken against Ms. Tuma represents a frightening step backward in terms of the exercise of competent and independent nursing thinking. Furthermore, we strongly support her valid struggle and attempts to thwart a legal decision which is a blatant sabotage of nursing practice. As we perceive her actions, Ms. Tuma was not interfering with the physician–client relationship, but rather responding to the client situation in an attempt to meet identified and voiced client needs. As we understand it, this is the goal of the health team.

As the situation has been described, we also reacted to the seeming lack of team functioning and accountability to each other. What could have been a situation allowing for the clarification of the client's goals was turned into a professional power struggle, again replacing the importance of client needs with irrelevant role defensiveness.—Carolyn Brose, R.N., Chairperson, Department of Nursing Education, William Jewell College, Liberty, Mo.
(*This letter was also signed by the 11 other members of the department.*)

The Idaho State Board of Nursing has, in my opinion, made an error that will go down in history to the shame of nursing.

I have studied the complete transcripts of the Tuma hearing, and have reviewed the Idaho State Nurse Practice Act as well. I have talked at length with Jolene Tuma and have found her to be young, idealistic, soft spoken, articulate, and highly professional. More shocking than the verdict is the continued silence of the American Nurses' Association.

Finally, unlike the editor of *Outlook*, who asked innumerable questions in her editorial, I have just two: How shall I talk to the young about convictions? What shall I say about courage?

Respectfully, from a nurse who informs . . . — Frances J. Storlie, R.N., Vancouver, Wash.

I would like to comment on the recent ruling by the Idaho Supreme Court regarding Jolene Tuma, who was charged with unprofessional conduct by her state's Board of Nursing ("News and Reports," June). The main points of the court's findings were: (1) The Idaho Nurse Practice Act includes a listing of specific examples of unprofessional conduct, but this listing does not include the type of action alleged to have been committed by nurse Tuma; i.e., having a conversation with a patient concerning treatment after the patient had given informed consent for that treatment to the attending physician; (2) The Idaho State Board of Nursing has had the responsibility under the 1951 act which created the board to revise such rules and regulations as necessary in order to proceed with the implementation of the examination procedures for licensure, the award of licensure, and the removal of licensure. The court notes that the definition of unprofessional conduct has still not been extensively delineated; (3) The Idaho Supreme Court does take notice of the fact that the Board of Nursing is composed of a group of experts and that it is the position of the board that these experts are capable of deciding what is unprofessional conduct on a case-by-case basis. In the opinion of the court, however, such case-by-case decision making would be a intolerable situation and not legally permissible; (4) The court also notes that it was not the Board of Nursing that found Ms. Tuma guilty of unprofessional conduct. It was a hearing officer, a non-nurse, who made the decision. According to the Idaho Supreme Court, the hearing officer did not have the knowledge and experience to determine that Tuma had acted unprofessionally; and (5) The court reiterates its opinion that the board failed to supply members of the profession with a definition of unprofessional conduct.

In essence, the Tuma case was decided on a technical matter involving the lack of extensive delineation by the Board of Nursing about what constitutes unprofessional conduct. Without such extensive delineation, which should have included the specifics charged against nurse Tuma, the court finds that Tuma cannot be guilty as charged.

The major implications which may be drawn from this decision by the Supreme Court of Idaho are:

1. The Idaho Board of Nursing needs to develop an exhaustive list of actions which may be considered unprofessional conduct. This need could conceivably be applicable to the other 49 state boards of nursing. The development of such a list would be an overwhelming task.

2. The original question would have to be answered: Does a conversation between a nurse and a patient concerning prescribed medical treatment after a patient has given informed consent to his physician interfere with the physician–patient relationship and thereby constitute unprofessional conduct? Nurses in Idaho are placed in a particularly difficult bind on this matter of discussing prescribed medical treatments with patients because of a provision within the medical consent law of that state. Specifically, Idaho Code 39-4304 states that "consent for the furnishing of hospital, medical, dental or surgical care, treatment or procedure shall be valid

in all respects if the person giving it is sufficiently aware of pertinent facts respecting the need for, the nature of and the significant risk ordinarily attendant upon such a patient receiving such care, as to permit the giving or withholding of such consent to be a reasonably informed decision. Any such consent shall be deemed valid and so informed if the physician or dentist to whom it is given or by whom it is procured has made such disclosures and given such advice respecting pertinent facts and consideration as would ordinarily be made and given upon the same or similar circumstances, by a like physician or dentist in good standing practice in the same community. As used in this section, the term 'in the same community' refers to the geographical area ordinarily served by the licensed general hospital at or nearest to which such consent is given."

In the Tuma case, according to the transcript of the hearing, the patient's physician did indeed fulfill his legal responsibility as prescribed in the above code. It is apparent from the transcript of the hearing that the patient did give consent for treatment with chemotherapy on the preceding day; however, on the day the treatment was actually to begin, when nurse Tuma was in attendance, the patient appeared to have second thoughts. Ms. Tuma then advised the patient about an alternative therapy—a natural approach which included nutrition, herbs, touch therapy, and Laetrile. One question, then, that still remains unanswered is, "What is the appropriate role of the nurse when confronted with such a situation?"

3. This case raises at least one additional question: What would have been the outcome of the case if Ms. Tuma had been charged with interfering with the physician's fulfillment of his legal duty under Idaho Code 39-4304? It appears that an answer to this question would reach to the core of the matter concerning such issues as the nurse's right to inform patients, to act as patient advocate, and to function in a collegial relationship with physicians.—Jo Ann T. Vahey, R.N., Boise, Idaho

Ethical Reflections on the Tuma Case:
Is It Part of the Nurse's Role to Advise on
Alternate Forms of Therapy or Treatment?

FACTS OF THE CASE

The client, Ms. W, was 59 years old and acutely ill with myelogenous leukemia, a cancer of the blood cells. Through diet and medication the client had kept the disease under control for 12 years. On March 3, 1976, the client was told by the physician that she was dying. She was informed that the only hope for prolonging her life was chemotherapy. The possibility of doing nothing was also discussed. The physician was frank in describing the unfavorable features of the treatment. He explained that Adriamycin and cytosine arabinoside destroy the rapidly multiplying cancer cells. They also kill the cells which form the blood and the cells which line the body's organs from the mouth to the anus. Ulcerations appear on all lining surfaces of the body, hair falls out, and the individual is especially susceptible to infection. A person who is subjected to chemotherapy must be placed in reverse isolation to avoid infection. The chemotherapeutic drugs are life-threatening in themselves. They are used only as a last resort, and cannot be expected to bring about a remission of leukemia in adult patients in more than 20 percent of the cases. Although the client had begun to suffer some degree of toxic delirium or mental impairment due to her terminal condition, the physician felt she was rational, so he obtained her and her family's consent.

Jolene Tuma, the nurse instructor from a local junior college nursing program, and who held a BS and MS in nursing with an emphasis on public health teaching, asked to care for the client so that one of her nursing students could learn about chemotherapy. Ms. Tuma had the dual role of nurse to the client and instructor to the student. When the student went to bathe Ms. W, Ms. W was upset and crying; the student reported this to nurse Tuma, who was preparing to administer the first chemotherapy dosage prescribed by the physician.

Ms. Tuma went to the client's room to talk with her and comfort her. Ms. W said she had fought leukemia successfully for 12 years with God's help, and that she attributed the success to her relationship with God and her faithful practice of her Mormon religion. She explained to nurse Tuma that she had always avoided drugs and stimulants in favor of natural foods and a healthy diet. Ms. Tuma and Ms. W then discussed natural remedies for the treatment of cancer.

After determining that Ms. W fully understood and consented to chemotherapy, the nurse started the treatment intravenously. The client pleaded with Ms. Tuma to return that evening to talk with her son and daughter-in-law about the natural remedies they had discussed. Ms. Tuma finally agreed. Later in the day, Ms. W's daughter-in-law telephoned to check on Ms. W, at which time Ms. W told her she was having second thoughts about chemotherapy and wanted the family to visit that evening to discuss alternatives with Ms. Tuma. The daughter-in-law called the physician and reported Ms. W's change of attitude. He told her to go to the meeting, but to be sure to get the name of the nurse.

The meeting was held in Ms. W's room at 8:00 PM and at the same time, the physician phoned in an order to suspend the chemotherapy because of the client's change of attitude. The content of the family discussion with Ms. Tuma was reported in the court proceedings from various viewpoints, namely: Ms. Tuma and the daughter-in-law who reported what Ms. W had told her on the phone. The chemotherapy and its side effects, the alternatives of natural foods and herbs, the fact that US doctors do not prescribe Laetrile, and the fact that the client would have trouble obtaining blood transfusions if she were to leave the hospital and terminate the chemotherapy, were all discussed. It was agreed by all that it was probably best for Ms. W to continue the chemotherapy. Upon orders of the physician, the chemotherapy, which was discontinued at 8:00 PM, was resumed at 9:15 PM. The daughter-in-law gave Ms. Tuma's name to the physician who next day demanded that she be removed from her position as clinical instructor of nursing by the College of Southern Idaho at Twin Falls. She was suspended on the basis of the physician's original complaint which was that the course of treatment had been interrupted. Later the accusation was changed to interruption of the physician–patient relationship.

In March 1976, on a request from the Twin Falls Clinic and Hospital which, in turn, had received a complaint from the physician, the board of nursing initiated an investigation. On April 30, 1976, a petition for the suspension or revocation of license was initiated against Ms. Tuma by the board of nursing of the state of Idaho.

On August 24, 1976, the hearing officer filed his *Findings of Fact and Conclusions of Law*, and his determination that the licensee violated Idaho code section 54-1422(a)(7) by interfering with the physician–patient relationship, which constituted unprofessional conduct. Ms. Tuma was accused of behavior which the Hearing Office clarified in his *Findings of Fact and Conclusions of Law* as follows:

> That during the conversations, discussions, and informational meetings on March 4, 1976, the Licensee specifically did the following:
>
> (a) While the Licensee may have further elaborated on the life-threatening effects of chemotherapy, Licensee did not tell the patient that chemotherapy would kill the patient;
>
> (b) While the Licensee did discuss with the patient as an alternative form of treatment the patient's discharging herself from the hospital,

> Licensee did not say to the patient that she *should* discharge herself;
>
> (c) While the Licensee did discuss with the patient as an alternative form of treatment the use of Laetrile, natural foods and herbs, Licensee did not tell the patient that such treatment would cure said patient;
>
> (d) The Licensee did state to the patient that the care of a "reflexologist" (Licensee's terminology) or a masseur (terminology of patient's son and daughter-in-law) would be arranged in the event that the patient did decide to accept the alternative treatments described by Licensee. That the name Wilma Benson was provided to the patient and the circumstantial evidence indicates that the Licensee would have made the arrangements had the patient elected to assume the alternative treatment described by Licensee.

Ms. Tuma defended herself on the basis of freedom of speech and the clients' right to have the information she requested. She did not admit nor was she accused of trying to influence Ms. W contrary to the physician's advice. Based on the hearing officer's findings, the board of nursing suspended Ms. Tuma's license for six months commencing September 14, 1976.

In her appeal, Ms. Tuma moved for a trial *de nova*, a new trial, which was denied by the district court. On February 4, 1977, the district court affirmed the board of nursing and the suspension.

Ms. Tuma won vindication in the Idaho Supreme Court. In a decision handed down April 17, 1979, the high court ruled that Ms. Tuma could not be found guilty of unprofessional conduct because the Idaho Nurse Practice Act neither defines unprofessional conduct, nor gives guidelines for providing warnings [13].

Ms. W died on March 18, 1976, two weeks after the chemotherapy began. As the treatment progressed small sores developed in her mouth so that she had difficulty swallowing, and she was comatose much of the time.

ADVISING VS GIVING ADVICE

The Tuma case has created much controversy in the nursing profession as is evidenced by the editorial [10], the letters to the editor of *Nursing Outlook* [9], the reactions of state nurses' associations, and the numerous lecture classes and discussions on the case [22]. Some nurses are adamant that what Tuma did was unprofessional and was not within her role; others contended that her discussion was within the nurses' professional responsibility because nurses engage in informing and advising clients every day and because clients have a right to know alternative approaches to treatment.

The crucial question here is: Is it part of the nurse's role to advise on alternate forms of therapy or treatment? For purposes of this discussion, advising is defined as sharing information as to the nature of treatment, pro and con. It is the contention of this paper that it is within the professional nurse's role to engage in advising or sharing information with clients on alternate forms of therapy or treatment.

Giving advice, on the other hand, is making specific recommendations as to which course of therapy or treatment the client should choose. This function is more in line with the role of the physician than the role of the nurse. Each discipline has its focus, although there are undefined "gray" areas in which both may have a role.

There are numerous ways in which the nurse is involved in informing and advising on therapy or treatment. For example, if the nurse detects a lump on the client's breast, but the client refuses to go to a physician, the nurse may discuss various forms of treatment in order to persuade the client to get medical care. For instance, that the physician may be able to determine that the lump is only a cyst or if he did a biopsy it may indicate that she will not need surgery, but if she does she still can decide not to have the surgery. Would a community health nurse not discuss insulin increases and diet control with a diabetic client? Advising is very much a part of the nurse's role in regard to diet therapy. If a client needed psychiatric therapy but would not seek it because of fear of shock treatment, would a nurse not share information on other forms of treatment such as medication and psychotherapy? One might argue that these are cases in which the person is not yet under medical care so there would not be a conflict.

There are many other situations in which the nurse may advise on therapy. If a client is scheduled for surgery but is frightened, the nurse may reassure the client by describing to him/her exactly what will happen, how the surgery will be conducted, and what the effects may be. This may be referred to as reassurance, in that the physician may be assumed to have provided this information already, but the nurse may also give the client information not given by the physician. It is obvious that nurses do advise or share information on therapy in many situations, within the limits of their knowledge.

APPROACHES TO ANALYZING THE ROLE OF THE NURSE

There are a number of ways one might explore the role of the nurse in advising patients on therapy or treatment. For instance, one might give examples of the common practices of nurses in this regard, study the nurse practice acts to determine the limits of the nurses' role. Another approach would be to view the situation according to the ANA *Code for Nurses*. This was done by the ANA ethics committee. The analysis of the committee will be presented. A *fourth alternative* would be to study how various authors or theorists define the role of the nurse. A nursing theory framework will be used for analysis in this paper.

THE ANA ETHICS COMMITTEE APPROACH

Because of the national interest generated in the Tuma case and the request by the Western executives that ANA investigate and take appropriate action on the case, the ANA ethics committee examined all the documents. The committee believed it inappropriate to comment on the legal merits of the case while it was still under appeal. However, the committee made general comments on ethical concerns in four areas and related them to statements in the Code.

One had to do with a nurse's authority and responsibility in her role at the time of the action. Was Ms. Tuma's primary function that of educator, an employee of a service institution, or an independent practitioner functioning within the policies of the institution? The client had a right to information, the nurse had this information, and made a conscious decision to become involved and to share it.

The ANA's second comment had to do with the nurse as patient advocate. The ANA ethics committee statement seemed to imply that Ms. Tuma may have filled the role of patient advocate to a minimal degree and only to protect her own integrity. A third statement referred to the collegial relationship which the Code emphasizes between the nurse and the physician, and that collaboration is a two-way process. Emphasis was placed on the Code statements which relate to the nurse exercising informed judgment and discretion before intervening in diagnostic or therapeutic matters.

The final comment of the committee stressed the responsibility and accountability of nurses for communicating with members of the health team and the recording of significant information. Reference was also made to the nurse's responsibility to utilize the nursing process and to be accountable for all aspects of that process.

The Ethics Committee reaffirmed ANA's long-standing operating policy that investigation of complaints of alleged violations of the Code by individual nurses should be handled at the state nurses' association level [7]. Therefore, it planned to take no further action on the case. The committee implied in their statements that Ms. Tuma had violated the Code as they proceeded to specify the Codes she violated. The Code could have been used to support some of Tuma's actions, if not all of her actions.

The committee gave two reasons for not taking further action: the case was in litigation, and the state nurses' association should handle it. I think the committee's actions in this issue are questionable. They ought to have analyzed the case from an ethical perspective rather than from a procedural and etiquette point of view. The committee did not respond to or protest the fact that the Code was not allowed as evidence because the board of nurse examiners of Idaho had not officially adopted it. Is one free as a professional nurse not to accept the profession's official Code? It is understood that the Code is not a legal document, but it should provide a framework as a guide for making ethical decisions. How can a nurse violate a Code if he or she is free to accept or not accept a professional Code?

A THEORETICAL FRAMEWORK ANALYSIS

One theoretical approach to nursing will be used for analysis and an effort made to define the legitimate role of the nurse within that theoretical framework. Most decisions in nursing have ethical implications; therefore, a nursing theory should provide a guide for ethical decision-making.

In this author's view, Orem's self-care theory provides the most comprehensive and well-defined nursing theory. It is logical, clear, and used as the curriculum framework in a number of schools of nursing and in many practice settings. Therefore, this theory will be used as a framework to define the legitimate role of the nurse.

According to Orem, nursing has as its special concern:

> the individual's need for self-care action and the provision and management of it on a continuous basis in order to sustain life and health, recover from disease or injury, and cope with their effects [14].

Self-care means consistent, controlled, effective action taken by a mature person to maintain health. If a person cannot provide self-care to himself and it is not provided by others, illness may result.

When is it legitimate for a nurse to provide nursing for those in need? When persons are unable "to maintain continuously that amount of quality of self-care which is therapeutic in sustaining life and health, in recovering from disease or injury, or in coping with their effects [15]." With children the inability may be with the parents or guardian. Persons unable to provide self-care to themselves need help or assistance which can be provided by nursing.

If nursing care is to be rendered, there must be some contact and communication with those who are in need of this service. This is done in private or group practice or within an institutional setting such as a health agency or hospital. Ideally nurses establish a contractual relationship with their clients. The relationship should include at least a verbal or implied agreement or contract to provide services within the domain of nursing for a specified time. Orem contended that when nurses are employed in health care institutions providing care to clients, there should be "verbal agreements between the nurse and each patient or individuals acting for the patient about the nurse's willingness to provide nursing and the patient's willingness to receive nursing from assigned nurses [16]." It is preferable if this agreement is explicit in verbal or in written form.

Many institutions have initiated primary nursing where one nurse assesses and diagnoses the client's need for nursing and designs a plan of action with the client to meet that need. This nurse assumes primary responsibility for continuous care, although she may be assisted by others.

What methods may be used by the nurse in meeting the self-care needs of clients? Orem identified five methods of helping or assisting others:

1. Acting for or doing for another.
2. Guiding another.

3. Providing physical or psychological support for another.

4. Providing an atmosphere or an environment that promotes personal development and independence so that the client is able to meet present or future demands for action.

5. Teaching others [18].

ANALYSIS OF THE TUMA CASE

In analyzing the Tuma case it may be helpful to view the situation from the patient's and the nurse's perspective, and from the physician's perspective.

The Patient's Perspective

Ms. W was her own self-care agent prior to her admission, even though she had had leukemia for 12 years. A change in her health state now made her dependent on others, a receiver of care. Her capacity was impaired, although not completely. She still wanted control and to be allowed to make decisions about her body and future well-being.

Ms. W needed the assistance of others to meet her self-care needs. Chemotherapy would introduce self-care requirements as well as hazards to Ms. W's situation. For example, the ulcerations in the mouth caused by the chemotherapy would create a special need for mouth care and a need to make adjustment in food consistency. The psychological impact of being told she was dying would give rise to further demands for care. She was upset and crying in this situation. Ms. W was a deeply religious person; in this time of crisis, while it would seem that her beliefs would be a source of strength and would enhance her power of agency, they in fact came into conflict with scientific, medical and family advice and gave rise to further need for nursing assistance. Ms. W had more faith in miracles, in proper diet and food, and in the avoidance of drugs and medication, than in the powers of scientific medicine. She had a married son who was distressed about her condition and wanted her to take the chemotherapy. The only alternative to chemotherapy presented by the physician was to do nothing. Hence, she was confronted by a dilemma which could be addressed through nursing.

According to Orem, generally the person or client in need of help will accept such help if he or she believes that "the helper has a right to give help, has sufficient knowledge and ability to help, is aware of the requirements of the situation, and will act prudently [18]."

Ms. W needed the nurse to support her in her anxious state, to respond to her inquiries and questions, and to assist her in making her decision whether to continue with the chemotherapy, to have another form of treatment, or to have no treatment. She asked the nurse if there were other forms of treatment. She seemed to lack trust in the treatment being given. What was Ms. W's role in this situation? It would seem that it was to be in control and use her power of self-agency to its fullest capacity.

The Nurse's Perspective

What was the situation from the nurse's perspective? Jolene Tuma had a master's degree in nursing, and as an instructor she was qualified as a professional and had the knowledge and ability to give care. She obviously had knowledge about the chemotherapy, its effects and administration. She was functioning in the accepted dual role of nurse for the client and teacher for the student. She had the knowledge and abilities required in this situation.

What agreement did nurse Tuma have with Ms. W? The nurse had known the client for two days. There did not seem to be any formal agreement, just an implicit one to give the needed nursing care. Did the client have a need or requirement that the nurse could legitimately meet? To answer this question, it might be helpful to analyze the methods of assistance used by nurse Tuma in caring for Ms. W. She may have used several methods of assistance, such as guiding, supporting, teaching, and providing a developmental environment. Guiding a client may be considered valid if the person has to make choices such as choosing one course of treatment in preference to another. Ms. W had doubts about her decision to have chemotherapy. "The guidance given must be appropriate, whether in the form of suggestions, instructions, directions, or supervision [19]." The nurse is expected to act prudently.

Supporting another may mean sustaining him or her in an effort and "thereby preventing the person from failing or from avoiding an unpleasant situation or decision [20]." Obviously Ms. W was in a stressful situation. She needed support in perhaps deciding to refuse the chemotherapy and/or to follow other measures or to accept and to live through the unpleasant consequences of the chemotherapy.

She needed support in knowing that it was all right to question the therapy or to be in control or to have this knowledge to make a reasoned choice. The client needed a basic support to exercise her right of self-determination.

Teaching as a method of assistance may also have been said to be used in this situation. In providing knowledge, did Ms. Tuma consider Ms. W's background and experience, life-style and habits of daily living, her mode of perceiving and thinking in her present stressful state, and whether her need was one related to self-care as opposed to medical care? How might Ms. Tuma, if she was to stay within the limits of nursing, have diagnosed the abilities of Ms. W to engage in self-care? What was Ms. W's self-care agency? What were her abilities and capacities for engaging in continuous and effective self-care? In Ms. W's case, self-care and self-management of a physical nature was unrealistic; therefore, the teaching role of the nurse would be comprised primarily of creating an atmosphere for psychological and spiritual self-care. In this teaching and supporting situation, the nurse's role would include such actions as providing information concerning Ms. W's therapy and affirming her right to a role in decisions about her care.

Was Ms. Tuma aware of the domain and boundaries of nursing? Did she keep her professional actions within these boundaries? Did the patient have a need that the nurse could legitimately meet? It would seem that Ms. W had limited capacity to engage in self-care because she was very sick. However, although she was delirious at times, she was rational both when she made the decision to consent to chemotherapy and when she questioned having made it. As a moral agent she was capable of making decisions. It would seem that Ms. W and Ms. Tuma had an effective nurse–client relationship. The client's unburdening of her concerns would give evidence of a certain trust and respect: The client asked the nurse rather than the physician for alternatives and the opportunity to weigh these.

The Physician's Perspective

If the focus of nursing is on the individual's capability or need for self-care action, what is the focus of medicine? Traditionally, medicine has as its focus the illness or disease states of individuals. Physicians assess states of health, and diagnose deviations or the presence or absence of disease. Physicians are also concerned with prevention and the correcting of defects and disabilities. They prescribe and give treatment to cure or alleviate the illness condition and to restore health. Physicians give advice or specific recommendations as to which course of therapy or treatment should be engaged in by the client.

In this situation the physician, who had not known the patient prior to this admission—approximately two days prior to the incident—diagnosed the patient as dying with leukemia. He saw only one possible therapy, chemotherapy, for which he obtained the patient's and family's consent. He was responsible in discussing all the side effects of chemotherapy, which was considered the best scientifically tested therapy available. The physician disclosed at the hearing that he was not knowledgeable about natural approaches, and was not concerned about the patient's religion. The legal definitions of the practice of medicine support the idea that discussion of medical diagnosis, prognosis, and treatment is the exclusive prerogative of the physician. The authority of the physician as the main decision-maker and as having exclusive rights to knowledge on treatment is being questioned with the emphasis on patient's rights.

The Role of the Nurse in Advising the Client

Some nurses would contend that Ms. Tuma was acting outside the boundaries and domain of nursing in giving information on alternative therapy. The question is, does the patient have the right to such information from whatever source it can be obtained, whether from minister, social worker, nurse, medical doctor, or former patient? Carpenter and Langsner contended that the informed consent process in which the physician assumes full responsibility for informing and advocating for the patient is severely limited. They said, "it is no longer legally or socially acceptable that this burden resides solely with the medical profession. The patient needs to share in the decision-making function; but is poorly prepared to do so [4]."

The nurse has a significant role in assisting the patient in making decisions. The potential of the nurse for guiding, supporting, and helping the patient is not being realized. Are there moral or legal reasons why clients cannot assume control of their own medical destinies if they desire and have the ability? Some physicians, but not all, acknowledge the client's rights. Clients may not be ready or willing, or even aware that they have the right or ability to make these decisions, but should they not be given the option if they are willing and capable? Do nurses not have a moral responsibility to assist patients to become aware of their right to make decisions?

Bandman asked if the nurse is supposed to remain silent when the client is bewildered by unexplained treatments, confused by technical terms, ignorant of alternatives, and seeking information on diagnosis and proposed therapies [2]. Clients have a right to refuse treatment and nurses have supported clients in that refusal. Is this not advising an alternative therapy? Meyer supported a patient in her expressed wish to have no more blood transfusions because she was ready to die. The nurse told the physician she could not give any more blood transfusions [12]. There are hundreds of such instances in everyday nursing practice. Unless nurses advocate patients, who will? According to the *Code for Nurses*, "the primary commitment of the nurse is to the client's care and safety [6]."

A nurse or any other health professional should not discuss a diagnosis or treatment unless they have sufficient knowledge on the subject, but in many instances it is not factual knowledge that is at issue, but the value judgments that may be made in relation to information. Value judgments are apparent in such words and phrases as: chemotherapy is the "best" or the "only" treatment or chemotherapy "will kill you."

The nurse's "demonstrating leadership in traditionally medical areas will often be reacted to by the physician as a challenge to and invasion upon the privacy, trust, and confidence of his relationship with his patients [5]." This was obvious in the Tuma case and, of course, she was not supported by her peers in nursing. Kelly speaks of the autonomous independent nurse decision-maker responsible to the client who may indeed put herself on the line but finds no support system in nursing. She called for nurses (like Tuma), who would stand up and be counted and be willing to fight back. Kelly said, "It may be that as the nurse asserts her right to be a colleague in health care, the physician and administrator will be educated to the value and responsibility of the nurse as patient advocate [8]." It is time nurses were recognized as professional peers, accorded due respect, and allowed to assume responsibility. Nurses need support and nursing leaders have a moral responsibility to support nurses.

In speaking to the issues of patients' rights and the doctor–patient relationship, Pellegrino contended that humaneness and compassion are dimensions of care neglected today and that the patient must be respected as a unique person. Individuals cannot be given standardized explanations. They need answers to questions in the context of their own life situation. He said, "physicians who have neither time nor inclination for this degree of personalization are bound by the first role of humaneness to see that other members of the health care team are permitted to answer the personal questions that lie at the root of the patient's plea for help [21]." Ms. W was asking questions, not about the scientifically proven methods of treatment, but about something deeper affecting her unique life situation, her religion, and former self-care practices. Self-care education must consider the knowledge and skill a person already has in the area of traditional family health practices or home remedies—or self-healing capabilities [11]. Lewis asked if the implication of the Tuma case was that, "unless the nurse first secures the physician's consent, she must not discuss treatment alternatives with the patient [10]."

The patient does have a moral right to information on medical care. Who should give this information as a procedural matter? Does one professional group have a right to limit the information another professional group may share? It would seem that this would depend on the need and request of the patient. The patient should make the decision. In the Tuma case the patient did request this information and only requested this information from the nurse.

Besch wondered if nurses have the freedom to inform patients of the risks and benefits involved in a treatment that they are considering. After a discussion on informed consent she concluded that the patient is not owned by any one professional, and so if a professional, presumably the physician, does not meet the patient's need for sufficient information to make a decision, it is the responsibility of another professional to do this. She advocated that the nursing profession study and act upon their values and beliefs regarding patients' rights and autonomy [3]. Annas argued that while the nurse has the potential to be the patient advocate, there are problems because of the traditional image of the nurse as physician–helper rather than as partner. Many physicians, nurses, and patients have this image and just giving a title does not change attitudes [1].

In conclusion, is advising the client on alternate forms of therapy or treatment part of the role of the nurse? In the self-care theory framework—advising or sharing information on treatment or alternate therapy may be referred to as assisting a client to develop his or her self-care agency—the ability to make decisions regarding his or her own care. Self-care is a concept that strongly supports the values of self-determination, self-control, and self-fulfillment. The client is the agent of his or her own actions and has the right to make decisions or to be assisted in making decisions regarding his or her therapy or care. The nurse who has the knowledge and competence to meet the client's need for information on therapy has an ethical obligation to provide such assistance.

REFERENCES

1. Annas, G. The patient rights advocate, can nurses effectively fill the role? *Supervisor Nurse* 5:20, 1979.
2. Bandman, E.L. The rights of nurses and patients: A case for advocacy. In E.L. Bandman and B. Bandman, (Eds.). *Bioethics and Human Rights*. Boston: Little, Brown, 1978. P. 332.
3. Besch, L.B. Informed consent: A patient's right. *Nurs. Outlook* 32, January, 1979.
4. Carpenter, W.T. and Langsner, C.A. The nurses' role in informed consent. *Nurs. Times* 71:1049, 1975.
5. Carpenter, W.T. and Langsner, C.A. The nurses' role in informed consent. *Nurs. Times* 71:1079, 1975.
6. *Code for Nurses with Interpretive Statements.* Kansas City: American Nurses' Association, 1976.
7. Ethical aspects of the Jolene Lucile Beverly Tuma Case. *Colorado Nurse* 15, August 1978.
8. Kelly, L.Y. The patient's right to know. *Nurs. Outlook* 24:26, 1976.
9. Letters to the Editor. *Nurs. Outlook* 25:596, 1977 and 27:8, 78, 1978.
10. Lewis, E. Editorial. *Nurs. Outlook* 25:561, 1977.
11. Levin, L.S. Patient education and self-care: How do they differ? *Nurs. Outlook* 26:170, 1978.
12. Meyer, C.A. Compassion in nursing. *Supervisor Nurse* 9:40, 1978.
13. News and reports, Jolene Tuma wins; court rules practice act did not define "unprofessional conduct." *Nurs. Outlook* 27:376, 1979.
14. Orem, D. *Nursing: Concepts of Practice.* New York: McGraw-Hill, 1979. P. 6.
15. Ibid., P. 7.
16. Ibid., P. 10.
17. Ibid., P. 11.
18. Ibid., P. 61.
19. Ibid., P. 64.
20. Ibid., P. 65.
21. Pellegrino, E.D. Protection of patients' rights and the doctor–patient relationship. *Prev. Med.* 4:398, 1975.
22. Stanley, A.T. Is it ethical to give hope to a dying person. *Nurs. Clin. North Am.* 14:69, 1979.

STUDY AND DISCUSSION QUESTIONS
THE NURSE–PHYSICIAN RELATIONSHIP: II. SOMERA AND TUMA

1. How would you account for the fact that only the nurse was convicted in the death of Anastacia Clemente?

2. Do you agree with Grennan's opinion that this tragedy worked to the benefit of the nursing profession—making nurses responsible for the orders followed?

3. Is Jolene Tuma guilty of unprofessional conduct? Did she interfere with the doctor–patient relationship?

4. Some of the letters critical of Tuma mention the lack of Tuma's collegiality. Is this a fair criticism? Was the doctor involved collegial?

5. An underlying assumption of some criticisms of Tuma is a certain view of the nurse–physician relationship and the subordinate status of the nursing profession. How do you see this issue?

6. Did Mrs. G.W. (the leukemia patient) have a right to know the information she requested from Tuma?

7. Did Tuma "promote" an illegal therapy as the Idaho Nurses' Association contends? (See Bejsovec)

8. What should the controlling factor be in the amount and kind of information the patient should receive—the patient's right to know, the physician's opinion of what is in the patient's best interest (additionally limited by mentioning only medically approved therapies and options), or something else?

9. If a social worker, a pastor, or a knowledgeable friend had provided the same information that Mrs. G.W. requested of Tuma, would this have been interference in the doctor–patient relationship?

10. Is a nurse under the same professional obligations as a physician to suggest as options only medically approved therapies?

11. Tuma stated that what she was doing wasn't "exactly legal" or "exactly ethical." The Idaho Nurses' Association (INA) was inclined to view these statements as admissions of guilt. The Idaho Supreme Court rejected this as evidence of professional misconduct. Which view is correct? Did Tuma do something illegal or unethical?

12. Do you think the ANA Code for Nurses supports Tuma's actions or the reverse?

13. In Idaho, professional misconduct was determined by a non-nurse hearing officer in the absence of guidance from the ANA Code for Nurses. Is this something the INA and the ANA should have protested or was the procedure nevertheless fair?

14. Stanley (as well as Storlie and Partridge) is critical of the lack of action on the part of the ANA committee on ethics. Do you agree with her assessment? What was or should have been the role of that committee?

15. Stanley argues that a nurse has an ethical obligation to meet a client's informational needs and to assist the client in making his or her own autonomous decision. Do you agree?

16. How does what happened to Jolene Tuma affect your views about patient advocacy?

6

The Nurse–Physician Relationship: III. Whistleblowing

INTRODUCTION

What should the nurse do in the face of physician errors, negligence, or mistreatment of clients? Again, how a nurse views the role of the nurse has a significant bearing on what action, if any, the nurse will take. The articles in this chapter begin with some historically extreme examples of how doctors and surgeons relied on and exploited the loyalty of nurses or failed to be mutually loyal. In 1910, under the title "Where Does Loyalty End?", The *American Journal of Nursing* published an editorial that lamented incidents reported in its letter pages. Nurses were being scapegoated to cover for medical mistakes and to preserve the reputations of doctors, and were not being given the same support they were expected to give. Both the editorial and letters averse to this are presented here.

In 1979, the popular journal *RN* published a survey, in "Dangerous Doctors: What to Do when the MD Is Wrong," of almost 300 readers on the issue of when they would intervene and how they would go about it. On the positive side, 96 percent said that they would intervene if the error were life-threatening; 93 percent if it were to prevent a risk of permanent injury; and 85 percent would speak to the doctor about it. But these percentages drop off considerably when it is a question of effectiveness of the therapy or just a matter of protecting the financial interests of the patient.[1] One reason for the decrease in intervention is the reception it receives. Nurses report that they often face hostility, lack of support from colleagues, and political hassles. Hence, nurses are making careful assessment of the worth of risks and benefits of such intervention.

As mentioned in the *RN* survey, the ANA Code for Nurses requires nurses to take action when they become aware of "instances of incompetent, unethical or illegal practice by any member of the health care team or the health care system, or any action on the part of others that places the rights or best interests of the client in jeopardy."[2] According to this survey, it would seem that nurses have not been as vigilant of client interests or rights as the code would hold forth as ideal.

In addition to the Code for Nurses, the law is giving a greater incentive for nurses to report medical negligence. Helen Creighton, a well-known nurse-lawyer, discusses a number of legal cases that underscores the nurses' obligation to report medical negligence in "Should Nurses Report Negligence in Medical Treatment?"

Freda Baron Friedman, in "The 'Joy' of Telling a Physician He's Wrong," reports a survey of 400 nurses that indicates the nurses' perception of the extent of physician mistakes and nurses' attitudes regarding this watchdog role. More than 80 percent thought that "most" of the physicians they work with are competent. Eight percent thought a "substantial" number were incompetent. Forty percent thought that hospitals placed too much responsibility on nurses for policing routine orders and procedures, although 81 percent reported that physicians took correction of errors in a professional manner.

The ANA Code for Nurses recommends that concerns about inappropriate or questionable practices be expressed to the person carrying out the practice, and that there should be an established procedure for reporting and handling of incompetent, unethical, or illegal practice within the employment setting that protects the reporting person. The code also recognizes that if the objectionable practices are to go uncorrected it may be necessary to go outside the employment setting to protect the welfare and safety of clients.[3]

Alfred Feliu in two articles, "The Risks of Blowing the Whistle" and "Thinking of Blowing the Whistle?", gives a general account of the rights of those who report unethical and illegal practice and advice on how to do it effectively.

Whistleblowing and ardent patient advocacy are not to be undertaken lightly. The cases of Christine Spahn Smith and Pat Witt are sobering illustrations of the terrible cost that can be extracted from nurses for acting according to the highest ideals of the profession. Smith, in "Outrageous or Outraged: A Nurse Advocate Story," discovered that when she became an outspoken patient advocate she had "little or no support from the medical or nursing community." Ultimately faced with retention of her job or her professional values, she chose resignation.

Like the nurses mentioned in the Feliu article, Smith was unsuccessful in bringing about the desired change, but nevertheless claims that "I would not have done anything differently." Pat Witt, on the other hand, was successful in bringing about reforms at the hospital she complained about. Paradoxically, she says, "I would never do it again." Her article, "Notes of a Whistleblower," appears to be a success story since she won her case against the hospital and the appeals were exhausted. As reported in the *Chicago Tribune* article, "Whistleblower Saved Lives, Lost Everything Else," Witt was not awarded damages due to a technicality in the law.

Finally, the article by Mary A. Kiely and Dierdre C. Kiely, "Whistleblowing: Disclosure and Its Consequences for the Professional Nurse and Management," presents a general characterization of whistleblowing and management responses to it. Of particular interest is their review of nursing literature on the topic.

NOTES

1. A larger survey of 12,500 nurses by Ronni Sandroff ["Protect the MD . . . or the Patient? Nursing's Unequivocal Answer." *RN* 43 (February 1981): 28–33] also address the issue of the nurses' perception of unnecessary hospitalization and surgery.
2. American Nurses' Association, *Code for Nurses with Interpretive Statements* (Kansas City, Mo.: American Nurses' Association, 1985) p. 6.
3. Ibid., pp. 6–7.

Where Does Loyalty End?

Under this heading, "Where does Loyalty End?" we are printing this month three letters in which are involved principles of fair dealing to the patient and justice to the nurse. These letters are characteristic of many that come to our desk in the course of a year in which, accepting the facts as presented by the writers, the question is constantly brought to us, Where does the nurse's loyalty to the doctor end? and is she required to be untruthful or to practice deceit in order to uphold the reputation of a physician at her own expense or that of the patient?

We know we are treading upon dangerous ground when we approach this subject, but so frequently do we hear of cases where nurses have been subjected to unjust accusations, amounting almost to persecution, that we feel the time has come when the entire nursing profession must dispassionately consider this very vital point upon which the two professions come together.

Where the physician is a man of the highest character we hardly think this question can arise, but there are in the medical profession men whose moral and medical standards are of such a low order that they do not hesitate to make a scapegoat of the nurse to protect themselves against their own mistakes.

We believe the time has come when, through our state boards of examiners, there should be established what we will term a board of arbitration between the two professions. It would seem to us that the nurse board and the medical board of examiners of a state could properly enter into affiliation and constitute such a tribunal, which would serve not only to afford protection and justice to nurses who feel themselves unjustly treated by physicians, but would also give opportunity to members of the medical profession to enter complaints against nurses who, they have had reason to believe, are disloyal both to them and to their patients.

Such a joint board would have other uses. Plans for the care of the great middle class, for a sliding scale, etc., would naturally be discussed, and suggestions be carried from one profession to the other for consideration at their state meetings.

These boards are already in existence in the majority of our states, the members are carefully selected according to standards fixed by law, their appointments are similar, and to utilize these for such a purpose would not add any amount of expense or new machinery, such as would be entailed in the appointment of new committees; and possibly such a tribunal, we whisper it with great caution, might lead to the establishment of a code of ethics which should apply to the mutual relations of the two professions, and loyalty to the nurse by the physician might be placed on the same footing as loyalty to the physician by the nurse.

We believe this plan for a conference on ethics would bring the two professions into closer unity and better understanding and would in every way promote the welfare of the patients served by both.

Where does loyalty end? (1910). *American Journal of Nursing, 10*, 230–231. Reprinted with permission of © American Journal of Nursing Company. All rights reserved.

Where Does Loyalty to the Physician End?: Letters to the Editor of *American Journal of Nursing*

I.

DEAR EDITOR: I had a most unfortunate experience recently when caring for a man who was ill with typhoid. The doctor, in passing the catheter, let it slip into the bladder and had to telegraph to a nearby city for a surgeon. The next day at noon an incision, one and a half inches long, was made in the suprapubic region and the catheter was removed. Of course the patient was desperately weak and for several days his life hung in the balance, but I am thankful to say he lived.

A few days before this operation, the doctor had ordered me to put the patient into the tub (a sitz bath tub), hoping to make him urinate, which I refused to do unless the doctor was present, as the patient's heart was not in the best shape and he was sufficiently rational not to wish me to do it alone. His old mother was the only other person in the house and she could not have helped.

When the surgeon came he brought another nurse with him, but I was given no help and had to prepare for the operation alone, with only a two-burner gasoline stove to use for boiling water and instruments, and I had to keep stopping to sponge the patient whose temperature was high. After the operation, the doctor told me the surgeon wanted the other nurse to stay on the case, which I gladly left in her hands.

The patient's people wanted to discharge the doctor, but being ignorant folks and not realizing their power, he talked them over into keeping him, and has since circulated all over town the story that if I had given him better help the accident would not have happened. What kind of a man must he be to need help with such a simple operation when the patient was perfectly sane?

H. S.

II.
(CONDENSED)

DEAR EDITOR: Some time ago I was called to a patient who had attempted suicide by taking "fifty cents' worth of paregoric, a pint of alcohol, and eight tablets." She was unconscious when I arrived; how long she had been so I do not know. Hot-water bottles had been used before my arrival and were cold when I removed them. A steam pack was ordered, which I gave with great care. There were burns at the points from which I had removed the bottles.

I was able to remain with the patient only twenty-four hours because of an obstetrical case then due, but I was asked to return and dress the burns. The patient was finally taken to a hospital and died after two weeks of "ulcer of the stomach, caused by burns."

Several weeks after her death her husband accused me of having caused the burns, in which the doctor sustained him, asserting that there was no hot water in the house until after my arrival. A neighbor woman, the only other witness, was silent.

I am a comparative stranger in a small city where the doctor, whose word is law, is making a scapegoat of me. My professional reputation seems to be ruined. I cannot run away, because I am not guilty.

What redress has a nurse in the face of such injustice and disloyalty on the part of a doctor?

M. T.

III.

DEAR EDITOR: I wish to make a statement regarding a nurse and a doctor who were, I am sorry to say, on opposite sides in a lawsuit over a patient they had taken care of. Has a nurse any right to defend her reputation in a case of this kind when the doctor tries to place all the blame on her shoulders? Is it a nurse's duty to remove vaginal or uterine gauze after an operation, or is it the duty of the doctor?

I was called in July, 1908, to take care of a woman who was suffering from extra-uterine pregnancy. I stayed with her for three weeks, when it became apparent that an operation must be submitted to in order to save her life. I followed the doctor's directions and recorded everything faithfully on the sheet I was keeping. I took the patient to the hospital where she underwent the operation and stayed with her for four weeks more, until she left the hospital.

It turned out to be a pus case and the woman did not seem to get well or gain strength as fast as she should have done. She had a great deal of trouble with her bowels and could not get a natural action without taking physic or injections and sometimes both. She left the hospital after four weeks, the doctor telling her what to do in regard to her health and what to take for her bowels. She asked if she might go to the country where she could be with her sister and would not have to worry or work about the house until she was stronger. She went to the country and I left her and took a rest.

Before I went to work again, being interested in my patient, I went to see her and to my surprise found her quite ill. I tried to find out what the trouble was and learned that she could not get any passage of the bowels and was suffering intense pain. I immediately tried to move the bowels with an injection but with no result. Then I gave her, separately, salts and castor oil, but she could not retain them on the stomach. Knowing that she had just gone through this operation, I advised her husband to get her back home as soon as possible and have her own physician take care of her. I don't know how we ever did it or how the patient ever stood it, for the pain was so intense that I shall never forget the suffering that poor woman went through. We got her home and up to her own room and then I immediately telephoned the doctor to come, telling him of her condition. He came at once and the first thing he did was to order an olive oil enema to be given at once. In the first place he made an examination and stated that there was an impaction of the bowels. She retained the oil, and from that time on there was no action of the bowels for fourteen days except the water that returned from the injections. He used all kinds of laxatives and cathartics, but with no effect.

At the end of the fourteenth day, while giving her an injection, I found that I could not insert the rectal tube as high up in the bowel as I had been doing. There seemed to be some pressure there that would not let the tube go any higher. The patient complained of great pain and said that she felt as if her bowels were going to move. I brought a slop jar that was thoroughly clean and assisted her to it, so that we could see what kind of an operation she would have. There was a large report of gas expelled and the patient and myself both heard something drop into the jar with great force and a loud thud. The patient, thinking her bowels had moved, got up from the jar with my assistance and we both looked into it to see how the passage looked. Her husband was standing there at the time and he also looked into the jar. We all noticed that it was a very peculiar movement and said so. I picked up the jar and carried it into the bath-room, the husband following, for he said that he wanted to know what that was. I took a burnt match and examined it and to my horror I found it was a hospital sponge. The husband immediately said that it looked like a rag and asked me what it was and I told him. What could I have done otherwise and be honest? It never entered my head that there would be a lawsuit.

I immediately telephoned to the doctor who had charge of the case and he came right over, as he lived only a couple of blocks away. I showed him the sponge just as it had passed into the slop jar and he examined it thoroughly. Then the family asked him what it was and he told them that it was a hospital sponge. The doctor told me to keep it until the next day. The next morning he came, and the woman's bowels were moving freely by that time, but her husband had decided that he would sue the surgeon because of the intense suffering through which his wife had passed, and he kept the sponge to offer as evidence.

I had a talk with the surgeon in regard to the sponge and he told me that I should have thrown it away and not told the family. The husband saw it at the same time that I did, so how could I have done so? When I was asked right out what it was, should I have lied to them?

I should always have had it on my mind, and if the story had ever come out, where would my reputation have been? And still I felt that I must defend the doctor; that I am always willing to do and will stand by the doctors through thick and thin and will be strictly honest with them, but I will not tell a lie for any one, and if nurses must do so to defend the doctor then I don't care for the profession and I do not consider that I can do so and be as true and noble a woman as Florence Nightingale was. She is my ideal as to what a nurse should be. The nurses are taught that they must stand by the doctor whether he is in the right or wrong, but when a doctor will have his lawyers and insinuate, himself, that the blame belongs on the nurse's shoulders, I think it is time for her to defend herself and have some voice in the matter. To my mind in this case, it was merely an accident and I am very sorry that it happened. The case has been tried twice and in both instances the jury awarded the woman damages and a larger amount the second time than the first. I should like to know if I did the right thing in regard to the case all through and what other nurses would have done had they been in my place.

What is the nurse to do when she is asked a question, lie or speak the truth? Especially if it goes against the doctor, must she tell a lie to defend him? I tried to keep out of the way of meeting the lawyers, but it was of no use, I was called into court to testify as to when the sponge passed and how.

E. C.

Dangerous Doctors:
What to Do When the MD Is Wrong

Linda Stanley

Cardiac arrest!

The cardiovascular surgeon begins CPR instantly. The situation seems under control.

But—incredibly—you suddenly realize he's performing it at twice the normal rate—with one hand placed to the left of the sternum. He can't be circulating any blood at all; and he's probably fracturing the patient's ribs.

What on earth can you do?

If you warn this doctor of the danger, there's a chance the patient can be saved. But there's an equally good chance that you'll merely earn yourself a derisive reprimand, and gain a powerful enemy in the bargain. If you intervene and the patient lives, the doctor may thank you—or curse you. If you intervene and the patient dies, the doctor will surely hate you. And if you *don't* intervene, you may well be dragged into court by the bereaved family of the deceased.

When a physician makes a mistake, the deck is definitely stacked against the nurse who tries to correct him. But nurses' increased clinical know-how and expertise in patient management have eased the "stacking" effect. And RNs today are more willing to stand up and be heard. Virtually all the nurses responding to a recent *RN* survey said they *would* take action when faced with a life-threatening physician-error. And 85% would confront the offending physician himself.

FACING UP TO THE DOCTOR

It's clear from the *RN* survey that most nurses feel they *must* take action, no matter how unfair the terms may be. But survey respondents also offered a number of suggestions for improving your odds. Your approach to the physician, for instance, can make a big difference in the outcome of the confrontation. *Do not* tell him he's making a mistake. Instead, ask questions: "Is this order what you meant?" "Could you explain something I don't understand?" "Could you discuss my patient's care with me?" or suggest, "We've had good results with . . . ." The common thread in all these methods is questioning instead of accusing, asking for a rationale for the doctor's action, and letting the doctor know your opinion or experience, backed with facts. One nurse said she would vary her approach, depending on the doctor, her rapport with him, and the situation.

You might ask if all this psychological planning doesn't amount to game-playing and manipulation, and, indeed, on one level it does. But you're in a tough political situation in the hospital, having to answer to three equally demanding bosses—the patient, the doctor, and the nursing supervisor.

For one thing, doctors' attitudes about mistakes make your task that much more difficult. In her book, *The Unkindest Cut*, Marcia Millman reports on her two-year observation of the hospital scene: "At every stop and turn of medical work, there are built-in professional protections for the doctor against having to recognize and take responsibility for mistakes made on patients. The defenses against acknowledging mistakes reside in the very heart of medical philosophy and organization."

On top of this, nurses are inexperienced at wielding power. While doctors have carved out unassailable positions in the hospital hierarchy, nursing administrators are often on the defensive, and may

Stanley, L. (1979, March). Dangerous doctors: What to do when the MD is wrong. *RN, 42,* 23–30. Reprinted with permission of © Medical Economics Company Inc., Oradell, NJ. All rights reserved.

seem unsympathetic if you approach them with a potentially volatile problem.

What, then, is your ideal course of action when you're faced with a doctor's mistake? We asked a number of nursing leaders this question, and they all agree it's best to go to the physician himself for starters. Anne Rose, RN, MS chairman of the Empire State Nurses Association, says, "To talk about someone behind his back is not only unprofessional but also unfair. You have to challenge him, give him a chance to answer."

Keep your goal in mind, however, when you challenge a physician, or you may find yourself involved in a game of point-proving that doesn't benefit you or the patient. Using some basic psychology can help get a dialogue going. Ms. Rose comments, "There are some basic approaches to all human beings that will keep them from becoming angry. Be honest and open about your question and don't display hostility yourself. Otherwise you're not going to get the information or response you want." She suggests saying, "I don't understand your procedure or order and I would feel more confident if you'd explain it to me."

If you *are* met with hostility you can try again, but it's important to keep cool and remain unflustered. A defensive doctor isn't using good communication skills, so you have to—for the patient's sake. That doesn't mean you should turn into a doormat. Simply remember what you are trying to get out of the conversation.

Try telling the doctor that you aren't threatening him. You can get that message across, according to Ms. Rose, by saying, "I wasn't making a value judgment about your action; I just want to understand what you did so that I can give better patient care."

"You almost have to become insensitive to hostility," adds Ms. Rose. "That's hard, because we all like to be accepted and valued. If you question a physician and he tells you, 'That's none of your business,' you should turn the situation around. Ask the doctor, 'Why isn't that nursing business? Aren't we all working for the same result—to make the patient healthier?' The point is, try to get a dialogue going in which he sees you as a reasonable person, not just as someone who is questioning him."

Unfortunately, even facing down the physician may not be enough. If he ignores you, you can *still* be held liable. It happened to several nurses found negligent in a 1977 malpractice case in West Virginia.* Their trouble began in 1973 when, in a fall from a

ladder, the plaintiff has sustained a comminuted compound fracture of the right wrist, a posterior dislocation of the right elbow, and a compression fracture of the second lumbar vertebra. A cast was applied from the knuckles to above the elbow, and he was admitted to the hospital for observation.

Two days later, the nurses on the day shift noticed that the patient's arm was edematous, black, and exuding foul-smelling drainage. He had a high temperature and was occasionally delirious. The charge nurse called the doctor and told him about the patient's condition, and that he couldn't hold down oral antibiotics. But when the physician took no action, she did not pursue the matter.

After two more days the patient was transferred to a university hospital, and then to a hospital in another state where he received seven hyperbaric oxygen treatments. Despite these efforts, the patient's right arm had to be amputated at the shoulder, and the patient brought a suit against the doctor and the hospital from whom he received his first treatment.

A jury ruled for the patient to the tune of $333,000, and when the hospital appealed to the State Supreme Court, the verdict was upheld because the *nurses* had been negligent. They had deviated from hospital policy, which required not only that RNs notify the attending physician if they suspected a medical problem, but that they bring it to the attention of the departmental chairman if it remained unsolved.

TACKLING THE CHAIN OF COMMAND

This is a lot easier said than done. Jane Hirsch, RN, MS, staff development instructor and former head nurse at the University of California Hospital, San Francisco, says a head nurse would probably feel more confident about doing this. "She has more experience and works more often with the physician, giving her a chance for a better rapport," she explains.

Karin Williamson, RN, BSN, assistant director of nursing services (staff development) at the University of Kansas Hospital, and an *RN* consultant, feels that going up the physician's chain of command may be easier in a teaching institution than elsewhere. If a doctor's reasoning doesn't make sense,

Utter v. United Hospital Center, Inc. and Lawrence Mills, 236 S.E. 2nd 213, W. Va. 1977.

When the MD is wrong

Though virtually all nurses would intervene in the event of life-threatening or injurious physician-mistakes, far fewer would involve themselves when the error is "minor." Roughly half might suggest a better alternative to acceptable therapy; but less than a third would risk severe political hassles merely to assure economical procedures.

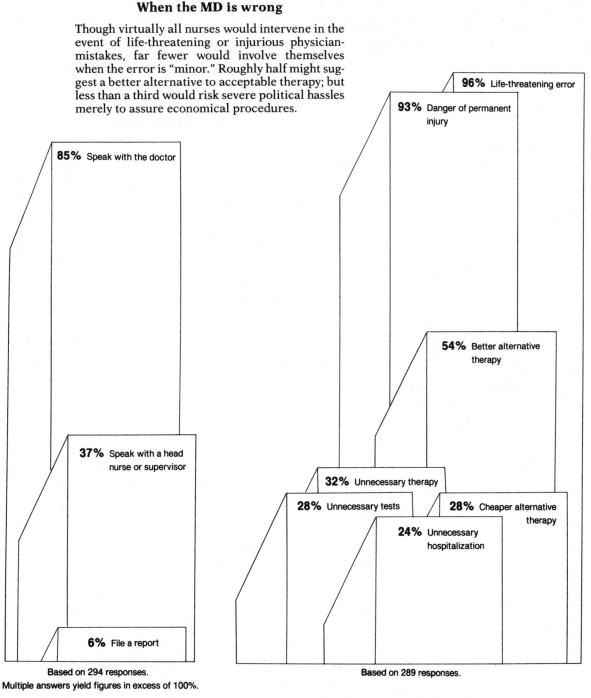

85% Speak with the doctor

37% Speak with a head nurse or supervisor

6% File a report

Based on 294 responses.
Multiple answers yield figures in excess of 100%.

What nurses would do about it . . .

96% Life-threatening error

93% Danger of permanent injury

54% Better alternative therapy

32% Unnecessary therapy

28% Unnecessary tests

28% Cheaper alternative therapy

24% Unnecessary hospitalization

Based on 289 responses.

. . . and when they'd take action

she suggests, try saying, "I'm concerned about the patient and would feel more comfortable if I clarified this with your chief." She adds, "Leave it that way and see how he responds. He may give you some information (which is what you wanted in the first place), ask you what your concern is, or tell you to go right ahead." Be prepared to actually go to the next level if the physician calls your bluff. Remember, you're not ratting on a doctor, you're trying to see that your patient gets the best care.

It's true that a teaching setting does give you more levels in the chain of command, but this also means it can be harder to know who to contact next. Ms. Williamson explains, "It is not uncommon for a patient to be treated by several different services at once. The plastic surgeon may not pay attention to what a certain medication is going to do to the patient's gastric ulcer, which is being treated by an internist."

When the system of checks and balances is too complicated in your hospital, or the physician's attitude is too difficult to deal with, go to your nursing superior. The *RN* survey indicated that 37% of the nurses would do this. Ms. Rose concurs: "I would stay away from the doctor's chain of command and deal with my own peer group, where I'd have a chance of finding more support." Still, your aim here should be to enlist help for another talk with the doctor; don't go off to the director of nurses before you've talked to the physician yourself.

If the situation is serious and your superior isn't doing anything, keep going. But if you plan to skip a link in the chain, let the person know. And don't be impulsive. Give your head nurse a chance to take care of the matter if she says she will. You can always check back with her to see what progress she has made. In fact, you should periodically ask what is happening, because passing the buck to someone else makes for a weak defense in court.

PROTECTIVE DOCUMENTATION

Keeping liability suits in mind, you should make every effort to document everything. You don't need to keep copious records, just an accurate account of what you did for the patient, as well as what you didn't do. For instance, if your patient were dehydrated and had a very poor oral intake it would be normal to be concerned if the physician discontinued the patient's IV. So if you were to talk to the doctor about the patient's condition and he

were to insist that you remove the IV, you would be wise to make a notation such as, "IV discontinued per Dr. Jones' order. Doctor made aware of patient's oral intake (100 cc over the last 24 hours) and inability to retain fluids (emesis × 2 during day shift)." Remember, though, that this type of notation still does not relieve you of the responsibility of notifying someone else of your concern about the order.

When extremely serious problems involve reporting to several levels of authority in the hospital, a different type of record might be advisable. One way to protect yourself is asking a neutral third person to witness your verbal report of the incident. Let the person know that you might ask her, in the future, to recount what was said.

Another suggestion comes from *RN* legal consultant Jack Horsley. He says that the nurse who contacts several levels of authority "should not chart her action, but should keep a detailed memorandum of whom she talked to and what was said."

In spite of all your planning, there are times that you will not get results, or the results you want. "If you don't get support from your director of nurses," warns Jane Hirsch, "you might have to grin and bear it, because it gets awfully cold out on a limb by yourself. But if the physician's error jeopardized my license or the patient's life, I would do everything I could to prevent it."

FIGHTING THE SYSTEM

Mary Ellen Mackert, RN, MSN, consultant in nursing service, assistant professor of nursing in a community college in Maryland, and coauthor of *Dynamics of Law in Nursing and Health Care*, goes further. She says, "If you go to your supervisor and the director of nurses, and the whole agency is unresponsive, then you might consider employment elsewhere. No one person can change the system."

Ms. Mackert's coauthor on the book is a nurse and a lawyer, Mary Hemelt, RN, MS, JD, a professor of nursing who is also chairman of the board of review of the Maryland Department of Health and Mental Hygiene. She cautions the nurse to look at the hierarchy before acting, commenting, "I hope that before taking on the whole hospital politically, you assess the potential for success. There is no point in putting your neck on the line without some possibility of getting results. It's important to plan strategy and for nurses to support one another in this. Some nurses think it's hypocrisy, but it's realistic."

Learn your hospital's standard procedure for reporting errors, and work, at least initially, within that structure. Try to determine your strongest ally. If you can't find results in the hospital and the situation is dangerous, you may have to go outside.

If you really want to press the point, contact your state's nursing association, medical society, or licensing and examining board for either profession (these boards usually handle discipline and investigations). But remember that this approach can progress very slowly, and once the hospital and doctor find out you may be harassed or sued—though most states have passed legislation giving health professionals immunity from civil suits brought for reporting a physician.

JUDGMENT AND CREDIBILITY

Of course, before you organize a small revolution you've got to consider just how great the danger is for the patient. Medical treatment has many gray areas, so you must ask *how* wrong the doctor is. "The term error implies a value judgment, and very often it is difficult to make one," says Ms. Hemelt. "You may be comparing the way Dr. Jones treats a patient with the way Dr. Smith would handle him. This is really not a matter of capabilities if you are comparing technique and personality instead of competency."

You must decide, however, and tailor the nature of your response to the situation. The *RN* survey shows that a nurse would be more likely to take action if the physician's mistake would lead to permanent injury or threaten the life of the patient, and nursing leaders agree that you must speak up in such a case on your legal and ethical responsibility. Certainly if the physician is asking you to take part you should refuse, telling him of your concern and being prepared to take the problem to the highest level.

When you aren't sure about your judgment, but you really question the physician's action, use the resources available to you. Ms. Hirsch suggests, "There are always libraries, pharmacists, and your colleagues to double-check yourself with. I have a strong background in physiology and want to know the physiological basis of orders. When something makes sense to me, I can accept it more easily." You can also go to another physician and ask his opinion, without mentioning names.

"You may be more likely to see life and death situations in the critical care areas," adds Ms. Hirsch. "There the nurse has standing orders that allow her to take action in, say, a cardiac arrest." Protocols don't provide absolute protection, though, because they are designed only to guide the nurse in the absence of a physician. Once he arrives on the scene, your hands may be tied.

An ICU setting gives you a chance to act quickly, notes Karin Williamson. "If you call the physician and say, 'I need a verbal order for this drug' or 'we need something quick and I'm ready with . . . .' then nine times out of ten he will say OK. It all boils down to your credibility with the physician. I see some staff nurses who can pull off all kinds of things like that, because of mutual respect. If I'm doing 15-minute neurological checks on a patient in the ICU and his condition starts deteriorating fast, I'll call the doctor. At three o'clock in the morning he may tell me the patient can wait until 6 A.M., but in this situation I would say, 'No, he can't. If you won't come, I'll call the staff man.' This will create a bad feeling only if you are crying 'wolf.'"

The problem is more complex when the physician orders therapy for which you think there is a better alternative. Basically, you just have to learn to live with different doctors' philosophies. One may be conservative and another radical, but they're both practicing medicine. "First think of how you would react if the physician came to you with a 'better' way of practicing nursing," says Ms. Mackert.

You're not in a good position to tell the physician what to do. That's not your role. But asking is perfectly legitimate and you're bound to learn something. You can always try putting an idea in the physician's head by suggesting something. Ms. Hirsch explains, "Our young doctors come from all over the country so they have different ideas, and I wouldn't hesitate to tell them about the success we have with certain methods."

WHEN IT'S NOT LIFE OR DEATH

If you think the patient would do just as well with less expensive therapy, ask the physician. Cheaper doesn't necessarily mean better, of course, but the strong consumer movement is sweeping everyone along and "the doctor might respond more to this type of problem because it affects his pocketbook," says Ms. Hemelt.

You'll have a stronger leg to stand on if you know the product you suggest. The doctor may want to use an expensive cream for the treatment of decubitus ulcers, when you have good results with Maalox and a heat lamp. "I usually ask him if he'll let us try our way for a few days," adds Ms. Hirsch.

One of the hardest problems to deal with is that of unnecessary therapy, tests, or even hospitalization. Unless there's a detailed history and physical on the chart, you may not have the faintest idea of what the physician is looking for, and without this guideline, you can't observe the patient for important signs and symptoms.

Utilization review committees monitor the length of hospital stays, and have been instrumental in setting standards for certain procedures. In the final analysis, though, it's the doctor's credibility that counts, and you may have to simply trust his judgment.

Ms. Hirsch uses patient management rounds to update ongoing patient care. "Once a week the physician, social worker, dietitian, and nurses sit down and discuss the patients. It's a good chance to ask about something like standing blood work orders."

What about the sensitive, and very serious, area of physician misconduct? If something about a physician's behavior leads you to believe that he is not functioning professionally your duty is clear cut, say the experts. If a doctor is drunk, abusing drugs, or even sexually molesting his patients, you cannot stand by and watch. Inform your superiors, tell his colleagues, and refuse to work with him until he is functioning appropriately. If you don't, you're definitely a party to his misconduct.

A CLIMATE OF COOPERATION

None of us consciously intends to allow a patient to suffer because of a physician's mistake, yet sometimes it happens because we're not sure of our ability to deal with our colleagues. There are some things you can do, however, to make that task easier.

Promote strong collegial relationships among doctors and nurses. Try to get nursing and medical support for joint meetings on communication problems. The National Joint Practice Commission has been defining new roles and relationships for doctors and nurses since 1972, and believes it is having success in testing the effectiveness of its concepts in several core demonstration hospitals. The commission recommends that nurses and doctors integrate their observations in the patient record in their progress notes. In addition, it encourages both doctors and nurses to openly challenge each other's clinical judgments, and resolve their differences on clinical grounds. William Schaffrath, Ph D, director of the commission, says, "Such a climate of collaboration makes the patient well safeguarded. This type of relationship leaves little room for error."

If you think the problem lies more with yourself than the hospital, pinpoint what you need to work on. Are you too timid, or too aggressive? Find a role model who manages confrontations well, and watch this person in action. Ask for hints on how to manage things smoothly.

Talk to a sympathetic superior for suggestions about courses to take. Assertiveness training for nurses is becoming increasingly popular, and you don't have to be suffering from the doormat syndrome to learn something from it. This type of instruction can also deal with the problem of toning yourself down. The point is to be constructively assertive.

Finally, enlist the patient's help whenever possible. You are trying to prevent a mistake that would affect him, so encourage him to speak up and ask the physician more questions. Health care teams are only as strong as their individual members, and informed patients are a vital part of the group process.

Despite all the pitfalls inherent in challenging a physician, the *RN* survey shows that nurses *are* doing it, and are getting results. About 80% of the respondents say they have actually taken some type of action at some time, and virtually all of these nurses say they feel it was effective. It may be difficult for you, but it's not impossible!

Should Nurses Report Negligence in Medical Treatment?

Helen Creighton

Many nurses have inquired as to whether they should report a physician who renders care in a negligent manner. Nurses continually work with physicians and, more than once, the conscientious nurse ponders her responsibility when she sees a medical bit of carelessness or negligence.

The problem is not a new one. Some twenty years ago in the case of *Farrel v. Kramer,*[1] a feud raged between a nurse and a doctor after the nurse was dismissed by the hospital for unprofessional conduct when she became openly critical of the postoperative treatment being given a patient by the doctor. The charges she brought against the doctor were dismissed by the Grievance Committee of the Aroostook County Medical Association. Some time later she was re-employed by the hospital on the stated condition that she should not discuss hospital business outside the hospital. When the physician learned that the nurse had been re-employed, he called the administrator and said: "I wanted to ask you if you would stoop so low as to hire that creep, that malignant son of a bitch, back to work for you in the hospital." He added: She was unfit for the care of patients . . . he could prove that . . . and he intended to make an issue of it.

The nurse learned of these remarks and brought suit against the doctor. If actual malice is shown, the plaintiff may recover compensatory damages and punitive damages. A jury verdict of $17,500 was reduced to $5,000 since provocation, although no excuse for slander, is a mitigating factor in assessing punitive damages.[2]

Following this celebrated case, many nurses have been careful to say comparatively little, if anything, when a doctor's care of a patient was less than the situation seemed to indicate necessary or desirable. The fear of being labeled a "stool pigeon" or a discontented nurse, *i.e.*, the threat to their job if they criticized the physician's work, minimized complaints. With the tightening of the economy and the concomitant rise in unemployment, jobs are scarce and nurses are even less likely to report a doctor for care which may seem to them less than adequate.

The recent case of the *Poor Sisters of St. Francis Seraph v. Catron*[3] brings the whole question up for review. There Catron was brought to the emergency room of the Hospital at about 3:40 A.M. in a comatose condition, apparently as a result of unintentional drug overdose, and her breathing was shallow. Knochel, the emergency room physician on duty, inserted an endotracheal tube to aid Catron's breathing. She was later admitted to the Intensive Care Unit (ICU) of the Hospital under the care of her family physician, Ralph Weller. Weller kept the tube in place in Catron's throat as Catron was still comatose and unable to breathe on her own.

Five days later, Weller ordered a nurse to remove the tube. When the nurse reported she was unable to remove the tube, Weller removed the tube. Later that day, when Catron began having difficulty breathing, Weller ordered a tracheostomy. Catron's condition improved and she was discharged after six more days. After her release, Catron experienced further breathing difficulties which necessitated her return for another tracheostomy. Catron also experienced difficulty in speaking and underwent several operations to remove scar tissue and open her voice box. At the time of trial, Catron could not speak above a whisper and she breathed partly

Creighton, H. (1983, January). Should nurses report negligence in medical treatment? *Nursing Management*, 1y, 47–49.

through her nose and partially through a hole in her throat created by the tracheostomy.[4]

After a trial, a verdict of $150,000 was rendered against the Hospital and the judgment was affirmed on appeal. The Court of Appeals held that: "(1) in view of testimony as to general rule that endotracheal tubes should not be left in patient longer than three or four days, jury could find that there was negligence in that nurses and inhalation therapist did not report treatment of hospital patient to their supervisor although they were aware that endotracheal tube was being left in patient longer than customary three to four day period."[5]

During the trial the hospital requested final instruction No. 7 given by the trial court read as follows: "Skilled hospital personnel have a duty to exercise reasonable care in administering services to patients in the hospital. If such personnel know that a licensed attending physician, without consultation, either by his failure to treat a patient or by treating a patient in a manner which is a substantial departure from accepted medical standards is endangering the health and life of said patient, then the hospital personnel have a duty to perform such acts as are within their authority to protect the health and life of said patient."[6]

The record in this case contains testimony by an expert witness that nurses who work in Intensive Care Units and inhalation therapists are specially trained to handle patients who have endotracheal tubes inserted. Several witnesses testified that as a general rule endotracheal tubes should not be left in a patient longer than three or four days. The head nurse in the ICU admitted that she knew the "rule of thumb" when working with endotracheal tubes was that the upper time limit for leaving them in place was three days. The inhalation therapist employed by the Hospital who handled Catron's respirator also testified he knew the recommended guideline for leaving in endotracheal tubes was 48 to 72 hours. Another nurse in ICU testified it is the duty of a nurse to report any critical condition to the doctor in charge and if he did nothing, to report the condition to her supervisor.[7]

Neither the nurses in ICU nor the inhalation therapists reported Weller's treatment of Catron to their supervisors although they were aware the endotracheal tube was being left in the patient longer than the customary three or four day period. Similarly, the nurses did not bring to Weller's attention the fact that the tube was being left in longer than usual.[8] These things the nurses and inhalation therapists should have done.

In *Brook v. St. John's Hickey Memorial Hospital*,[9] a radiologist injected a contrast medium into the calves of a patient. The injection, which was given in the presence of an x-ray technologist employed by St. John's, resulted in injury to the patient. In this case, the suit against the hospital was dismissed because of lack of evidence that the hospital employee who witnessed the injection was trained to recognize the proper injection sites. However, the Supreme Court did recognize in some cases the failure of hospital employees to "recognize and report any departure from normal practices" may amount to a breach of duty for which the hospital is liable.[10]

In *Utter v. United Hospital Center, Inc.*[11] the plaintiff was admitted to the hospital with a broken wrist and dislocated elbow. A cast was put on the wrist and the arm began to swell and turned black and the patient became delirious. Although the nurses observed the worsening condition of the patient and reported some of the symptoms to the physician, they did not report the delirium. When the doctor did nothing further, the nurses did not call the hospital authorities. The West Virginia Supreme Court restated the jury verdict against the hospital: " . . . The question of the propriety of action or inaction of the nurses is one to be decided by the jury under the evidence before it.

The tenor of the defendant's contentions indicates that the nurses are being treated unfairly and that they should not be expected to heal the patient's ills. While registered nurses certainly are not charged with the responsibility of curing patients, they are charged with duties clearly reflected in the record. Nurses are specialists in hospital care who, in the final analysis, hold the well-being, in fact, in some instances, the very lives of patients in their hands."[12]

In *Toth v. Community Hospital at Glen Cove*[13] where premature infants were blinded by too high a concentration of oxygen being administered for too long a period of time, the court said: "At that point it became the nurse's duty to inform the attending physician, and if he failed to act, to advise the hospital authorities so that appropriate action might be taken."

In *Darling v. Charleston Memorial Hospital*[14] a college football player sustained a broken leg and it was placed in a cast by a general practitioner at a community hospital. At first the foot was warm but became cold two days later and there was a foul smell in the room for two weeks. The nurses told the doctor of the condition and noted it on the chart. At first the doctor did nothing, but then he cut the cast and, in so doing, cut the leg. The leg eventually had to be amputated at a medical center to which the patient was transferred. The community hospital was held liable under the doctrine of *respondeat superior* because the nurses either did not observe or at least failed to report patient problems that were overlooked or not thought to be significant by the doctor. The court said: "Thus, if a nurse or other hospital employee fails to report changes in a patient's condition and/or to question a doctor's orders when they are not in accord with standard medical practice and the omission results in injury to the patient, the hospital will be liable for the employee's negligence."[15] The physician himself settled out of court; he had no specialty training and had not secured a consultation.

Nurses are recognized specialists in hospital care and ICU nurses as in the *Poor Sisters of St. Francis Seraph* are legally clinical specialists with special knowledge and skills and are responsible for reporting medical negligence through appropriate channels. It is emphasized that the reporting should be done professionally through appropriate channels. Tact as well as professionalism is useful. Failure to report negligence on the part of physicians is negligence by omission, *i.e.*, nonfeasance: the failure to do what another reasonable and prudent nurse of similar education and skill would do under comparable circumstances.[16]

REFERENCES

1. *Farrell v. Kramer*, 159 Maine 387, 35 A2d 218, 193 Atl. 560 (Maine 1963)

2. Creighton, Helen. *Law Every Nurse Should Know*, 4th ed., Philadelphia, W. B. Saunders Co., 1981, p. 212

3. *Poor Sisters of St. Francis Seraph v. Catron*, 435 N.E. 2d 305, 306 (Ct. App. Ind. 2nd Dist. 1982)

4. *Idem*

5. *Op.cit.*, supra, note 3, p. 305

6. *Ibid.* p. 307

7. *Ibid.* p. 308

8. *Idem*

9. *Brook v. St. John's Hickey Memorial Hospital*, 269 Ind. 270, 380 N.E. 3d 72, 74 (S. Ct. Ind. 1978)

10. *Ibid.*, p. 75

11. *Utter v. United Hospital Center, Inc.*, 236 S.E. 2d 213 (S. Ct. West Va. 1977)

12. *Ibid.*, p. 216

13. *Toth v. Community Hospital at Glen Cove*, 22 N.Y. 2d 255, 292 N.Y.S. 2d, 239 N.E. 2d 368 (Ct. App. N.Y. 1968)

14. *Darling v. Charleston Community Hospital*, 211 N.E. 253 (S. Ct. W. Va. 1965); Creighton, Helen. *Law Every Nurse Should Know*, 4th ed. *Op.cit.* supra, note 2, p. 163, 334

15. *Idem*

16. Cf. Regan, William A. Intensive Care Nursing: Doctor Problems, *Regan Rep. on Nursing Law*, 23:4, Sept. 1982

"The 'Joy' of Telling a Physician He's Wrong"

Freda Baron Friedman

How do *you* handle your everyday, nagging doubts about the appropriateness of an MD's orders or attitude? Suppose, for example, a doctor asks you to give a medication you know is not very effective for the patient's problem. It may not hurt the patient, but it won't do him much good, either.

Or, how about this situation: While you're explaining ostomy care procedures to a patient who is very nervous and worried about being able to manage on her own, her physician comes in. He abruptly announces that he has already explained the whole procedure to his patient. When you comment that she still seems anxious, he gives you an icy stare and says: "Don't you have anything else to do on the floor?"

Finally, a third: It is Saturday night and Mr. Zynt down the hall has become very agitated and insists on seeing his doctor. You phone the physician, but his answering service says he can't be reached all weekend.

What would you do in each of these cases?

The 400 nurses *RN* surveyed about RN/MD relations said they face such dilemmas all the time. These sticky little problems may not be as dramatic as the cases of outright physician incompetence that become legendary in hospitals—the doctor who amputates the wrong leg, leaves an instrument inside a patient, or prescribes medication that triggers a near-fatal reaction. But run-of-the-mill difficulties still can have many serious, long-term consequences for the patient and for the nurse—in whose lap they often land. What's the best approach to take when doctors don't fill out the proper paperwork for an order, fail to update a medication form, ignore

isolation procedures, or treat a patient or family brusquely?

At one time, nurses might have been more willing to go along with whatever a physician did or did not do in the line of duty. Many nurses simply assumed that the physician was always right. Even if they didn't, many were not willing to take the risks involved in correcting a doctor or calling him on the carpet for an oversight. Those attitudes are changing.

END OF INNOCENCE

First of all, most nurses now recognize the fallibility of physicians. Of those who responded to the *RN* survey, only 10% felt that *all* physicians are highly competent. More than eight out of ten said that while most of the physicians they work with are competent, there are "a few bad ones." Happily, the ranks of the totally disillusioned are small. Only 8% of the *RN* respondents felt a substantial number of MDs are incompetent.

A second reason for change is that the risks are too high to let errors and oversights slide by, no matter who on the health care team makes the mistakes. First, of course, the patient's welfare and well-being are at stake. In such instances, the nurse must decide what her moral responsibility is to patients who may suffer the effects of physicians' errors. But there are also legal strictures that weigh heavily on the decision. Nurse practice acts and many hospital policies spell out, in varying degrees

Friedman, F. B. (1982, April). The 'joy' of telling a physician he's wrong. *RN, 45,* 35–37, 96. Reprinted with permission of © Medical Economics Company, Inc., Oradell, NJ.

of detail, just what the nurse's duty is to the patient. Ignoring these dictates can lead to loss of license and personal reputation and, on a broader scale, the collective reputation of nurses—even if an error originates with a physician.

"Why should we always take the blame when a physician makes an error?" ask many nurses who feel this happens far too frequently. "This jeopardizes our personal integrity and puts our public image in a negative light. It can also jeopardize our jobs."

Nevertheless, many hospitals hold nurses responsible for incorrect actions, even if they're the result of following a doctor's orders. "We are told by the administration that policing is part of our job," says Genevieve Murtaugh, RN, of Tampa, Fla.

"In our hospital, there is no specific policy, but it's taken for granted that nurses will police the medical staff; if not, and a problem arises, it is usually the nurse who is told that she should have questioned the order," comments Lynne Sanson, RN, of Montclair, N.J. Another explanation is given by Virginia Colt, RN, of Boring, Ore.: "Our nurse practice act deems us responsible for our actions in following orders and we are liable for errors, so we have to police and judge doctors' orders carefully."

MIXED REVIEWS FOR THE ROLE

How do nurses feel about this watchdog role? Four out of ten respondents feel hospitals rely too heavily on nurses to double-check on doctors. "My time is too valuable and I resent having to spend it reminding MDs of their responsibilities," complains Susan Adams, RN, of Great Falls, Va. "I'm busy enough without doing their work," adds Alice Duke, RN, of New Bern, N.C. Another nurse points out the logistical problems in policing: "With the present shortage of nurses, it's very hard to check up on the doctors. Most floors have no charge nurse on the evening and night shifts."

But many nurses don't seem to mind. More than half of the *RN* sample said that the responsibility their facilities placed on nurses for double-checking MDs on routine orders and hospital procedures was about right. Says Claire Witte, RN, of Massapequa, N.Y., "My facility does not rely on RNs to double-check MDs' orders, but I do it for my satisfaction, contentment, and personal sense of responsibility." A nurse from Oregon echoes that sentiment: "As a

good RN, you should know the routine orders and should be checking them anyway for all your patients." Alice Hale, RN, of Massillon, Ohio, thinks the system of double-checks is a good one because "two heads are always better than one."

Some nurses feel that they should have an even larger role in policing MDs. Although few are looking for that added burden, the 4% of *RN*'s survey respondents who are willing to take it on have strong feelings about the subject. Says one nurse, "When it's for her own safety and her patient's safety, the nurse should be allowed to *triple-*check!" Another feels that nurses should be allowed to police MDs more, and, more importantly, that "our complaints should be taken seriously. As it now stands, no one will listen until something tragic happens."

WAYS THAT WORK

The nurse who comes right out and accuses a doctor of not knowing his business usually gets nowhere, except on the doctor's bad side. But correcting a specific oversight by a physician is usually relatively easy to handle. In the case of medication errors, for instance, 81% of the respondents said that doctors do take corrections in a professional manner. "It all depends on how the nurse presents the error to the physician," says Priscilla Moser, RN, of Reading, Pa.

And what *are* the best ways of approaching this ticklish situation? Claire Witte suggests presenting the correction as a question, not a challenge. Paula Willoughby, RN, of Davenport, Iowa, suggests another indirect approach: "Never tell a physician he is in error. Just say you can't understand the order and would appreciate his verifying it."

Attitude is everything, suggest several nurses. If a nurse wants to point out an error, it should be done diplomatically in a non-threatening and nonaccusatory manner.

Backing up the question with facts also seems to help. "I always check with the pharmacy to be sure of my facts," comments Catherine Joruby, RN, of Orange, Calif. In some hospitals, a nurse who suspects a medication error can ask the pharmacist to intervene directly. "This approach always works well," says Linda Russell, RN, of New Britain, Conn., since the pharmacist is always willing to clarify orders.

Most physicians appreciate having an order questioned if it is incorrect, report many nurses. "They feel you are aware of meds and are conscientious," says Rhonda Lawrence, RN, of Owosso, Mich.

There are, however, doctors who do not take any correction kindly, as some *RN* respondents pointed out, citing "unprofessional reactions" they have had to face.

"'Since when do you have a license to prescribe?' is the typical response I have gotten from one doctor when I've questioned the drug prescribed," relates Dianne Bennett, RN, of Chapman, Neb. But she adds that most doctors, including this one, don't mind if nurses question the frequency and dosage of a drug as long as they don't pass judgment on the *choice*.

Sarcasm, belligerence, annoyance, and even outright temper tantrums do occur occasionally, say some nurses, but doctors who respond this way are the exception.

When a doctor refuses to acknowledge a medication error and correct it, does a nurse have recourse? A number of respondents suggest referring the matter to the pharmacy department. One ED nurse simply turns the tables: "We have several physicians who often order doses that are too high. We generally ask *them* to give the medications they have ordered, explaining that we don't feel comfortable with the dosage they have prescribed. Very often they will then reduce the dosage."

PROBLEMS OF OMISSION
AND ATTITUDE

Policing medication errors is relatively easy compared to policing physician neglect or ignorance. High on the list are outdated orders; inadequate follow-up; insensitive reactions to patients, families, or nurses, particularly in geriatric settings; orders for diagnostic tests that nurses feel are excessive for the patient's condition; inadequate response to a nurse's request for information or orders; and inadequate recommendations for treatment.

Why do these problems occur? According to the nurses who have to live with the consequences, some develop because the doctors are just not available. "There's too much telephone medicine; it's hard to find doctors on weekends, holidays, and in the evenings, and they don't come around to see their patients enough," are the various complaints.

Nurses in long-term care facilities are particularly vehement about physician absenteeism. "Some doctors will not visit their patients regularly, in spite of constant reminders," comments Merilyn

Fisher, RN, of Upper Darby, Pa. This results in inadequate follow-up and inadequate orders to cover varying stages of the patient's condition, observes Evelyn Flock, RN, of Urbana, Ill.

"Some doctors are available, but are either too inexperienced or too insensitive to the patient's needs to do the right thing," observes one nurse. "Many are competent with simple problems, but do poorly with complex illnesses," adds another. "Many physicians are reluctant to bring in a specialist as a consultant," observes Carol Wells, RN, of Jacksonville, Fla.

Communication is also a problem. "They don't spend enough time with their patients, but they don't want nurses to give advice and educate the patients, even though they won't do it themselves," says Lavern Whitmire, RN, of St. Louis.

Physicians' attitudes toward patients, nurses, and life in general also create problems for some of the respondents. Some physicians "have not kept up on things and don't want to learn any new methods. In fact, they resent any kind of change," comments one nurse. Others feel that doctors just don't care about their patients. Connie Johnson, RN, of Bethlehem, Pa., relates an experience to illustrate her point. "I work in a nursing home and pointed out to one of the doctors a reddened area on what turned out to be the fractured arm of one patient. He quickly diagnosed it as an infected hair follicle, without having asked the patient much of anything. Three days later, the patient died of a pulmonary embolism."

"If doctors did an adequate job of policing themselves, we would not have to be put into this position," comments a nurse from Ohio. Just how well doctors do police themselves is a controversial topic, with respondents about equally divided on the question. Those who feel physicians are doing an adequate job often qualify their evaluation with some reservations. Others insist that doctors usually do not police themselves voluntarily—or very enthusiastically.

DOCTORS PRESSURED
TO SELF-POLICE

"Their policing is slow and, many times, subtle," comments a nurse from Michigan. "If a physician is barely competent, the word gets around. He'll stop getting referrals and start losing patients, but this usually takes time."

Sometimes the pressure to police comes from nurses themselves. Sagretta Labashosky, RN, of Rockford, Ill. says, "It usually takes a lot of incidents and complaining by nurses before something is done."

Susan Smith, RN, of Myrtle Beach, S.C., suggests that societal pressure is often the key factor. "It's adequate in the very small hospital and small town where I am because gossip spreads." Robin Lake, RN, of Helena, Ark., suggests the other side of the coin: "In a large facility with a reputation to maintain, policing is necessary."

Formal mechanisms, such as PSROs and tight monitoring of adherence to hospital policies, *do* encourage doctors to police themselves. But sometimes the policing backfires, observes Sharon McKinney, RN, of Columbus, Ohio: "A doctor will criticize a colleague or argue about treatments done or planned right in front of the patient. This creates a lot of animosity and is certainly not good for the patient." That may be why many doctors don't keep watch on each other. Among the respondents who feel that MDs don't do much in the way of "keeping their own house in order" is Priscilla Moser. She says, "they cover up for each other far too often." Comments Edward Johnson, RN, of Bay Village, Ohio, "I've heard their complaints about each other; some are serious, but no censure of MDs is involved. The problem is usually 'buried.'"

"There's not enough peer pressure," suggests Marge Van Asten, RN, of Little Chute, Wis. "There's no system for reporting incompetence," adds another nurse. "While nurses have to make out incident reports if they give vitamin pills to the wrong patient, most of the time Mds' mistakes—even serious ones—go unreported," observes Maryanne DiPrimio, RN, of Waterbury, Conn. "I've never known an MD to make out an incident report at any hospital."

Policies and procedures, as well as attitude, seem to vary from one facility to the next. Where the spirit of cooperation and professionalism runs high, high expectations are set for and by most members of the staff. That is when policing is viewed as a positive function rather than a negative one—and the attitude is one of "I'll help you, you help me, and the patient will get the best care possible."

This spirit does not eliminate all problems and potential for error, but, according to respondents who feel positive about their policing role, "Without this option, it would be hard to live with ourselves and to face our patients. This way, we feel we are doing what we can and what we should do to make sure our patients get high-quality care."

The Risks of Blowing the Whistle

Alfred G. Feliu

Patricia Lampe, head nurse in the intensive care unit at Presbyterian Medical Center in Colorado, objected to the reduction of her already over-worked staff at a time when the unit had an 80–90 percent occupancy rate. The response to her concern? A notice of termination(1).

Margaret Rookard, director of nursing at Harlem Hospital in New York City, refused to sign permits for foreign nurses who did not work for her and objected to other questionable practices. Rookard was transferred to headquarters, given a five-by-seven-foot cubicle office (which doubled as an employee clothes closet and kitchen), and, after a short while, was fired(2).

Nurse Alyce Rozier, who witnessed various patient abuses, was ordered to take a polygraph examination after an article appeared in a local newspaper detailing the incidents. She failed the test and was fired(3).

These three nurses each went to court seeking redress, and lost. Each discovered, to her chagrin, that the ethical response to a professional dilemma is not always protected by law—at least as the law stands today.

A strong and growing sense of professionalism has emboldened a number of nurses, like Lampe, Rookard and Rozier, to speak out against illegal or unethical practices. In fact, the ANA *Code for Nurses* demands that nurses serve as client advocates: "The nurse's primary commitment is to the client's care and safety. Hence, in the role of client advocate, the nurse must be alert to and take appropriate action regarding any instances of incompetent, unethical, or illegal practice(s) . . ."(4).

Yet, blowing the whistle guarantees neither correction of the ill nor protection against reprisal. A crucial question then is: What are the rights of a nurse who decides to expose illegal or unethical practices? Knowing the answer could help a nurse decide *whether* to blow the whistle, how best to do so, and how to prepare—legally—for any ramifications.

The law in this area is only beginning to develop. In the United States, under the century-old Employment-At-Will doctrine, employers have had the authority to fire employees for any or no reason. In recent decades, Congress, state legislatures and the courts have delineated circumstances that limit this broad right. For example, employers may not discriminate on the basis of race, sex, religion, place of origin, or because of an employee's union activity(5). These are significant limitations but, legally, employers are still free to fire employees for practically any other reason. While race may not be a basis for dismissal, a preference for the Beatles rather than Beethoven may be.

The only other substantial limitations on management's ability to fire employees are bargaining agreements with unions. Most union contracts require that management have "just cause" for disciplining or discharging an employee who is covered by the contract. For example, an employer has "just cause" for firing if an employee has been chronically absent, has been shown to be incompetent, or has stolen employer property. Less than one quarter of the American workforce, however, is unionized.

Public-sector employees are similarly protected against unjust dismissal, but they too make up only a small percentage of the workforce. The sad fact is that job security for most employees is subject, to a surprising extent, to the whims of management.

If this were the complete picture, a whistle-blower's prospects for vindication before a court would be bleak. Fortunately, some courts have

Feliu, A. G. (1983, October). The risks of blowing the whistle. *Americn Journal of Nursing, 83,* 1387–1388, 1390. Reprinted with permission of ©American Journal of Nursing Company. All rights reserved.

recognized exceptions to the dismissal-at-will rule. For example, courts have allowed ex-employees to sue former employers when the dismissals were based on an employee's refusal to commit perjury before a state legislative committee; an employee's willingness to fulfill jury duty; the filing of a workers' compensation claim; an employee's willingness to assist police in investigating theft by fellow employees; and a refusal to participate in an illegal price-fixing scheme, to name a few notable cases(6-10). While the number of courts willing to come to the defense of employees in this way has grown steadily in the last decade, they are still in the minority.

Another approach taken by some wrongfully discharged employees is to claim that management, by word or deed, had *promised* not to discharge them except for "just cause" even though there was no law or union contract. For example, the Michigan Supreme Court ruled that an employer would have to abide by a statement, found in the handbook issued to all employees, that employees would be dismissed only where "just cause" existed(11). In another case, the same court required that an employer abide by the promise made to a newly hired employee that he would not be dismissed so long as he "did his job"(12).

In a similar case, a nurse in an orthopedic hospital in Spokane, Washington, was discharged after she and a teenage patient engaged in playful water throwing(13). The patients and staff were reportedly amused by the horseplay, but the hospital viewed the nurse's behavior as gross neglect of her duties and, on that basis, fired her. She sued, and a Washington court ruled that the personnel handbook gave the impression of promising job security, for example by establishing a four-step termination process—oral counseling, written counseling, final warning and termination—that was not followed. The court concluded that the hospital both failed to live up to its promises and lacked good cause to fire the nurse. The nurse was awarded back wages and the value of her lost pension benefits.

But such decisions are few and so far have had limited impact on the wide-ranging ability of employers to fire.

PROTECTION FOR WHISTLEBLOWERS

In April 1981, Michigan became the first state to pass a law to help both government and private-sector employees who expose illegal or dangerous employer activity(14). This pioneering legislation was a result of two environmental catastrophes in the 1970s.

One incident was the accidental contamination of livestock feed with the fire-retarding chemical PBB (poly-brominate biphenyl). Employees at the Michigan chemical company responsible for the contamination were allegedly told by management that if they reported the problem to government officials they would lose their jobs. The delay in uncovering the contamination aggravated the disaster and cost the state economy over a billion dollars: Michigan farmers lost millions of dollars in poisoned livestock, and the state government had to spend $16.2 million in a highly publicized clean-up.

The Michigan whistleblower law also was triggered by widespread toxic waste dumping that contaminated ground water and exposed countless citizens to chemical poisoning.

Connecticut recently has followed Michigan's lead and enacted its own whistleblower protection legislation(15). So far, those two are the only states with laws designed to protect private- as well as public-sector whistleblowers. A number of other states and the U.S. Congress, however, have passed legislation that bars discrimination against government workers who expose illegal practices, fraud, gross waste of funds or abuse of public power(16).

In addition, government employees may seek First Amendment protection if they have been penalized for speaking out on a matter of public concern. For example, imagine that a nurse at a V.A. hospital writes to a government official or newspaper that she believes that the dioxin-containing herbicide, Agent Orange, is responsible for the high incidence of certain types of cancer in Vietnam War veterans. If the hospital retaliates, the nurse can persuasively assert in court that her First Amendment right to comment on a public issue has been violated. In fact, when city employee Margaret Rookard was fired, she framed her argument in First Amendment terms(2).

Finally, Congress has, in recent years, attached to certain safety, health and environmental protection acts provisions that bar reprisal against employees who report violations of those acts(17). For example, medical physicist and radiation safety officer Dr. Clifford Richter notified the Nuclear Regulatory Commission (NRC), as he was obligated to do, that a radioactive isotope, iridium-192, had been accidentally left in the body of a patient for approximately three months. The patient died as a result. The NRC found that the hospital had violated a condition of its license permitting it to use radioactive materials in treatment.

Dr. Richter, who had consistently received favorable ratings before reporting this incident, began to be excluded from meetings and found his position first downgraded, then eliminated. He filed a complaint with the Secretary of Labor under the antireprisal provision in the Energy Reorganization Act, and he was awarded back pay and attorneys' fees and was reinstated. The hospital appealed, but a federal court of appeals backed the secretary's determination in full(18).

In summary, legal protection for whistleblowers exists, but the laws and the situations they cover vary widely, depending on such factors as whether the employee works in the private or public sector, on the nature of the issue raised, on the employee's motives in raising the issue, and on how soon after the disciplining or dismissal the employee brings the matter to the attention of appropriate authorities.

Despite the limitations of available legal remedies, recent changes in the law are significant. Why? Because they show some recognition that an employee who puts the public's interest and welfare before that of the employer (even when those interests conflict on the job) may deserve society's support.

REFERENCES

1. Lampe v. Presbyterian Medical Center, 590 P.2d 513 (Colo. App. 1978).

2. Rookard v. Health and Hospitals Corp., No. 82-7739 (S.D.N.Y. 1982).

3. Rozier v. St. Mary's Hospital, 411, N.E.2d 50 (Ill. App. 1980).

4. American Nurses' Association. *Code For Nurses with Interpretive Statements.* Kansas City: ANA, 1976; p. 8.

5. 42 U.S.C. § 2000e; 29 U.S.C. § 58 (a)(1), (4).

6. Peterman v. Int. Bhd., 344, P2d 25 (Cal. App. 1959).

7. Nees v. Hocks, 536 P.2d 512 (Or. App. 1975).

8. Frampton v. Central Indiana Gas Co., 297, N.E.2d 425 (Ind. 1973).

9. Palmateer v. International Harvester Co., 421 N.E.2d 876 (Ill. 1981).

10. Tameny v. ARCO, 164 Cal. Rptr. 839 (1980).

11. Toussaint v. Blue Cross, 292 N.W.2d 880 (Mich. 1980).

12. Ebling v. Masco Corp., 292 N.W.2d 880 (Mich. 1980).

13. Voorhees v. Shriners Hospital, 590 P.2d 513 (Wash. App. 1980).

14. Mich. Comp. Laws §§ 15. 361-15.369 (1980).

15. 1982 Conn. Pub. Acts 82-289.

16. *See e.g.* Civil Service Reform Act of 1978, 5 U.S.C. § 2301 (b)(9) (1979).

17. *See e.g.* Clean Air Act Amendments of 1977, 42 U.S.C. §§ 7401, 7622; Energy Reorganization Act, 42 U.S.C. § 5851.

18. Ellis Fischel State Cancer Hospital v. Marshall, 629 F.2d 563 (8th Cir. 1980), Cert. denied, 101 S. Ct. 1757 (1981).

Thinking of Blowing the Whistle?

Alfred G. Feliu

What should you know before you blow the whistle on illegal or unethical practices? First and foremost, that your life will never be the same once you do. By definition, blowing the whistle is an *extraordinary* step. It is speaking out on your own initiative about activity within your organization that otherwise would not come to public attention.

It may require that you go over your supervisor's head. It may require naming names. It may mean hurting your colleagues, and it may very well cost you friends. None of this need happen, but if you are thinking about blowing the whistle you must be aware of the possible consequences. In short, yours must be an informed decision.

Your ability to avoid the harsh repercussions of blowing the whistle depends on a number of factors—your position in the organization, the substance of your complaint, the source of the problem within the organization, and the rigidity of the organization and its willingness to receive and act on employee complaints. In brief, the effectiveness of your whistleblowing and how likely you are to survive it can fairly be reduced to a question of *power*. How much do you have? Do you have enough to get your views heard and to counter any action against you?

Does this mean that a nurse with minimal power in the organization should refrain from blowing the whistle to protect a patient or the general public? Not necessarily, but it does mean that the decision to do so must be a thoughtful one. *How* one blows the whistle and the *motives* for doing so can be crucial, particularly in any litigation that may ensue. The following advice can help you choose your path:

1. Verify facts, document claims. Be sure you have the story straight. Misinterpretations and unverifiable leads may be fatal. Document your claims. Solicit witnesses where necessary and possible, and check to see how far they are willing to go with you. In short, lay a paper trail.

2. Begin to make your concerns known within the organization. This may be hazardous. Be careful how and to whom you raise the matter. Talk to your supervisor. If that person is unreceptive, or is the problem, seek out other authority figures, an employee relations or nursing official, for example. Try to solve the problem informally before whistleblowing.

3. Exhaust all internal remedies. Once you have tipped your hand, pursue all avenues within the organization. If there is an "open door" policy, use it to talk with the appropriate officials. If there are dispute resolution or counseling procedures, use them. If you are told the problem is being looked into or remedied, don't be hasty. Give the system a chance to work (as long as the danger you are pointing out is not imminent). Keep a close eye on what is being done. If you are not satisfied after a reasonable period of time, prepare to go public.

4. Get a lawyer. If you can afford to hire a lawyer who is familiar with this area of law, it may be in your best interest to do so. An attorney can give you some sense of the law in your state and your chances of success should your case ever go to court, and can guide you in resolving the problem internally.

FIGHTING REPRISALS

What if you have blown the whistle and suffered reprisal? Filing a lawsuit is not necessarily your next step. First, try nonlegal remedies:

Feliu, A. G. (1983, November). Thinking of blowing the whistle? *American Journal of Nursing, 83,* 1387–1388. Reprinted with permission of ©American Journal of Nursing Company. All rights reserved.

1. File a grievance. If you are a union member or a civil servant, your first formal means of appeal is the grievance system established by civil service law or in your union contract. While a union is not required to process your claim, it may not arbitrarily refuse to pursue an apparently meritorious grievance.

2. Contact the review board. Your organization, particularly if it is a hospital or educational facility, most likely has an institutional review board (IRB) that, for example, evaluates research plans and oversees the integrity of research involving human subjects. If your employer has an inspector general office (or an audit or anti-fraud group by some other name), contact it if fraud or malfeasance is involved.

3. Tell your professional society. If you are a member of a professional society, you should immediately inform the committee that oversees the profession's ethical code. Even when a professional society's attempts at persuasion fail, it still has a potent tool, namely, publicity. In the right situation, you may find the society willing to publicize and, in this way, aid your case.

LEGAL LAST RESORT

When your job has suffered as a result of your whistleblowing, and all other efforts have failed, you may need to turn to the law. But the victory, if you get it, will be hard-earned and won at great emotional and financial cost. The legal remedies that exist, limited as they may be, serve less as an efficient means of redress than as a statement of public policy; nevertheless, they promise a remedy for those daring and desperate enough to seek it. You may be able to challenge an employer's actions on the following legal bases.

1. Whistleblower protection laws. Check whether your state has passed a whistleblower protection act (such as those pioneered by Michigan and Connecticut) and see if you meet its requirements.* This is the most obvious and direct source of protection. Nonetheless, remedies tend to be limited under these laws.

2. Wrongful discharge lawsuit. If you can demonstrate that the action taken against you violates a clear and significant public policy—for example, if you were dismissed because you assisted in an investigation of a colleague's incompetence or malfeasance—you may be able to sue for wrongful discharge. In the end, you could be awarded damages for pain and suffering or injury to professional reputation, as well as back wages and lost benefits.

3. Breach-of-contract lawsuit. Were you promised, orally by a member of management or in your employee handbook, that you would not be discharged except for "good reason," "just cause" or "as long as you perform your job satisfactorily?" If so, you may be able to convince a court to require your employer to live up to its promise. If you win, the court will try to reinstate you.

4. Anti-reprisal protection. If you lose your job or your job position suffers because you are trying to encourage enforcement of public protection laws, you should check with the government agency responsible for enforcing the law in question. It is possible that you are entitled to protection. Protection is more often invoked under anti-discrimination and employee health and safety legislation than under environmental protection acts, though each offers some protection. Relief, though, is usually limited in scope.

5. First Amendment. If you are a public employee or work in a government-subsidized facility, and your position at work is harmed due to your speaking out on a matter of public interest, you may have a claim under the First Amendment. The recovery here tends to be limited to back wages, lost benefits and reinstatement to your former or an equivalent position.

In sum, the answer to the question "What are the legal rights of nursing professionals who blow the whistle?" is at present a disheartening "It depends." But the law is changing. In fact, two late developments should be noted: First, Margaret Rookard, the nursing director who was fired after questioning practices at a city hospital has won the right, under a federal court of appeals, to challenge her dismissal on First Amendment grounds.* Second, the New York State legislature has just passed an amendment to the labor law to include a subsection on "Licensed

*See *AJN*, Oct. 1983 Legal Side.

professionals' rights of refusal." It states: "It shall be unlawful for any employer . . . to discharge, demote or otherwise discipline or retaliate against any employee because such employee has refused to engage in conduct which would constitute professional misconduct."

The next subsection goes on to say that any licensed professional who believes an employer has violated this provision ". . . may commence an action in the Supreme Court for damages and other appropriate relief, including reinstatement and pay."

If, as Shakespeare wrote in *King Lear*, "ripeness is all," whistleblowing nursing professionals may find comfort in knowing that the time for legal protection may finally be ripe.

Outrageous or Outraged:
A Nurse Advocate Story

Christine Spahn Smith

Mojtabai, in describing an outrageous friend, said, "We need him. In some crazy way, we depend on him to do that outrageous thing. He has a way of speaking his mind. What the rest of us only dare to think silently, he blurts out top voice. We ought to cherish him."[1] To paraphrase that description and apply it to nursing, one can only wonder: How cherished is the outspoken nurse? What happens to the nurse who blows the whistle on questionable patient care practices? Does she speak the mind of others? For that matter, do they care?

I became an outspoken patient advocate, found I had little or no support from the medical or nursing community, and paid the price—I resigned before being fired. Some may say I was outrageous. I, on the other hand, feel outraged.

I was employed for several years during the late '70s as the director of nursing in a county health department that served a population of 350,000 people. In the course of my work, I reviewed statistical data concerning maternal and infant mortality and morbidity within the county. I was struck by the findings that in one large hospital where 554 women delivered 559 infants during a period of three months, 211 multiparous women had episiotomies with fourth-degree extension tears of the perineum. In addition, 10 percent of the infants born to primiparous women had Apgar scores of zero at one minute and at five minutes, and ten of the infants had a score of zero at ten minutes. All of these infants were born of women who had a no-risk factor pregnancy, no significant problems in pregnancy, and an uneventful labor which fell within the norm for the primagravida on the Friedman labor scale.[2]

During the postpartum period, there was a 10.3 percent infection rate among the total group of 559 mothers. Since the infection rate in postpartum women for the United States about that time was 3.8 percent, this rate is significant and would warrant investigation.[3]

In reviewing these data and the medical literature, it was ascertained that episiotomies with extended maternal injuries can be caused by a number of variables which would have to be studied to determine ways to reduce the incidence. However, in reviewing high-risk factors for infants, we found that vacuum extraction was identified as a significant factor in newborn morbidity.[4,5] This method of delivery had been used in delivering all the newborns with zero Apgar scores at the hospital.

I presented these findings to nurses and physicians in the health department and in the community. Although they agreed that the findings suggested problems that needed to be dealt with, they merely raised their eyebrows, shrugged their shoulders, and did nothing. The maternal-child health nurse from the health department, who served as a liaison between the hospital and the department, continued to compile data for the next three-month period. The results were almost identical.

We again discussed all this information with key individuals in medicine and nursing, and again there was agreement that the data indicated that problems existed in the delivery care at this hospital. But those who could take action did not. We then tried to speak with hospital representatives who had decision-making power to suggest combining our efforts to study the problem. Communication with the hospital had always been poor and now the channels closed completely: physicians, nursing administrators, and nursing supervisors did not think it was necessary to pursue the matter further. One doctor patted the liaison nurse's head and told her not to worry her pretty little head with such matters!

When the liaison nurse initially requested setting up a referral system, those in authority at the hospital agreed she could gather data from the charts if she did it herself. Eventually, the hospital clinic, unit, and nursery nurses started to fill out the forms; in no time, the interns and residents were also writing on them. It was at this point that both the public health nurses receiving the forms and the hospital nurses filling them out became aware of the significance of the information they were recording and talked to me about the questionable maternity care at the hospital.

I conferred with the medical director and other key people repeatedly, and became discouraged when no intervention was made on behalf of the clients. I also conferred with a university nurse faculty member who used the hospital for students' clinical practice. Unaware of our concern, she had written to HEW and received no reply. She and her students then collected objective data and sent it to consumer advocate, Ralph Nader, with no reply.

I finally made a decision to be an advocate for the clients. I explained my position to my staff and asked for their support. Everyone agreed, believing it was important that we voice our concern about the care women were receiving at this hospital. I also spoke to the advisory board for the public health nursing department. One member supported me wholeheartedly and encouraged me to speak out in behalf of the women clients.

My advocacy position on the issues became open knowledge to key people in the community. They confronted the hospital medical staff, who became very angry and denied all of the findings on the basis that their infection rate "was comparable to any other hospital"; that the Apgar scores had " . . . the meaning of water"; and that " . . . the interns and residents needed experience with all types of interventions for delivery of a baby and the vacuum extractor was a safe procedure."

How did this come about? For years before I came to the agency, information about maternity patients was gathered in an almost clandestine manner. A volunteer who admitted maternity patients wrote their names and addresses on slips of paper and put them in a desk drawer in a hall. A public health nurse picked them up. These slips comprised the only information the public health nurses obtained. Hospital postpartum referrals were sent to our department after a woman had her six-week checkup, but the information they contained was sparse.

I had tried to introduce a systematic and more informative referral system at the hospital without success. After three years, I tried a new approach. A prepared nurse in maternal-child health within the department was assigned as a liaison to the hospital to obtain the needed data. She developed a referral form that included the kind of "delivery" information that would be helpful to the field nurses in the department. These nurses had long complained about the inadequacy of the data they received and the time they lost making home visits to clients who didn't need them while missing clients who did.

Sometimes a referral was received for a high-risk woman that contained little information about her condition and/or instructions about her care. As a result, the nurse had no information before the home visit, and the client often could not tell her why she had been referred.

We had also changed to primary nursing and needed better information when newborns were registered in our newly developed comprehensive child health care nursing clinics. We matched client needs with the expertise of individual nurses. At the clinic, the pediatric nurse practitioners, using various assessment tools, were identifying many newborn problems. They were also learning about maternal problems that occurred during pregnancy that should have been referred to them for teaching and counseling at that time.

The result: the liaison nurse was denied further entry to the hospital, the hospital nurses were no longer allowed to give us any information, and I resigned my position to retain my principles and because I was told I was "to be punished." I also paused and took stock: everyone had deserted me, including the board member who had given me much support. The supervisor within the health department who had supported me on behalf of her field nurses was in conference with the medical personnel. She was immediately made director of nursing and rewarded with a potted plant and new drapes in her office.

At this point, I could speak about the theories of problem solving, the power to effect change, hierarchy stratification of the health professions, the psychological mind set of nurses, and advocacy. But readers are familiar with the literature; the problems lie in putting these theories into practice.

I would not have done anything differently. In any situation there are always questions to ask and to answer. Having spent so many years in maternity nursing—as a supervisor, teacher, and, above all, practitioner—I too have had questions, but I still come up with the same conclusions. Vigier reminds us that, as professionals, we must hold to principles to safeguard and uphold the values in our society and our profession. We must believe in these values and not let others compromise our beliefs.[6]

Hott reports that when one body of performers cannot advocate, inquire, and question the performance of another body of performers, we are allocating privileges to one group which can then override and dominate the privileges of the other group.[7] If this occurs in professional groups performing a unified service for a group of people, the people receiving the services suffer.

As practicing professionals in any society, we not only have a responsibility to know what we need to know to practice, but also a responsibility to act as advocates for those who cannot speak for themselves. As professionals, we carry a commitment and responsibility to all the people in the community in which we practice.

REFERENCES

1. Mojtabai, A. G. *The Four Hundred Eels of Sigmund Freud.* New York, Simon and Schuster, 1976, p. 236.
2. Friedman, E. A., and Sachtleben, M. R. Station of the fetal presenting. Part 1. Pattern of descent. *Am. J. Obstet. Gynecol.* 93:522–529, Oct. 15, 1965.
3. Sweet, R. L., and Ledger, W. J. Puerperal infectious morbidity: a two-year review. *Am. J. Obstet. Gynecol.* 117: 1093–1100, Dec. 15, 1973.
4. Hobel, C. J., and Others. Prenatal and intrapartum high-risk screening, Part 1. *Am. J. Obstet. Gynecol.* 117: 1–9, Sept. 1, 1973.
5. Scipien, G. M. and Others. *Comprehensive Pediatric Nursing.* New York, McGraw-Hill Book Co., 1975.
6. Vigier, Francois. *Change and Apathy.* Cambridge, Mass., MIT Press, 1970.
7. Hott, J. R. The struggles inside nursing's body politic. *Nurs. Forum* 15(4):325–340, 1976.

Notes of a Whistleblower

Pat Witt

I had never before been in a situation in which I felt no one, absolutely no one, would support me.

I saw patients abused and I reported it. The abuses continued. Physicians prescribed bizarre, and what seemed to me potentially harmful treatments—I questioned and objected. Nothing changed. I stayed a year, in the hope things would improve. A crisis made me realize that they wouldn't, not without outside pressure. This is what happened.

September 1979. Started working as a head nurse at a 150-bed private psychiatric facility. Responsible for a unit with three experimental programs: one for patients who had not responded to any other psychiatric treatment, one for hearing-impaired psychiatric patients, and one using orthomolecular therapy. Each program had a physician team leader; in addition to the 30 to 35 hospital-employed nurses, assistants, and clerks, each physician had a primary therapist and a nurse. It all sounded very exciting and interesting.

October 1979. Found out what the physicians' "primary therapists" do. They do the therapy and the physicians bill for it. At least that's what the person who does the billing said. We had lunch, and I commented that I never saw the physician in charge of the hearing-impaired program do any therapy. He refused to learn sign language and never asked for an interpreter. She responded that she knew for a fact that this physician was billing 80 dollars an hour for sessions.

December 1979. Saw the orthomolecular physician abuse a patient. The patient was agitated and grabbed at the physician's jacket. He struck her and then shoved her into a room. When she started out of the room, he slammed the door on her hand. I jumped up as soon as I heard the commotion, and the physician briskly walked away. That the woman was agitated and paranoid didn't seem abnormal to me, considering that she was being starved in this orthomolecular "treatment."

I was beginning to think the whole orthomolecular program was abusive. Based on the belief that psychiatric illness is due to cerebral allergies, patients were taken off food and medications and given only bottled water for four to seven days. Then, one by one, foods were introduced; the patient's blood pressure and pulse checked before and after each feeding to determine if the patient was allergic. Patients were not allowed to smoke or leave the unit, even for occupational therapy, to prevent cheating.

Nevertheless, some tried to cheat: I caught patients digging through garbage cans for food, and I saw some seriously disturbed patients attempt to eat anything, including Kleenex and Tampax. Some patients, while in restraints, chewed through the mattress to feast on the stuffing.

I took my objections to the director of nursing and to the weekly grand rounds. By one, I was reassured and by the other, overruled.

January 1980. By this time, I was thinking that I was the crazy one. I heard the orthomolecular physician claim that he could cure nine out of ten "last resort" cases with this starvation treatment. Meanwhile, I was looking at a bunch of emaciated patients walking around like zombies, and felt like I was working in a concentration camp.

The orthomolecular physician had an article published on his "success," and we started getting a big influx of patients from gullible, weary families looking for the "last resort cure." I sensed things were very wrong, but found it terribly hard to challenge a "noted authority."

February 1980. The orthomolecular physician admitted a young woman with a diagnosis of cerebral allergy. He neglected to tell me she was a drug addict who had been taking drugs just before she was admitted. After I explained the unit routine and told her she would be confined to that unit, she dived through a plate glass window, fortunately acquiring only minor lacerations. Another woman with "cerebral allergy" turned out to be an alcoholic. She went into withdrawal, becoming very agitated and combative.

By far the worst example of what I again labeled patient abuse was when the physician ate an apple in front of a fasting patient. First, she begged for food: then she went into a rage—at which point, the physician called for me to put her in restraints and start a vitamin IV.* I refused to do either and went directly to the director of nursing. The administrator, who was also the medical director, was called. He voided the restraints order and admitted the physician had been out of line.

Nevertheless, I began to suspect there would be no changes. I had been documenting such incidents in written memos at the weekly grand rounds. To protect myself, I began keeping copies.

March 1980. The public health department made its survey. Beforehand, I was told to hide the orthomolecular records and not to discuss the program. If I ever considered (which I did) not obeying the "gag order," the way the survey was conducted dissuaded me. The surveyors interviewed me in front of an audience that included the director of nursing and the administrator.

May 1980. I was also disappointed by the JCAH survey. One of the administrators told me that the orthomolecular patients' charts in medical records had been "stored" in the basement during the survey. As in public health department surveys, there was an audience during the surveyors' interview. Before the surveyors arrived, some patients were taken off the unit.

June 1980. I kept reporting to the director of nursing and writing up the incidents on the daily report sheets and in memos for discussion at grand rounds. Nothing changed. I began to fantasize that surveyors would arrive unannounced and speak to me privately. I would tell them how to find the documentation of what was really going on, and everything would be made better. Then, I would wake up. I began seriously considering leaving.

July 1980. The owner of the hospital told me of his plans to open another facility in October, and he asked me to be the administrator there. I thought, "If only I can hang in here, I'll be in a position to set the standards there."

August 1980. Three of the most upsetting experiences in my career made me realize that I would never have made it till October.

First, a 34-year-old man was admitted to the orthomolecular program and his psychotropic medicines discontinued. He became agitated, confused, and combative. Several staff members were hurt. He was placed in restraints, and he begged for medication to calm him down. The physician refused, and the man was kept in restraints eight days and nights—screaming continually and urinating all over himself. I insisted the director of medical services come to the unit. At last he did, and the man was discharged from the program.

Then, a 24-year-old man who had been on the unit for several months and who was quite emaciated, fainted and struck his head. The physician was notified but did not come either to assess or treat the patient. Two days later, it happened again and again the physician was called. Nothing was done. At 8:00 AM the next day, the patient was found unconscious and unresponsive. The physician ordered a vitamin IV, stating that the problems of late were an allergic reaction to some milk the patient had drunk six days before.

Later the patient's mother asked me if I believed that, and I told her no. She asked me what she should do. I told her to get a medical opinion. She called her internist, who wanted to see the patient in the ER right away. An ambulance was ordered; but before it arrived, the director of medical services found out. I was reprimanded, and the ambulance was cancelled.

At about noon, the patient regained consciousness, but was very agitated and screamed constantly. Then at 11:00 that night, he began having continuous seizures. The internist on call administered IV

---

*The vitamin IV consisted of a 500 cc Ringers Lactate solution that, according to the physician, contained 1,000 mg pyridoxine, 60 cc sodium ascorbate, 10 cc calcium glycerophosphate/calcium lactate (Calphosan), 10 cc magnesium choride, 5 cc D-Panthothenol, and 5,000 units heparin. Additives not available in the U.S. were privately obtained and supplied by the physician.

Valium, glucose, and Dilantin. He left a TID order for Dilantin. The next morning the orthomolecular physician promptly discontinued the Dilantin. He told the family the patient was allergic to the drug.

The last straw was when a 36-year-old man, in the program one week, announced he didn't wish to continue and was threatened with commitment and a competency hearing. I was appalled when the physician sat at my desk with the family and asked them to "create reasons" (in my language, that means lies) in order to have the patient declared incompetent. The man clearly was not incompetent, but it appeared he was trapped. The physician cut off his phone privileges. I put the patient in the conference room and gave him telephone numbers where he might get help. He got it.

The following day a lawyer from the Illinois Guardianship and Advocacy (G&A) Commission came to the hospital. First he spoke to the patient, then he spoke to me. I told him about the program, the patient, and what I had seen and heard. He asked if I would be willing to say the same thing in court. I was stunned. Of course, I wanted things to change, but I had four children who depended as much as I did on my salary. I thought, "If I volunteer, I'll be fired. I know it." But I knew that I was at the end of my rope, so I said that I would if I were sent a subpoena. I also told him that I had other patients in trouble and I described them. He said I should talk to the Human Rights Authority about the others. I did.

September 1980. I was called to the office of the director of nursing. The administrator was there, and he announced that *he* was relieving me of my head nurse's position and offered me an entry-level position on another unit. I told him I wasn't interested. He asked if I would quit. I said no. When asked what I was going to do, I asked for a few days' sick leave.

While on sick leave, I was called to testify at the patient's hearing. A colleague who worked as the weekend supervisor came with me because she had never seen a competency hearing. The next day, she was called and told she wouldn't be needed for that weekend. The same happened the following weekend.

We realized we were in trouble. Together, we went to the Illinois Nurses Association and were told that we needed a statement of our employment status in writing. When we went to the hospital to obtain such a document we were threatened with arrest for trespassing. Apparently, we were unemployed.

When I tried to find another position, I discovered that the hospital was answering job-reference inquiries by describing me as "psychotic" and "incompetent because of psychosis." I suddenly had no income. When I tried to collect unemployment benefits, the hospital said I had not been fired, but had failed to report to work, and this denied my right to benefits. (After a bloody battle, I won my appeals to collect unemployment benefits.)

Staff began coming to my house to share their horror stories. Anything I didn't know before, I learned then. In fear, I went to as many agencies as possible. In case one was bought off, I wanted to make sure others were involved. I turned over copies of all my memos and other documentation to the public health department.

I also met with the local Health and Human Services office. They were the most responsive. After my presentation, they sent in a top team for a surprise survey right away.

October 1980. Unemployed, black-balled and running through the money I'd saved as though it were water, I decided to sue the hospital for reinstatement under a new, untested law that supposedly protects anyone from retribution who cooperates with a G&A commission investigation. I had had such bad luck with lawyers, though. Soon, I had no money to pay one anymore, and I decided to try to represent myself. Going through a divorce gave me some knowledge of motions, so I drafted my own legal motion.

August 1981. My case against the hospital and its administrator was heard in June. I represented myself and won. That month, the judge ordered reinstatement, compensatory damages, and punitive damages. Naturally, the hospital appealed. I was told an appeal would be too complicated for me to handle. Since I was working for a temporary agency, I was able to borrow money to hire a lawyer.

May 1983. The judge's decision was affirmed. Two years was a long wait. It seems the file for the appeals had been lost for a time. Then, the hospital took the case to the state supreme court.

September 1983. The supreme court refused to hear the case, saying it had been fully litigated. All that remains for this nightmare to end is for a judge to set the damages.

Whistle-blower Saved Lives, Lost Everything Else

Eric Zorn

Pat Witt, her moment of fame and courage long over, is down and out in Arlington Heights.

Witt, 47, was in all the papers in 1981 as the defiant head nurse who was fired for reporting controversial practices at the Des Plaines psychiatric hospital where she was employed, and she became the first person in Illinois to test a law designed to help protect whistle-blowers from retaliation.

She won the major court battles but has since lost nearly everything else, including her savings, her furniture and her $160,000 home in a Buffalo Grove subdivision.

"This is humiliating. I'm at the end," she said, speaking at the Arlington Heights home of a friend who, three weeks ago, agreed to put her up for several days. "No one in their right mind would do what I did."

What she did was to go in 1980 to the Illinois Guardianship and Advocacy Commission, which is mandated to protect the rights of disabled persons, with a roster of complaints. She called attention to a hospital treatment program in which patients were made to fast and were given large doses of vitamins.

Her information provoked a state investigation that led to reforms at the hospital, according to a psychiatrist who worked on the case for the Illinois Department of Public Health. "She saved lives, yes," said the psychiatrist, who requested anonymity.

But Witt, who has a nursing degree and graduate training in counseling and psychotherapy, was fired for being "uncooperative" and "disruptive," according to hospital officials who testified against her.

After extended litigation, the court ruled that Witt had been wrongfully terminated for speaking out, a violation of the 1979 Illinois Guardianship and Advocacy Act. She never received a cash settlement because of legal technicalities that closed her case.

But since her court appearances, Witt, a single parent of four with 15 years experience as a nurse, has been unable to find a regular job in her field.

"Hospitals would say, 'We admire what you did, but we can't hire you,'" she said. "No institution anywhere is 100 percent clean. Accidents happen. They don't want someone around who might tell on them."

Witt said she worked several temporary nursing jobs in senior citizens' homes and picked up odd work, telling stories at a Barrington apple orchard, packing boxes and caring for children. But she suffered debilitating emotional problems owing to stress in 1984, she said, and was unable to work.

"It certainly backfired on her," said Joan Bundley, nursing practice administrator of the Illinois Nurses Association. "Her case still comes up in conference workshops on whistle-blowing as an example of what can happen to a person."

Bundley said hospitals seem reluctant to hire workers who have taken their previous employers to court. "If you want to blow the whistle," she said, "you'd better be prepared to pay the consequences."

"Unfortunately, hers is a typical story," said Don Schlemmer, an attorney with the Government Accountability Project, an organization in Washington, D.C., that attempts to assist whistle-blowers.

"They try to keep their identities secret, but who can keep a secret anymore?" Schlemmer asked "The CIA can't even keep a secret."

Witt, who has appeared on syndicated and cable-television talk shows to discuss her plight and has written accounts of it in national nursing journals, has been living a nomadic life in the city and suburbs for 10 months.

She lost her mortgage and was evicted last summer from her two-story colonial home in the Cambridge neighborhood of Buffalo Grove. Until that time, she said, neighbors had been extremely sympathetic, giving her food and other supplies and offering rides when she could not afford gas for her 1977 Pontiac.

A service agency offered her a temporary room in a Palatine motel, but the place didn't look right to her and wouldn't allow the family dog, Kelo, a black Labrador. She moved in as a caretaker for a woman with physical and mental problems, and her children, now ages 18 to 24, stayed with friends or fended for themselves.

When Witt's job with the disabled woman ended, she began staying with a series of friends, her belongings in suitcases jammed into the trunk of her car. She said her car has been vandalized, her tires slashed and her typewriter and other possessions stolen.

"We almost always have a waiting list," said a worker at Northwest Community Services, an outreach organization in Mt. Prospect. "It's very tight. Very difficult."

Witt said she and Kelo have now worn out their welcome and cannot stay much longer in Arlington Heights. "My life has disintegrated," she said. "My career is over. I am literally facing the street."

She is trying to enlist legislators' help in getting her case reopeened so that she might receive a settlement, but she is having little luck.

"I don't think she has a case," said Geri Davis, caseworker in the office of U.S. Rep. Philip Crane (R., Ill.), but "I feel sorry for her."

Witt said: "I worked my way through college, nursing school and graduate school. I raised my kids alone for 18 years. Then all of a sudden I was punished for doing the right thing.

"I'd never do it again."

Whistleblowing: Disclosure and Its Consequences for the Professional Nurse and Management

Mary A. Kiely and Deirdre C. Kiely

The label "whistleblower" brings a variety of connotations and meanings to mind when it is used. To some, it is synonymous with informer, "squeal" or muckraker, and to many, it reeks of organizational disloyalty. To others, it is evidence of social conscience and commitment to ethical and moral thinking. The simplest definition of a whistleblower is "a person working in an agency who publicly criticizes that agency's administrative practices by disclosing pertinent information to the public."[1] This action has both positive and negative implications, both for the organization and the individuals within it, who must literally play a game of "truth or consequences."

DESCRIPTION OF THE PROBLEM

The phenomenon of whistleblowing is not new. In 1849, Henry David Thoreau wrote an essay entitled "On the Duty of Civil Disobedience." In his dissertation he stated: "The only obligation which I have a right to assume is to do at any time what I think right. It is truly enough said, that a corporation has no conscience; but a corporation of conscientious men is a corporation with conscience."[2]

The whistleblowing has continued into recent times with many highly publicized cases. In 1977, Snepp attempted to publish a book critical of CIA activities during the Vietnam war. The U.S. government retaliated with a civil action suit against the former CIA employee.[3] In 1982, a New York City social worker, Irwin Levine, publicized mishandling of child abuse cases by Human Resource Administration personnel. He was suspended and demoted from his position. Later, he was reinstated at the Mayor's request.[4] These two cases represent two types of "internal muckrakers" identified by Peters and Branch. The pure whistleblower attacks his institution while still employed there, as in the Levine incident. The "alumnus whistleblower," like Snepp, exposes what he finds as crimes against the public soon after leaving the service of the organization he accuses.[5]

According to Parmalee, Near, and Jensen, attempts to characterize whistleblowers are limited in the literature. In general, however, whistleblowers differ from other employees because they are not motivated by blind organizational loyalty and do not aspire to move vertically within the organizational structure. They are risk-takers who may feel little dependence on their employer since they can obtain employment easily. They tend to be younger, better educated, married and independent in nature.[6]

The issue of organizational loyalty or the lack of it is often addressed in relation to whistleblowing. According to Weinstein, obedience in organizations may be related to a sense of loyalty or obligation to a hierarchy that tends to color an individual's evaluation of its policies and actions.[7] The notion of being a traitor is abhorrent to a society that holds Benedict Arnold and others known as turncoats in such high disregard. This was illustrated by Whyte in his

Kiely, M. A., & Kiely, D. C. (1987, May). Whistleblowing: Disclosure and its consequences for the professional nurse and management. *Nursing Management, 18*, 41–42, 44–45. Reprinted with permission of © S-N Publications. All rights reserved.

description of the organizational man, in which he identified a new "social ethic." The consequences of this new work ethic are loss of individuality to the corporation or organization and total conformity to organizational demands.[8] In such an environment the notion that "to get along you have to go along" becomes the group norm.

One must also examine the concept of the bureaucracy and its response to dissent. The bureaucracy, as described by Weber in Weinstein's *Bureaucratic Opposition*, is a formal organization characterized by specific attributes, as identified in Table I. Rationality is a key assumption underlying the bureaucratic organization and its functions. Weinstein asserts that such conventional organizational theory excludes the phenomenon of dissent which bureaucrats constantly seek to eliminate. She concludes that "when subordinates disobey orders or attempt to change policies, managerial theorists view their actions as irrational because of assumptions that: 1) those in authority know and order appropriate means to reach universally shared goals, and 2) there is agreement on the goals themselves. . . . [10] These assumptions may indeed be invalid and this directive authoritarian structure can come into conflict with individual motivations and/ or perspectives. This view of dissent within the bureaucracy as irrational may be translated into accusations of mental instability, and labeling of the whistleblower as paranoid or neurotic.

According to Drucker, as quoted by Orr, "whistleblowing" is simply another word for informing and as such, "no mutual trust, no interdependence and no ethics are possible."[11] Whistleblowing may indeed become a dangerous occurrence if it is commonplace. Other authors suggest that whistleblowing is only legitimate under certain conditions: 1) It must deal with a very serious issue. 2) The individual must have competence to make a judgment and has consulted with others to confirm that judgment. 3) The individual has exhausted all internal

Table I
Specific Attributes of
Bureaucratic Organizations

- An authority structure in which loyalty is based upon impersonal hierarchical relationships.
- Existence of rational rules and regulations that control bureaucratic structure and processes.
- Highly developed division of labor and specialization of tasks.

mechanisms to solve the problem.[12] Whistleblowing, according to Mitchell, can be bad for morale, as it encourages workers to question policy and procedures in an organization and makes management generally uncomfortable.[13]

WHISTLEBLOWING IN NURSING

A recent review of the nursing literature reveals little about the occurrence of whistleblowing among professional nurses. Several articles do address the problem of conflicting loyalties of the nurse, which play a significant role in whistleblowing. The work environment sometimes creates conflict between loyalty to the patient and to the physician, according to some authors.[14] Problems arise when nursing staff perceive administrative policies contrary to the delivery of safe, competent practice. These authors cite the Lampe case as an example of this problem. In this case, an assistant head nurse in an intensive care unit refused to follow the nursing administrator's request to reduce staff overtime hours. Ms. Lampe was subsequently fired for failure to follow appropriate procedures and to adhere to budgetary constraints. This resulted in a highly publicized lawsuit in which the nurse sued for damages resulting from dismissal. The suit charged that the hospital violated Colorado public policy and tenets in the Colorado Nurse Practice Act. Ms. Lampe lost the lawsuit and the courts stated that she had no basis for a claim against her former employer. The authors concluded that "if nurses feel ethically bound to act in the interest of the patients rather than the employer, the nurse may have no legal recourse if they are dismissed."[15]

Hull addresses the question of accountability in nursing. He states that the nurse is accountable to her patient if the patient has contracted with the nurse to perform certain tasks and is capable of evaluating her performance of them. In the nurse-physician relationship, Hull states that accountability to the physician only exists "when the physician has the task-responsibility of supervising her and holding her answerable."[16] This role is not inherent in the nurse/physician relationship. Nurses also are accountable for professional standards established by licensing boards, and certification or peer review boards. McClure, in her discussion of nursing accountability, questions nursing's responsibility toward other nurses and members of the health team.[17] Hull translates this into the question, "Does the nurse have the responsibility for blowing the whistle on incompetent or careless practice by another member of her team?" He concludes that if such action is demanded by the nurse's professional code of ethics, then she is indeed accountable for such action.[18] The Canadian Nurses' Association's code of ethics would not advocate such action. It states: "The nurse must participate fully in the team effort and even when one member of the team is suspected of being incompetent or unethical, relationships between team members must not be affected 'unnecessarily,' for the sake of the patient."[19]

Another position is that "nurses have an obligation to report behavior when it endangers client welfare," although the practice of reporting medical malpractice is extremely risky.[20] Greenlaw, in her discussion of "cover-ups" by nurses, states that the consequences of such actions can be more damaging than the original incidents. Falsification of records can result in license revocation, malpractice suits, and even criminal charges. She advocates ethical decision-making and the assumption of full responsibility for whatever actions follow.[21]

GUIDELINES FOR THE WHISTLEBLOWER

There is little in the literature that provides direction for the person compelled to blow the whistle. There is a great deal of warning regarding the perils involved, yet there are few suggestions on how to avoid them. Raven-Hansen published such guidelines in an article in 1980.[22] They are summarized in Table II.

MANAGEMENT'S RESPONSE TO DISCLOSURE

Management may respond to whistleblowing in a variety of ways, which are sometimes unpredictable. If the whistleblower uses established mechanisms for investigation of problems and/or issues, appropriate action may be taken to remedy the situation. This is not always the case, however. In Westin's description of 10 cases, all the whistleblowers suffered some form of reprisal. Actions ranged from the

Table II
Guidelines for the Whistleblower According to Raven-Hansen

1. Focus on the disclosure itself, not on personalities
   A. Types of disclosures that control bureaucratic structure and processes
      1. Mandatory; required by law
      2. Prohibited; forbidden by contractual agreements signed upon employment.
   B. Disclosure format
      1. Write clear, short summary
      2. Demonstrate verification of data
      3. Identify the data source
      4. Force management to go on record about the issue.
2. Use internal channels before "going public"
   A. Management may respond with action.
   B. It may be required by agency regulations.
   C. It demonstrates willingness to work through the system.
3. Disclosure should be simple and convincing
   A. Do not use agency time or resources to make disclosure.
   B. Avoid anonymity
   C. A civil authority or regulatory agency is the most appropriate recipient of the information disclosed.
4. Anticipate and document retaliation
   A. Challenge retaliatory actions
   B. Consult a lawyer before "going public"
   C. Be prepared to go to court
   D. Be prepared to look for a new job

dismissal and black listing to threats of physical violence.[23] Ewing has identified other suppressive techniques used with bureaucratic dissidents.[24] These include:

1) reassignment of the individual to an obscure department;

2) elimination of the dissenter's job within the agency;

3) voiding evidence that supports the whistleblower's claims;

4) harassment to unnerve the dissident;

5) removal of resources necessary for whistleblowers to perform their jobs;

6) termination.

Retaliation serves the purpose of threatening or warning other potential whistleblowers. According to Parmalee, Near, and Jensen, it represents an organizational control measure over its members. The comprehensiveness of the retaliation reflects the organization's overall response to discredit or silence the whistleblower.[25]

The whistleblower may be isolated and shunned by peers and colleagues after the incident, as group norms found in the workplace may have been violated by the whistleblower. The greater the cohesiveness in the group, the less tolerance it will have for a dissident.[26] Carr describes this reaction after he blew the whistle on an incompetent, alcoholic physician. House staff refused to speak with him, and many nursing staff were cool and demonstrated resentment toward him for months.[27]

The decision to blow the whistle cannot be made lightly. It has serious ramifications for both the individual making the disclosure and the organization involved. Occasionally, it results in effective action and remedy of the problem. Often, however, it is an exercise in frustration which leaves the whistleblower unrewarded and unpopular. There are times when the best action is to leave the situation and/or agency. It is a difficult decision and this, too, was recognized by Thoreau in his discussion of civil disobedience. He reminds us:

"It is not a man's (or woman's) duty, as a matter of course, to devote himself (herself) to the eradication of any, even the most enormous wrong; he (she) may still properly have other concerns to engage him; but it is his (her) duty, at least, to wash his hands of it, and if he gives it no thought longer, not to give it practically his support."[30]

PROTECTING THE WHISTLEBLOWER

The First Amendment of the Constitution guarantees freedom of speech to Americans, yet the whistleblower may remain at risk of organizational reprisal. The federal government recognized this problem and in 1978, the Civil Service Reform Act was passed. It assigned responsibility for safeguarding merit systems in the federal government to the Merit Systems Protection Board. In addition to this, it created a special counsel position responsible for investigating charges of reprisal for whistleblowing in federal agencies. This reprisal is prohibited under Title I of this act.[28] The public employee also has the benefit of the Privacy Act and the Freedom of Information Act to obtain information regarding personnel action.

The employee in the private sector is not as well protected, however. Union membership may afford some protection, as many unions specify in contracts prohibition of discharge or discipline except for just cause. For the nonunion worker, some other form of protection against arbitrary dismissal is needed. St. Antoine is a proponent of state statutes prohibiting dismissal. He suggests that existing administrative agencies such as labor relations boards or civil rights commissions could act as enforcement agents.[29] In 1981, Michigan became the first state to pass a law protecting the whistleblower; Connecticut followed suit in 1982. In states without laws, charges of harassment or unfair dismissal must be decided in the local courts.

REFERENCES

1. Chandler, Ralph C., and Plano, Jack C., *The Public Administration Dictionary* (New York: John Wiley and Sons, 1982), p. 380.
2. Thoreau, Henry David, "On the Duty of Civil Disobedience," in *The Rhetoric of No*, (eds.) Ray Fabrizio, Edith Karas, Ruth Menmum (New York: Holt, Rinehart and Winston, Inc., 1970), p. 245.
3. Richman, David, "The CIA Silences a Whistleblower," *Human Rights*, 10:1 (Winter, 1982): 25.
4. Van Gelder, Lindsey, "Blowing in the Wind," *Daily News Magazine* (December 2, 1984): 8.
5. Peters, Charles and Branch, Taylor, *Blowing the Whistle* (New York: Praeger Publishers, 1972), pp. 4–5.
6. Parmalee, Marcia A., Near, Janet P., Jensen, Tamila C., "Correlates of Whistleblowers' Perceptions of Organizational Retaliation," *Administrative Science Quarterly* 27 (March, 1982): 33.
7. Weinstein, Deena, *Bureaucratic Opposition* (New York: Pergamon Press, 1979), p. 38.
8. Whyte, William H., *The Organizational Man* (New York: Doubleday 1956).
9. Mouzelis, Nicos P., "The Character of Bureaucracy and Bureaucratization," in *New Readings in Public Administration*, (ed.) Jae T. Kim (Dubuque, Iowa: Kendall-Hunt Publishing Co., 1980), p. 151.
10. Weinstein, Deena, *op. cit.*, p. 4.

11. Orr, Leonard, "Is Whistleblowing the Same as Informing?", *Business and Society Review* (Fall, 1981): 4.
12. *Ibid.*, p. 6.
13. Mitchell, Greg, *Truth . . . and Consequences* (New York: Dembner Books, 1981).
14. Trandel-Korenchuk, Keith, and Trandel-Korenchuk, Darlene M., "Conflicting Loyalties of the Nurse," *Nursing Administration Quarterly*, 6:2 (Winter, 1982): 63.
15. *Ibid.*, p. 65.
16. Hull, Richard T., "Responsibility and Accountability, Analyzed," *Nursing Outlook*, 29:12 (December 1981): 711–712.
17. McClure, Margaret, "The Long Road to Accountability," *Nursing Outlook*, 26:1 (January, 1978): 49–50.
18. Hull, Richard T., *op cit.*, p. 7112.
19. Wilson, Jane, "A New Code of Ethics in Nursing," *Canadian Medical Association Journal*, 130 (April 1, 1984): 721.
20. Wilson, Jane, "Ethics and the Physician-Nurse Relationship," *Canadian Medical Association Journal*, 129 (August 1, 1983): 292.
21. Greenlaw, Jane, "What to Do If Your Supervisor Orders a Cover-Up," *R.N. Magazine* 45:12 (October, 1982): 82.
22. Raven-Hansen, Peter, "Do's and Dont's for Whistleblowers: Planning for Trouble," *Technology Review*, (May 1980): 34–44.
23. Westin, Allan F., *Whistleblowing!* (New York: McGraw-Hill Book Co., 1981).
24. Ewing, David, "How Bureaucrats Deal with Dissidents," in *Organizational Shock*, (ed.) W. Clay Hamner (New York: John Wiley and Sons, 1980), pp. 328–331.
25. Parmalee, Marcia A., *et al.*, *op. cit.*, p. 20.
26. Waters, James A., "Catch 20.5: Corporate Morality as an Organizational Phenomenon," in *Organizational Shock*, (ed.) W. Clay Hamner (New York: John Wiley and Sons, 1980), pp. 375–376.
27. Carr, Anthony, "Should a Nurse Report a Nurse?", *Nursing Mirror*, 156:12 (March, 1983): 26.
28. Bellis, Jonathan P., "The 1978 Civil Service Reform Act: Meeting the Needs of Public Management," in *New Readings in Public Administration*, (ed.) Jae T. Kim (DuBuque, Iowa: Kendall/Hunt Publishing Co., 1980), p. 216.
29. St. Antoine, Theodore J., "You're Fired!," *Human Rights*, 10:1 (Winter, 1982): 36–37.
30. Thoreau, Henry David., *op cit.*, p. 248.

BIBLIOGRAPHY

American Nurses' Association. Code for Nurses with Interpretive Statements. *ANA*. Kansas City, Missouri: 1976.

Allison, Graham T. *Essence of Decision-Making: Explaining the Cuban Missile Crisis*. (Boston: Little, Brown and Co.) 1971.

Felin, Alfred G. "The Risks of Blowing the Whistle." *American Journal of Nursing*. 10 (October 1983): 1387–1390.

Joint Commission on Accreditation of Hospitals. *Accreditation Manual for Hospitals*, 1982 Edition. JCAH. Chicago, Illinois, 1981.

Lorenz, Fred J. "Nursing Administration and Undivided Loyalty." *Nursing Administration Quarterly*. 6:2 (Winter, 1982): 67–73.

Perrucci, Robert, Anderson, Robert M., Schendel, Dan E., Trachtman, Leon E. "Whistle-Blowing: Professionals' Resistance to Organizational Authority." *Social Problems*. 28:2 (December, 1980): 149–163.

Sandroff, Ronni. "Protect the M.D. . . . or the Patient?" *R.N. Magazine*. 44:12 (February, 1981): 28–33.

STUDY AND DISCUSSION QUESTIONS
THE NURSE–PHYSICIAN RELATIONSHIP: III. WHISTLEBLOWING

1. Compare the 1910 letters to the editor of the *American Journal of Nursing* and the 1979 *RN* survey. How has the situation of the nurse changed?

2. The *American Journal of Nursing* editor in 1910 suggested a joint medical and nursing board to redress injustices against nurses and also complaints by physicians against nurses. Would a proposal such as this have merit today?

3. E.C. wrote in her 1910 letter to the editor that, "The nurses are taught that they must stand by the doctor whether he is in the right or wrong . . ." In what sense does the nurse owe loyalty to the physician today?

4. According to the 1979 *RN* survey, 96 percent would intervene if they thought that a life-threatening error was being made. This implies that 4 percent would do nothing to prevent what they believe to be a life-threatening error. How do you read these statistics? Do you find it admirable that so many would intervene or are you shocked that 4 percent would do nothing?

5. The ANA Code for Nurses indicates the primary commitment of the nurse is to the "health, welfare, and safety of the client," and burdens the nurse with safeguarding the client from instances of "incompetent, unethical, or illegal practice" or the jeopardizing of "the rights or best interests of the client." Which of the following do you think would require intervention according to the code?: life-threatening error, error causing risk of permanent injury, better or cheaper therapy, unnecessary therapy, unnecessary tests, unnecessary hospitalization, early hospital discharge, or failure to order diagnostic tests.

6. Do you agree that concerns or objectionable practices should be made known first to those carrying them out?

7. According to Creighton, what is the legal responsibility of nurses regarding medical negligence?

8. What is your view of the percentages presented in the Friedman *RN* survey? How much medical incompetence do you believe occurs?

   How do you account for 40 percent of the nurses disdaining the watchdog role? Is this shirking professional responsibilities or something else?

9. Consider the recommended ways of telling a doctor that he or she is wrong. Is this the doctor–nurse game?

10. According to Feliu, what legal protection does the whistleblower have? Should there be more legislation of the sort described?

11. Did Christine Smith do the right thing?

12. Why do you think board members and the supervisor withdrew support from Christine Smith? Were they right to do so?

13. Did Pat Witt do the right thing?

14. How do the Smith and Witt cases make you feel about advocacy? the nursing profession? physicians? hospitals?

15. Does the profile of whistleblowers described by Kiely and Kiely fit many nurses? Should it?

7

The Nurse–Nurse Relationship

INTRODUCTION

As witnessed in the previous chapter, nurses have often complained that whistleblowing or raising concerns about questionable practices resulted in their feeling deserted by nursing colleagues. As such, the readings in this chapter highlight the difficulties in the nurse–nurse relationship. Leah Curtin and M. Josephine Flaherty, in "The Nurse–Nurse Relationship," set the agenda here. Describing the importance of intraprofessional relationships and their ethical foundations, Curtin and Flaherty conjecture about why the professional bonds in nursing are weak, and blame in large measure the educational model used. Curtin and Flaherty also offer some interesting and suggestive remarks about revitalizing the notions of professional character traits and virtues.

The articles by Morrison and Flaherty serve as commentary on these latter points. Ian Morrison, in "Power Brings Out the Worst in Women," suggests a different interpretation of why the professional bond in nursing is weak, locating the difficulty in the socialization of females.

M. Josephine Flaherty, in "Guilt By Association?", raises questions about the private behavior of nurses and further explores the implications of insisting upon professional character traits and virtues.

Before discussing these articles, however, Curtin and Flaherty's argument deserves some commentary.

CURTIN AND FLAHERTY

Curtin and Flaherty argue that a moral commitment to the profession of nursing involves a commitment to the care of and for patients *and* fellow nurses. Underlying the ethics of intraprofessional relationship are the recognition of human rights, the profession's obligations to serve the public welfare, and the development of a professional bond.

This professional bond encompasses more than duties nurses owe each other, and involves commitment to the profession's ideals and obligations. However, Curtin and Flaherty believe that the professional bond must run much deeper than an outward conformity to certain modes of behavior—it must form part of the character of the nurse. Indeed, Curtin and Flaherty believe that nurses need to cultivate certain professional character traits: fidelity to the promises of the profession; respect for human rights and the profession's ideals and obligations; and intellectual honesty and integrity.

In the course of their article, Curtin and Flaherty diagnose some problems in the nurse–nurse relationship. Chief among problems is a weakness of the professional bond among nurses. According to Curtin and Flaherty, nursing needs to regain and nurture a sense of professional identity, commitment, and responsibility in its members; it needs to heighten its sense of obligation to one another. Nurses must "nurture, support, guide, and correct one another." In addition "nursing must address the systems, institutions, and structures that shape the environment in which nurses practice."

For Curtin and Flaherty, nursing has been inadequate to these tasks. Nursing education has not done enough to provide the skills for critical inquiry into the values shaping society and the profession. The socialization process in nursing has not developed strong professional bonds. Nor has nursing been critical enough of the institutions and values that shape nursing practice. Although Curtin and Flaherty do not offer any specific solutions to these problems, they do intimate the general form such solutions would take. For instance, they identify the role model who embodies the ideals of the profession as the preeminent transmitter of values. Even so, it is still unfortunate that nursing education has chosen an educational model that keeps nursing students "apart from the mainstream of the work world of nurses" because of negative associations with apprenticeship training. As educators, Curtin and Flaherty believe nurses must be models of scholarly behavior and inculcate these values to students. Their solution here would also entail some modification of the nursing curriculum so as to provide tools of critical intelligence (i.e., study how to critically evaluate the values, attitudes, and goals of nursing, and the institutions and systems within which it exists). However, this measure would not be satisfied by the mere inclusion of a course or two from a discipline like philosophy. Rather, the tools of the discipline itself (philosophical reflection) would be infused into nursing education and carried on in all levels of nursing practice.

Although Curtin and Flaherty wish to enhance and strengthen the commitment of nurses to the profession and to each other, they do not describe such goals as ends in themselves. Nursing exists as a profession to serve the public welfare. In their view, an increased commitment to the profession and to each other would not allow issues of professional welfare to override nursing's commitment to society. Nor does this imply that a strong professional bond means shielding fellow nurses from charges of incompetence or negligence. Such has been the historic stance of nursing. The suggested code of 1926 made this clear when it stated:

The "Golden Rule" embodies all that could be written in many pages on the relation of the nurse to nurse. This should be one of fine loyalty, of appreciation for work conscientiously done, and of respect for persons of authority. On the other hand, loyalty to the motive which inspires nursing should make the nurse fearless to bring to light any serious violation of the ideals herein expressed; the larger loyalty is that to the community, for loyalty to an ideal is higher than any personal loyalty.[1]

MORRISON—THE WEAKNESS OF PROFESSIONAL BONDS

Ian Morrison offers another explanation for the weakness of the social bond among nurses that differs from that offered by Curtin and Flaherty. Whereas Curtin and Flaherty mention the lack of role modeling, Morrison believes the issue goes deeper. In a somewhat ironic manner he says: "It is my opinion, as a male, that hospitals bring out the worst in women. They cannot help it of course. It is something to do with their philosophy." Morrison complains that, in the context of the British system of nursing education, female nurses tend to flaunt newly acquired power. Such behavior isolates them from other nurses, degrades mutual respect, and lessens cooperation. Morrison finds the root of this problem in the socializing styles of men and women. In his experience, new male nursing students quickly develop a comraderie, but females tend to be critical of each other.

Morrison's remarks may be the embittered product of an unfortunate incident, but other nurses have made similar complaints about the weakness of intraprofessional bonds among nurses.[2] The situation is quite paradoxical. How can a profession so devoted to caring be so apparently deficient in caring for and nurturing other nurses? Are the educational models at fault as Curtin and Flaherty suggest? On a deeper level, does the problem concern socialization of male and female roles as Morrison believes? Are males generally more accustomed and practiced in exercising power, working cooperatively in groups, and devoted to professional ideals? Or could it be that this perception of weak professional bonds is a misconception and that nurses are as mutually supportive of professional ideals and other nurses as other professionals? Whatever the answers to these questions are it remains true that professional bonds are a key element in fulfilling the ethical obligations of the nursing profession.

FLAHERTY—PROFESSIONAL CHARACTER TRAITS

Flaherty, in "Guilt by Association," presents a case of a nurse who was convicted of allowing illegal activities to take place on her premises (her home). Her husband was found guilty of growing and selling marijuana. Although she was given a suspended sentence, the hospital where she worked discharged her claiming she had "lost her professionalism."

This account presents some difficulty for those like Curtin and Flaherty who advocate the development of professional character traits and virtues. Possessing certain virtues and traits of character speaks to who you *are* not merely what you *do*. To be a good professional nurse requires that you be a certain type of person, not just that you perform certain actions while doing nursing. If this is so, then quite clearly a nurse's behavior outside the professional context may have a bearing on whether that nurse has the requisite professional character. It may be difficult, if not impossible here, to draw clear lines of demarcation between one's private and professional life since both have a bearing on what one is.

An alternative is to reconstrue talk of character traits as ideals, and restrict professional behavior to actions performed in the professional context. In this way, *anything* done outside the nursing context would have no bearing on whether a nurse performs professionally. What a person does outside of nursing is a private affair.

VIRTUE AND THE CODES

Significant changes have taken place in nursing's professional stance toward the nurse's private life. In nursing's first professional code in 1950, the following statements were made:

> The nurse in private life adheres to standards of personal ethics which reflect credit upon the profession.
>
> In personal conduct nurses should not knowingly disregard the accepted patterns of the community in which they live and work.[3]

The ANA Committee on Ethical Standards published a commentary on the code in which they drew no hard and fast lines between the personal and professional life. The committee said, "the well-integrated person is not two people—one on the job, another away from it—but the same person in either situation."[4] It also warned nurses that failure to conform to community values including those concerning "dancing, smoking, drinking, cardplaying, keeping late hours," and how one dresses may bring discredit to the profession.[5] In the 1960 code, these admonitions were reduced to "The nurse adheres to standards of personal ethics which reflect credit upon the profession."[6] By 1968, however, references to personal ethics and general duties of citizenship were eliminated and have not reappeared in subsequent revisions.[7]

The trend, historically illustrated by the codes, has been to enlarge and isolate the private lives of nursing professionals. And yet those articulating moral visions of the appropriate role conception of nursing have not shied away from the language of virtue and character in their depictions. For instance, who can doubt that courage and risk-taking are central to the concept of the nurse as advocate? How to reconcile a desire for privacy and the nagging suspicion that nursing needs professionals of a certain character is difficult to imagine. Both are appealing but, perhaps, incompatible ideals. On which side would it be better to err? Would it be permissible, for example, to dismiss a student from a nursing degree program because it is believed that the student is not a courageous risk taker and is far too submissive to authority figures? How far will nursing progress as an autonomous profession if it does nothing to discourage such individuals from becoming nurses? Questions of this sort remain to be answered.

SUMMARY

Many of the typical dilemmas and problems in the nurse–nurse relationship (such as should a nurse cover up mistakes for another nurse, favoritism, lack of support and solidarity, and denigration of nurses seeking advanced degrees) stem from a weak professional bond. This chapter addresses the nature and source of intraprofessional obligations and raises two interrelated issues: views on why the professional bond is weak and the implications of revitalizing the idea of virtues and professional character traits.

NOTES

1. American Nurses' Association, Committee on Ethical Standards. "A Code for Nurses," *American Journal of Nursing* 26(August 1926):601. References to the Golden Rule were retained in the Code up until the 1960 revision—American Nurses' Association. "The Code for Professional Nurses," *American Journal of Nursing* 60(1960):1287. It is interesting to note that in the 1926 Code proposal there were different standards for reporting the misconduct of professionals. Nurses were to be "fearless" with regard to other nurses, but nothing was mentioned about physician misconduct. The first official nursing code [American Nurses' Association Committee on Ethical Standards, "A Code for Nurses," *American Journal of Nursing* 50(1950):196] makes no distinction among professions when it comes to the exposure of incompetent or unethical conduct.
2. A recurring theme in Chapters 5 and 6 was the sense of isolation and non-support nurses felt from other nurses when pursuing a professional mandate.
3. ANA, "A Code for Nurses," 1950, p. 196.
4. American Nurses' Association, Committee on Ethical Standards, "What's in Our Code?", *American Journal of Nursing* 53(November 1953):1358.
5. Ibid., p. 1359.
6. American Nurses' Association, "The Code for Professional Nurses," *American Journal of Nursing* 60(September 1960):1287.
7. American Nurses' Association, "Code for Nurses," *American Journal of Nursing* 68(December 1968):2581–2585.

The Nurse–Nurse Relationship

Leah Curtin and M. Josephine Flaherty

"The greatest trust between men is the trust of giving counsel."

Francis Bacon

Among the basic commitments for nurses who practice according to generally accepted standards is that they participate as members of the health care team. This involves collaboration with other health professionals, including other nurses. Hence, it is essential for nurses to understand fully how they are embedded personally in the body of their profession. Each nurse is an active and intimate part of nursing—a profession that every nurse both practices and helps to create.

The ethics of a profession not only delimit the role and scope of its activities and prescribe the nature of the relationship that should exist between its members and the lay public, but also establish the duties that professionals owe to one another and to the profession. That the ancients recognized the unique nature of the professional relationship is demonstrated in the Hippocratic Oath: "I swear . . . to hold him who has taught me this art as equal to my parents and to live my life in partnership with him . . .".[1] Codes of professional ethics usually included a pledge to exert one's best efforts to maintain the honor of the profession, to uphold its public standing and to extend the bounds of its usefulness.[2] Nurses, then, as they assume their professional identities, are pledged to: (1) the work of understanding, interpreting, and expanding the body of the profession's knowledge; (2) the equally disciplined work of criticism and self-regulation; and (3) the work of developing and cultivating in themselves and in their colleagues the character traits on which personal and professional excellence depend. The deep-seated relationship between a profession and its individual members and the relationships among the professionals cannot be forced into conformity with a model; rather, they should be described in terms of the practitioners' actual experiences of the profession.

The moral commitments of nurses to their profession and to one another form a foundation for professional life. The practitioners' perceptions of and fidelity to these moral commitments will affect and, to a large extent, will create the structure of their intraprofessional relationships.

To the extent that nurses recognize their commitment to common goals, the similarity of their knowledge base and their indebtedness to the nurses who went before them, to their teachers and to their peers, they will devote themselves to the advancement of the profession and to the growth of their colleagues. Hence, nursing as a caring profession involves not only care for and of patients but also care for and of fellow nurses. It is on this base that the significance of the nurse–nurse relationship rests. In the fulfillment of nurses' contracts with society, with patients and families and with employing institutions, their relationships with their fellow nurses are crucial.

The importance of intraprofessional relationships in nursing may not be appreciated fully by nurses if they focus their ethical concern solely on the well-being of patients and their families. Mature recognition of their own limits and capabilities leads nurses to rely on and incorporate the knowledge, the experience and the research of other professionals in their own practice. Clearly, the structure of work in most facilities requires nurses to function interdependently, that is, to trust in the professional expertise of colleagues, both in and outside of nursing, as each member of the health care team strives to achieve personal and professional goals. That nurses work collaboratively with members of other professions is obvious. What may be overlooked is the fact that nurses' professional interdependence demands special—even fraternal—relationships *among nurses.* Reflection on these relationships reveals interesting and challenging dimensions.

THE PROFESSIONAL RELATIONSHIP: AN ETHICAL IMPERATIVE

The ethical principles that underlie the formulation of professional relationships derive from several sources.[3] The first source is comprised of the universally applicable concepts of human rights and the duties attached to those rights. Nurses are human beings and they deserve to be treated as such by all persons, including other nurses. As is the case with all other human relationships, nurses' mutual humanity forms the fundamental framework for relationships among the people who belong to the same profession. Therefore, the relationships that obtain among nurses should be characterized first and foremost by respect for one another's human rights. Nurses should guard against behaving in ways that could threaten those rights. Such attention will help nurses to avoid demonstrating a lack of consideration for other nurses as both strive to fulfill professional duties and responsibilities.

A second source of the ethical principles that underlie professional relationships is in nurses' obligations to promote the public's welfare. Because nurses are professionals, they are responsible to the public for the services rendered by all members of the profession. As professionals, nurses assume a duty to practice in accord with established standards and to improve standards as knowledge increases.[4] One of the most effective ways to promote excellence in nursing practice and to disseminate new information is for nurses to offer support, guidance, criticism, and direction to one another. To fail or to refuse to offer this kind of assistance actually constitutes a breach of faith—not just with colleagues, but also with the public because it will affect negatively the quality of nursing service offered. It could result in nurses, in their professional care of patients, displaying a lack of knowledge, skill or judgment, or a disregard for the welfare of a patient. In some statutes, such behavior constitutes professional incompetence.[5] Hence, ethical nurses cannot ignore the practice of colleagues but most assume some responsibility for

the promotion of excellence in the practice of fellow nurses. Because all nurses share this corporate responsibility for the work of the profession as a whole, as it fulfills its contracts with society, with patients, and with other individuals and groups, they must look beyond their own specific patient assignments in order to fulfill their duties as members of the nursing discipline.

While human rights and concern for the public welfare form a basic framework for the special nature of intraprofessional relationships, a third source of the underlying ethical principles breathes life into them. When nurses enter the profession, they figuratively "adopt" their colleagues as brothers or sisters.[6] The ethical obligations flowing from this source derive from the professional bond rather than from blood ties or mutual liking. Typically, the duties ascribed to the "fraternal" aspects of the professional relationship are formalized in rules regarding the handling of incompetent colleagues, canons of loyalty and professional courtesies. The superficial manifestations of the professional bond only begin to approach the realities of the human experience that is the professional relationship. It is incumbent on nurses to examine how the professional bond affects the behavior in their professional lives and to decide whether what they see is acceptable.

Professional relationships enable one to be a professional (specifically a nursing professional) through identification with others and through recognition of the dilemmas of others within oneself. Such relationships do not tell one how to act as much as how to be. The discovery and understanding of oneself as a professional stems from one's perception and knowledge of other professionals. This means that each nurse discovers the outline of herself/himself in the human totality of nursing colleagues: each recognizes himself or herself in others and sees the characteristics of others in herself. More precisely and powerfully, between their first experience of the professional relationship and their last, professionals actually exchange characters. The exchange of characters between self and others creates what one is as a nurse and, at the same time, the ideal of what one should be as a nurse—in general and in particular.

In terms of the sociology of the profession, the function of the professional bond may be described as that of role modeling and role internalization. The latter occurs when individuals begin to identify with their role models and to adopt their behavior patterns, both consciously and unconsciously. It has been said that nurses of today may have difficulty with such identification and that role models in nursing practice, in all types of venues, may be conspicuous by their absence. This creates a void for practicing nurses who need competence figures. "Ironically, the deficits in role inculcation probably relate to the educational model adopted by the nursing discipline. In misguided attempts to improve the educational status of nursing, students often have been 'protected' from interaction with practicing nurses, with the rationalization that such interaction smacks of apprenticeship."[7] However, all experts were apprentices or beginners at one time who were taught and guided by master craftsmen. If nursing students remain apart from the mainstream of the work world of nurses, they will be like spectators who sample the practice field but never really feel that they are significant parts of it. As a result, the professional bond in nursing is weak for nursing students; it may remain this way for registered nurses because their professional identity does not develop, either during student experience or after their entry to professional practice following graduation.

The lack of professional identity is evidenced by the large number of nurses who leave the field and by those who practice at subprofessional levels (regardless of what degrees or credentials they earn).[8] Such nurses do not see that their concern, commitment, and genuine involvement in the profession and its development are what makes the profession viable. They do not appreciate the true interdependence of all members of a profession.

Only as nurses discover and create their own practices and identities as nurses, and only as they understand the roles that these play in the viability of nursing will they discover, add to, and create their profession. In the end, the sources of the ethical principles underlying intraprofessional relationships—human rights, commitment to the public welfare, and the professional bond—give structure and life to the practitioner's experience of the profession. This, in turn, revitalizes the profession itself. It follows that where positive professional relationships are weak or absent, both the profession and the professionals suffer. It is incumbent on nurse educators and nurse leaders to ensure that professional relationships are fostered and maintained. This is a challenge that forms an essential part of the daily professional life of a nurse.

PROFESSIONAL PREROGATIVES

When one becomes a professional, one assumes a number of obligations and earned rights. Earned rights, as distinct from human rights, encompass those prerogatives that are necessary to the fulfillment of professional obligations. They are not privileges in the sense of mere courtesies (although the importance of true courtesy never should be underestimated) because they are essential to the practice of the profession. They are not rights in the sense of something that automatically is owed to all persons; rather, they are enabling qualities that one merits through effort, education and experience, that is, they are earned. If one proves unworthy of them, one no longer has them: they can be removed formally by a statutory body, by an institution or by the profession, and informally by fellow professionals or by patients or clients and their families.

Earned rights are not extras, pleasantries, or even behavioral expectations of other professionals and members of the public, because they are necessary—indeed, integral—to the practice of a profession. Among the earned rights of nurses are:

1. The right to practice nursing in accord with professionally defined standards

2. The right to participate in and to promote the growth and direction of the profession

3. The right to be trusted by members of the public

4. The right to intervene when necessary to protect patients, clients or the public

5. The right to testify authoritatively to the community about the health care needs of people

6. The right to be believed when one is speaking in the area of his/her expertise

7. The right to be respected by those inside and outside the profession for one's knowledge, abilities, experience and contributions

8. The right to be trusted by colleagues

9. The right to give to and to receive from colleagues support, guidance and correction

10. The right to be compensated fairly for services rendered.

These earned *rights* are, in fact, accurate reflections of the *duties* of nurses, all of whom have the duty to:

1. Practice nursing in accord with the standards of the profession

2. Participate in and promote the direction and growth of the profession

3. Fulfill the promises the profession has made to the public
4. Intervene to protect patients or clients from the unethical or illegal actions of any person
5. Testify to the public regarding the health care needs of people
6. Speak out accurately and honestly in one's area of expertise
7. Strive constantly to increase one's knowledge and experience
8. Give to and to receive from one's colleagues guidance, support and correction
9. Render adequate and safe nursing services within professionally defined standards and institutional or agency policies.

Failure by nurses to fulfill these duties cancels the rights that are attached to them. However, failure by both nurses and others to recognize that rights are attached to these duties leaves nurses powerless in the face of awesome responsibilities. Germane to the nurse-nurse relationship are nurses' rights: (1) to be trusted by their colleagues; (2) to give to and to receive from their colleagues support, guidance, and correction; and (3) to be respected for their knowledge, experience, and contributions to the profession. These earned rights of nurses translate into guidelines—actually, behavioral imperatives that are well grounded in ethical principles—for their professional relationships. Nurses should be treated and should treat one another in congruence with these professional imperatives.

These rights and responsibilities of nurses make it incumbent on nurses at all levels to ensure not only that nurses *do* fulfill their duties and responsibilities but also that conditions in the work situation are such that nurses *can* fulfill them. Failure of nurses and others—including employers, fellow professionals, and society—to provide conditions that make it possible for nurses to fulfill their duties constitutes infringement of the human and professional rights of nurses and it is unethical behavior. Hence, the rights and duties of nurses are inseparable and are essential to each other.

PROFESSIONAL CHARACTER TRAITS

Contemporary nurses appear to have been far less interested than were their predecessors in the identification and cultivation of the character traits that are necessary to the life of a profession. This may be due in part to a reaction to the almost monastic life that used to be required of nurses and in part to the fact that this area may seem to be subjective and elusive. Whatever the reason, the result is that too little thought has been given to the question of the virtues that are appropriate to the development of professional character.

For a person to enter fully into professional relationships with peers requires:

1. Fidelity to the promises of the profession: a shared commitment to the profession's goals provides identity for the group and forms a solid foundation for cooperative effort. Nurses must decide what are the basic beliefs and values of the profession and adhere to them so that practice can be sufficiently predictable and consistent that both nurses and the public can be confident that the behavior of members of the profession will fulfill nursing's contracts with society, patients, colleagues *et al*.

2. Respect for the human and earned rights of oneself and of one's colleagues: self-respect enables one to stand up for one's beliefs; respect for others infers openness to discussion and debate in order to clarify differences of opinion, fact, and intent; both are essential to healthy relationships. Nurses must be prepared to articulate their beliefs and values and to submit them to the scrutiny of their peers. Failure to appreciate that colleagues have opinions and values and to give consideration to them connotes lack of respect that will hinder the development of effective professional relationships.

3. Honesty and intellectual integrity: these virtues are at the very heart of a "community of scholars"; they are essential to sound relationships within the profession and between the profession and the public; they infer a willingness to share knowledge and to work with others toward mutually defined goals. Shakespeare has noted that one who is true to himself cannot be false to others, and so it is with nurses in their professional relationships with one another.

If these character traits are appropriate to professional life, the virtues that nurses must seek and nurture in themselves and in others are benevolence, honesty, respect, fidelity, and integrity. Without these virtues, the moral fiber of the profession will be weakened and the activities of the profession itself will be reduced to commercial transactions at best. The dictum, *caveat emptor* (let the buyer beware) certainly is not an appropriate motto for the nursing profession. If matters of professional virtue—and the presence or absence of it in each nurse—are not addressed, the vast resources of the profession will be for sale to the highest bidder.

THE GROWTH OF THE PROFESSION AND THE PROFESSIONAL

If nursing is to become and is to continue to be a justifiable and viable profession, three developments must take place. All are possible because all exist today, although in muted form.

First, the profession must regain and must nurture a sense of commitment—of vocation—in its members. The knowledge that nurses possess and the skills that they acquire are more a public trust than a private acquisition to be prized and sold on the open market. Nurses' current concern with their economic status can be salutary but, if it becomes a preoccupation, nursing will be placed in an extraordinarily vulnerable position because money is far too narcissistic a focus for a profession. Opportunities for financial gain and personal advancement within a profession flourish only in the context of the valuable services that the profession provides to the public; the utility and the advancement of a profession depend on the individual members who have some sense of professional identity, commitment, and responsibility. When the professional bond is weak and each practitioner thinks of himself or herself as an entrepreneur—alone, unencumbered by a public and professional trust—the profession is wounded, perhaps mortally. By virtue of its traditions and its contract with society, nursing can ill afford to deny its public function, the interdependence of its practitioners, or its inherently altruistic goals. However, to engage in critical inquiry into the tension between adequate remuneration and altruistic service is, itself, a social act that infers accountability and responsibility for judgments and decisions and that assumes that these actions can be evaluated by others. "Critical inquiry is part of the public life of the mind, an indispensable ingredient to a professional life that has more to offer than the technical services for personal gain."[9] Such inquiry necessarily includes a weighing and weighting of the values, obligations and goals of the practitioner and of the profession. The sense of commitment to the profession and to the public trust is embodied in professional and ethical codes for nurses[10,11] and in standards of nursing practice,[12,13,14] in both Canada and the United States, some of which are covered by statute.[15,16]

The second development is that members of the nursing profession must become far more aware of their responsibilities to one another. Nurses must recognize, more fully than they have done to date, their duty to nurture, support, guide, and correct one another.[17] Cooperation and mutual growth must be recognized widely as norms in professional relationships—instead of competition or acquisition of power. Practically speaking, one's own success depends largely on the knowledge and skill of one's colleagues as well as on their willingness to share information and insights and to engage in the constructive criticism that is part of collaboration, cooperation and peer review. The nurse-nurse relationship is one vital factor that is notorious for being inexplicably weak. However, without a strong intraprofessional relationship, nurses will be unable to fulfill their commitments to the public and to achieve their personal and professional goals. Hence, nurses must take action to improve their relationships with one another.

The third development that must take place is that nursing must address the systems, institutions and structures that shape the environment in which nurses practice. Indeed, the ethical spirit of the profession today has been shaped largely by institutions—both schools and work places. In the eighties, perhaps more than ever before, health care professionals, including nurses, must go beyond direct patient care to consider and act on factors associated with the nature and shape of the health care system and the practice of members of the health care team.[18] Nurses are required by ethics and by law to question directions, including direct orders of other health professionals such as physicians and supervisory and management nurses, as well as policies and practices of institutions, about which they have concern.[19]

Therefore, it is appropriate and necessary for nurses to examine health-related institutions and systems and to strive to improve them. Such examination includes scrutiny of the customs and taboos of the situations in which they find themselves, including their own behavior and that of their colleagues, to identify whether what they see is consonant with the standards of practice for which they stand accountable.[20] Efforts to improve health care situations include the making of suggestions about and the testing of new methods and patterns of practice and of organization and willingness to be open to the ideas of other participants in the health care enterprise, including fellow nurses.

Do schools of nursing prepare students to engage in critical inquiry into the values that shape society and the profession? Do they provide opportunities for students to become skilled at such inquiry? Are they developing the kind of professional who can function effectively to meet the needs of the public and to advance the profession? Do nurses' workplaces provide environments that are conducive to excellence in nursing practice? Does the socialization process in both schools and workplaces promote the development of the professional bond? The answer to all of these questions is no—or at least not to the degree necessary to advance the profession.[21]

Nursing's institutions of higher learning, reflecting the general trend in higher education after World War II,[22] have concentrated chiefly on the development of operational and technical intelligence. "For example, in adopting the behavioral objective many nursing programs have eliminated all attempts to inculcate values, attitudes, thought processes, that defy a simplistic behavioral translation."[23] Although, in contrast, the counter-culture movement of the late sixties and early seventies stressed the affective component to learning,[24] both of these approaches reflect a far too narrow concept of intelligence. The result is a constellation of nurses who define themselves in terms of the technical tasks that they perform and who discuss values, goals, and ethics in terms of how they feel rather than what they think.

Development of operational intelligence helps the learner to determine how to get from here to there. It deals with means but it does not criticize ends. On the other hand, critical intelligence involves the making of judgments about the worth and value of the ends and the means that are appropriate for achievement of the ends. The word critical has its roots in the Greek verb, *kritikos*, that means "to judge, to discern, to separate, to distinguish."[25] The intellectual activity that is demanded in professional life includes the task of normative as well as descriptive inquiry—the use of critical as well as operational intelligence. If nursing's institutions of higher learning are to develop fully the intelligence of their students, nurses must take seriously the proposition that they constitute a community of scholars, learn how to behave in a scholarly fashion and then do so. Nursing educators in particular must demonstrate scholarly behavior and demand that students question and challenge nursing's propositions, methods, and goals. Thus, reasoned discourse and debate can take place and discriminating judgments can be made about ends and values. This will create the atmosphere of open and critical inquiry that is essential to the task of giving to and

receiving from one's colleagues criticism, support, direction, and guidance. Such discussion and debate should be an ongoing part of nursing practice at all levels, from the daily nursing care conference to the highest level nursing boards and councils in the profession. This type of activity will provide the opportunity and the basis for critical inquiry into the development and utility of the profession's goals and activities. If nurses are to be the change agents that their profession mandates them to be, they must define goals clearly and judge critically the value of those goals. It is the responsibility of nursing leaders and managers to create environments in which such activity can and will take place.

Sociologists and economists may offer valuable services to the nursing profession by describing the systems within which nurses work,[26] but they cannot offer nursing the conceptual tools that are necessary for critical analysis of the values and goals either of the systems or of the profession. The value or disvalue of hierarchical structures, interprofessional relationships, dependent versus interdependent and independent practice, social attitudes toward women, remuneration for nursing services, specialization and diversification among nurses and the like must be addressed by the profession as a whole—and this will be achieved only if nurses recognize and cherish their professional bond and work together within it. By and large, the institutions and systems in which nurses work were designed to serve laudable utilitarian ends and have functioned to provide services to the community. Their destruction is unlikely to serve the public's interests. Hence, nursing must weigh the social impact of its strivings for change if its struggles to reform "the system" are to serve the health needs of the populace as well as the aspirations of the profession. The enhancement of the profession and the strengthening of the professional bond among nurses must never become more important to nurses than their commitment to public well-being. Rather, these two elements of nurses' professionalism must be directed specifically toward fulfillment of nursing's commitment to society. Otherwise the profession will degenerate into a self-serving occupation and the professional bond will become an excuse for protection of professionals rather than a relationship that enhances practice.

In short, a profession that derives its authority and its influence from the fact that people need its services can become exploitative unless its members possess a high degree of altruism and work together to promote and foster high ideals in themselves and in their colleagues. People need to trust nurses, and to maintain this trust, nurses need to trust and to rely on one another. In fact, the very nature of nursing supports the claim that to be a nurse is to be a part of creative, constructive, professional relationships that involve being a partner in the development of a profession, the primary goal of which is to serve the needs of others. The extent to which each nurse demonstrates a caring quality in nurse-nurse relationships is proof of the extent to which the claim "to be a nurse" is being realized by the profession through the behavior of its members.

NOTES

1. "Appendix: Codes of the Health Care Professions," in Warren T. Reich, ed. *Encyclopedia of Bioethics* (The Free Press, New York, 1978) p. 1731.
2. *Ibid.*, pp. 1732–1815.
3. Veatch, Robert. "The Ethics of Professional Relations," in Warren T. Reich, ed. *Encyclopedia of Bioethics* (The Free Press, New York, 1978) pp. 178–179.
4. American Nurses' Association. *Code for Nurses with Interpretative Statements* (American Nurses' Association, Kansas City, Missouri, 1976) Statement No. 8.
5. Ontario. *The Health Disciplines Act, 1974, Part IV, Nursing.* 1974 c. 47, s. 84(4), as amended by 1975, c. 63 (Toronto, 1975).
6. Veatch, *op. cit.*, p. 178.
7. Stevens Barbara J. *Research in Nursing Education: Perspectives for the Future* (Teacher's College, Columbia University, New York, 1979) pp. 12–13.
8. *Ibid.*, p. 12.
9. May, William F. "Normative Inquiry and Medical Ethics in Our Colleges and Universities," in David Smith and Linda Bernstein, eds. *No Rush to Judgment* (Indiana University Foundation, Bloomington, Indiana, 1978) p. 334.
10. American Nurses' Association. 1973, *op. cit.*
11. College of Nurses of Ontario. *Guidelines for Ethical Behavior in Nursing* (College of Nurses of Ontario, Toronto, 1980).
12. American Nurses' Association. *Standards of Nursing Practice* (American Nurses' Association, Kansas City, Missouri, 1973).
13. College of Nurses of Ontario. *Standards of Nursing Practice: for Registered Nurses and Registered Nursing Assistants.* Revised, May 1979 (College of Nurses of Ontario, Toronto, 1979).
14. Canadian Nurses Association. *A Definition of Nursing Practice. Standards for Nursing Practice* (Canadian Nurses Association, Ottawa, 1980).
15. College of Nurses of Ontario, 1979, *op. cit.*
16. Ontario. *Regulation made under The Health Disciplines Act, 1974, Part IV, Nursing.* Ontario Regulation 578/75, s. 24 (Queen's Printer, Toronto, 1975).
17. *Ibid.*, s. 21, i.j.
18. Flaherty, M. Josephine, "Accountability in Health Care Practice: Ethical Implications for Nurses." Chapter 23, in Davis, John W., *et. al.*, eds. *Contemporary Issues in Biomedical Ethics* (The Humana Press, Clifton, New Jersey, 1979) p. 273.
19. *Ibid.*, p. 271.
20. *Ibid.*, p. 276.
21. Many sources could be cited here. For example, see Fromm, Linda, "The Problem in Nursing, Nurses!" *Supervisor Nurse*, Vol. 8, No. 10 (October 1977) p. 15.
22. May, *op. cit.*, p. 338.
23. Stevens, *op. cit.*, p. 12.
24. Alinsky, Saul D. *Rules for Radicals* (Vintage Books, New York, 1971) pp. i-xxvi.
25. *Webster's New World Dictionary.* Unabridged, Second Edition (World Publishing Company, New York, 1968).
26. For example, see Dachelet, Christy Z. "Nursing's Bid for Increased Status," *Nursing Forum*, Vol. XVII, No. 1 (1978) pp. 19–45.

Power Brings Out the Worst in Women

Ian Morrison

Like many other third-year students, Nurse Maxwell was not too keen on staff nurses, and nurses who had recently been promoted were even more disliked. She had a fairly logical mind and, quite naturally, wondered how a nurse a mere four months ahead of her as far as training was concerned could suddenly wield so much power; how a nurse who was friendly one day, could overnight change her personality. She thought about the words of her boyfriend, who often said: "Girls are strange creatures."

A nurse whom she regarded as a colleague one week would suddenly look the other way in the canteen, all because she had the keys to the drug cabinet hanging from her bosom. The new staff nurse was now in demand from registrars and consultants, when previously the lowly houseman was sufficient fodder for her attentions.

Nurse Maxwell was undecided whether it was a good thing to pass her finals, but declared that if she did she would remain as she was now—a girl in her early twenties who was happy with life and was even happier giving out bed-pans and ruffling pillows. She would never change.

It is my opinion, as a male, that hospitals bring out the worst in women. They cannot help it of course. It is something to do with their physiology. Give me an introductory training school, and I guarantee that after four hours the males would be discussing mutual interests, and the women would be silently criticizing each other's modes of dress, hair styles and choice of deodorant.

At the end of the first day in school, the men would meet in the local pub while the girls would be scribbling letters to their parents, telling them of the horrid girls they would be expected to work with.

However, it is when the prospect of real power looms that the trouble starts. A girl of 18, on the threshold of a career in nursing, quite naturally is in awe of everybody she meets, from ward clerk to second-year nurse, from domestic to laboratory technician. I remember my first day on the ward. I was taken to one side by the kitchen domestic who told me in motherly terms: "Don't worry, love, if you've any problems, come and see me." But I digress.

SUDDEN POWER

I was introduced to the phenomenon of sudden power on the male surgical ward. A third-year student had been going to discos and dances with a male nurse who had started his training four months after her. The girl passed her finals and applied for a staff nurse post on the same ward. Wearing her new staff nurse's uniform, she passed the male nurse who had been her dancing companion two nights' earlier. The brief conversation went as follows:

"Make sure the sluice is tidy, nurse."
"But Mary, I wanted to ask . . ."
"Make sure you call me staff nurse. The sluice, please."

From that moment I resolved that if I ever passed my finals I would never humiliate a student, and I don't think I ever have.

There is something about a sudden rise to power that is highly unpleasant. From innocent adolescent, young girls are transformed overnight into

Morrison, I. (1984, April 25). Power brings out the worst in women. *Nursing Mirror, 158*, (17) 26–27. Reprinted with permission of © *Nursing Times*. All rights reserved.

talented but obnoxious beings. They quickly learn how easy it is to lose friends.

Patients can always tell a newly qualified nurse. She is the one who openly hunts junior nurses, making sure that she has an audience before demonstrating her new powers. Fortunately, this action has the effect of immediately ensuring that any sympathy is given to the victim of the verbal assault. Patients and more mature nurses are not deceived by newly qualified nurses. Frankly, some of them are a pain in the neck.

The sensible staff nurse, newly qualified, will seek the help of other nurses on the ward. She should realize that there will be other nurses who will know far more than her, and the relationship should be one of mutual respect. One cannot function without the other. The new staff nurse may be able to count the pethidine, but she will find difficulty when it is apparent that nobody wants to witness the act.

The art of being a good staff nurse is a subject which takes years, and which is never completed.

Too many think that, because they have passed their finals, they can now sit in the office, thinking that their work ended when SRN was placed after their name. They see their task as delegating work, occasionally popping out of the office, and making tea for the registrar.

Yes, it's amazing how nurses can change their personality in a matter of days. I sometimes think it would be a good idea if training took place over 10 years and not three. It certainly takes that length of time to reach the maturity required.

The point I am trying to make is that the nursing profession is in danger of becoming less efficient than it should, all because of what can happen in a single week . . . the period of transition between student and SRN.

I often wonder whether Florence Nightingale was ever in charge of the dangerous drugs cupboard. If she ever was, then I think she would have treated her junior nurses with respect and dignity, at all times.

Guilt by Association?

M. Josephine Flaherty

A story in the local newspaper noted that a citizen had been charged by federal police authorities with a drug offense. He had been growing marijuana, he was in possession of a supply of it and he had sold some of it. His wife, the joint owner of their family home, was charged with being a contributor to his crime because she was aware of his activities. Although she did not approve of them and took no part in them, she had failed to notify federal officials of his contravention of the drug laws; hence, she was allowing illegal activities to occur in premises of which she was a part owner.

The wife is a registered nurse who was employed in the town's general hospital. The director of nursing telephoned her, confirmed that she was the same person named in the newspaper story (that did not identify her as a nurse or as an employee of the hospital) and suspended her from her nursing position pending the outcome of the court trial. When the latter took place, both husband and wife were found guilty. The wife was given a suspended sentence.

However, her employer, the hospital, discharged her on the grounds that she had "lost her professionalism" and hence would not be a suitable employee. Some hospital authorities believed, apparently, that the hospital would be in a difficult position in the future if a drug offense "incident" took place in the agency because of the presence of a "known drug offender" on the staff. Was the hospital's action justified? Why or why not?

ANALYSIS

Organized nursing of the eighties has declared that nursing is a profession and that its members want to embrace the privileges and responsibilities of professional people. These include the expectation that nurses, in the performance of nursing services as registered nurses, shall exercise generally accepted standards of practice for the performance of the nursing services. The standards of nursing practice in the jurisdiction in which the drug offense situation took place include the requirement that the nursing practitioner will function in accordance with a code of nursing ethics that outlines expectations for nurses in their nursing practice behavior.

Early in this century, statements about nursing ethics and nursing practice standards in Canada and in the United States made reference to nurses' personal virtues and their behavior in their personal lives.

Today, however, such statements and codes refer to actions in the practice of the profession without reference to behavior outside nurses' job situations. One would wonder, then, how an error or an indiscretion in one's home, in one's private life, that bears no direct relationship to behavior in the professional context, can become grounds for dismissal from a job in nursing.

In the situation cited above, the employer did not identify the aspect of the undefined "professionalism" that had been "lost" by the nurse. It can be assumed that the nurse was aware that her husband was breaking the law. Apparently she discussed this with him and tried to persuade him to cease and desist, and this was to no avail. She refused to have any part of his drug-related activities, even to the extent that she would not go into the part of the house where the illicit drug was kept. One would suppose that she could have uprooted the marijuana plants and destroyed them and that she could have destroyed the drug material that was to be sold. She could have refused to remain in the family home, but perhaps she had notified federal authorities of her husband's behavior.

One would suppose that she gave thought to some or all of these options and that she decided, in her wisdom or lack of it, to do none of these and instead, to continue to try to persuade her husband to change his behavior. This may have been a poor judgment. However, in light of the other alternatives, that probably included the break-up of her marriage, her home and her family, in which there were children, perhaps she believed that she had chosen the least of several evils.

Hospital authorities noted that because she had made a bad judgment in this instance, she no longer could be trusted to make sound judgments related to drugs in her professional work. Perhaps this could be the case if the nurse's offense were relevant to her suitability to practice, that is, relevant to the performance of nursing services. With regard to drugs, this could include her misappropriation of a patient's or of the employer's drugs, particularly this action involved the denying of a drug to a patient for the purpose of the trafficking of it or mis-use of a drug for herself or for another person. Should the fact that a nurse shared a home with a person who broke a law, albeit a serious one, and failed to take direct action either to interfere physically with the other person's action or to report the action to the police, necessarily be considered evidence that the nurse cannot be trusted to make sound professional judgments? If this were the case, how many health professionals could be found who had never made even one wrong or questionable judgment in their personal lives? Are many of us totally without blemish with regard to traffic regulations, speeding laws, customs declarations, income tax violations, truth telling, occupational health and safety rules and so forth, violations of law all of which could result in court convictions? Should we be dismissed from our nursing positions for even the first "wrong judgment" we make, even in terms of an omission such

as the failure to report our families or neighbors for violations of federal or state laws? Should we be regarded as having lost our professionalism and hence to be unsuitable nursing employees?

Should a hospital feel that any conviction of an employee, even one of being "found in," so to speak, in his own home during improper conduct by another member of the household, would reflect so negatively on the hospital's credibility that the public would be concerned about the professional competence of hospital employees?

The statutory (registering) body for nurses in the jurisdiction in which this incident took place was aware of the events because the nurse involved had reported them herself. No action had been taken by the registrar up to the time of writing, that is, up to four months after the court trial and conviction. This suggests that the registering authority had not decided that this nurse was unsafe for professional practice.

The job description for the nurse in question was never tabled as evidence of the nurse's failure to fulfill the requirements of her position. One can question whether there was a specific job description for this nurse. When such descriptions do exist, do they include expectations for personal behavior outside the work situation? Should such expectations be included in professional job descriptions? Why or why not?

The nurse in this situation filed a grievance as a result of her dismissal. The grievance was denied. The nurses' union took the case to arbitration where it was at the time of writing.

How should the arbitration board rule on this case? If readers believe that the nurse should be dismissed, what would be the grounds for such action? If the nurse should not be dismissed, what action, if any, should or could nurse managers take on this issue? To what extent is it legitimate for employers to monitor the private lives of nurse employees? Is a case such as this one the beginning of a new trend in employee employer relationships? If it is, should nurse managers support this trend? What are we going to do about it?

STUDY AND DISCUSSION QUESTIONS
THE NURSE–NURSE RELATIONSHIP

1. According to Curtin and Flaherty, what are the three sources for the ethical principles underlying the nurse–nurse relationship?

2. Curtin and Flaherty believe that part of the development of the professional bond occurs in "role modeling" and "role internalization." It is by identification with role models and the conscious and unconscious adoption and imitation of their behavior patterns that creates a professional bond. Do you agree? Who or what do you perceive as models for your practice of nursing?

3. Curtin and Flaherty believe that one reason the professional bond in nurses is weak is because nursing students are isolated from working professionals. Do you think this is so?

4. Would the "earned rights" described by Curtin and Flaherty qualify as rights according to our discussion in Chapter 3? That is, would these rights pass the prerogative test (they may be exercised or not without injustice at the agent's prerogative) and the corollary thesis test (they impose duties on someone to see that they are fulfilled)?

5. Do you believe nurses ought to have certain traits of character? If so, which ones? Does your list differ from Curtin and Flaherty's?

6. Do you agree with Curtin and Flaherty that nursing curricula do not focus enough on the development of critical intelligence?

7. Curtin and Flaherty argue that "the enhancement of the profession and the strengthening of the professional bond among nurses must never become more important to nurses than their commitment to public well-being." Do you agree? Should loyalty to other nurses ever be placed above reporting mistakes that may affect the health or welfare of patients?

8. Ian Morrison implies that the weakness of intraprofessional bonds in nursing relates to the fact that nurses are mostly women. Is this true? Is there caring, support, and solidarity among nurses? If not, why do you suppose this is the case?

9. Assuming there is a problem of weak professional bonds in nursing, who is more accurate in determining the cause—Morrison? Curtin and Flaherty? Neither?

10. In the case presented by Flaherty, do you agree that the nurse "lost her professionalism" when she was convicted of failing to notify the authorities of the illegal activities of her husband—possessing and selling homegrown marijuana?

11. Flaherty mentions that early in this century statements about nursing ethics and nursing practice standards in Canada and the United States

made reference to nurses' personal virtues and their personal behavior, but that recent statements and codes have omitted such references. Do you think this is a good idea?

12. Can private conduct reflect badly on the profession? Should the ethical codes require a standard of moral conduct that reflects credit on the profession?

13. Is it possible to maintain both (a) what a nurse does outside nursing is nobody's business and (b) there are some professional character traits all nurses ought to have? If so, how? If not, what is better for the nursing profession to emphasize—character or privacy?

8

Professional Obligations of Nurses

INTRODUCTION

This chapter begins with a discussion by Leah Curtin about the nature and source of professional obligations. The Muyskens article presents the concept of collective responsibility as a means of understanding the problem of nurses caught in the middle—that is, being responsible for their own actions and yet compelled to support policies and carry out actions that violate their sense of professional obligations. Muyskens wishes to plot a middle course between two judgments on this situation. On the one hand, it may be said that, if required, nurses ought to put their jobs on the line and are morally remiss if they do not. On the other hand, it may be argued that nurses have pushed the issue as far as morality and good conscience would require. Muyskens believes that, while the first judgment is too harsh, the second would perpetuate a system that fosters substandard medical care.

The following articles represent dissents to the Muyskens view. "Engineers as Moral Heroes" reports on a paper by Ken Alpern, which implies that it is not too much to ask of nurses to fulfill their professional obligations even if that means risk to their jobs. On the contrary, the selection by Hayes, Hayes, and Kelly argues that such situations present a morally excusable reason for failing in one's moral and professional obligations.

A more complete account of these articles plus a note on hospital liability for failure to protect patients from negligent or incompetent acts follows.

CURTIN—THE NATURE AND SOURCE OF PROFESSIONAL OBLIGATIONS

Leah Curtin conceives of nursing as a moral art whose professional obligations stem from promises it has made to the public. The basic promise is to meet a fundamental need for care that involves a commitment to improve the quality of living of those seeking or receiving nursing services. From this basic promise, Curtin derives others.[1] The actualization of these promises depends on the moral commitments of the practitioners, their perception of their role, and their willingness to maintain standards of excellence.

Curtin is particularly critical of two things. First, nurses have not been so diligent in developing systems of prevention, chronic care, and maintenance. Nor have nurses been particularly effective in testifying against a system that fails to meet fundamental health needs of its citizenry.

Second, the ethical issues nurses have chosen to consider focus too exclusively on "specific, individual problems"—a case orientation that overlooks questions of social justice and the larger implications of our moral decisions. Curtin believes that:

> The commitment of nursing demands that nurses develop an approach to ethics that is proactive rather than reactive; that nurses concentrate on the deeper aspects of preventive, chronic, and maintenance care rather than acute care; and that nurses direct attention to the milieu in which they must make decisions, that is, environmental and personal factors that inhibit or advance the ability of individual providers to implement decisions.

Some of the obligations mentioned by Curtin are by their very nature collective. That is to say, no single nurse could fulfill all the promises that nursing has made to the public. No single nurse must do research, engage in the assessment of public health delivery systems, ensure that standards of nursing education and practice are met, improve the quality of life of the dying, and so on. These are promises that nursing has made collectively and, therefore, although an individual nurse need not engage in all of these activities, the profession as a whole remains responsible for their fulfillment. Nevertheless, if a nurse is to be faithful to the promises of the profession, he or she must provide support for the actions nursing organizations take to fulfill these public promises.

THE MORAL REQUIREMENTS TO FULFILL PROFESSIONAL OBLIGATIONS

James L. Muyskens is a philosopher. The selection here, "The Nurse as a Member of a Profession," is a chapter from his book, *Moral Problems in Nursing: A Philosophical Investigation*, in which he defends an advocacy ethic.[2] The difficulty he sees in nursing is that nurses are accountable for their individual actions, and yet they work in systems where the individual client's interests are sacrificed to policy and orders that must be obeyed. Nurses are sometimes pressured by physicians and hospital administrations by threats against their job. The endemic problem of blame avoidance behavior is a natural consequence of such a situation. The feeling is, "You do what you can, but you cannot fight the system." On the one hand, if no one fights the system, then substandard health care will continue unabated. On the other hand, can it be required of persons to take on the system? We have seen in previous chapters the cost extracted from individuals like Tuma, Smith, and Witt. To be a hero is by definition a supererogatory act—that is, one that is above and beyond the call of duty. Hence, the dilemma: to require heroism is too strong a duty, but to exonerate nurses from fighting the system perpetuates substandard care and violates professional obligations.

Muyskens introduces the concept of collective responsibility as a means of analyzing this situation. He wishes to preserve the intuitions that would exonerate the nurse from the charge of moral failure (if the nurse has done all that can reasonably be expected) *and* nevertheless find fault with the profession for allowing the situation to continue.

He notes that we often assign blame to groups of individuals. He argues that the conditions under which it is appropriate to assign collective responsibility to a group are met by the nursing profession. A key feature of this concept is that fault may be ascribed to a group without it being the case that every member of the group is at fault. Thus, it would be possible to blame the group or profession without attaching personal liability to blame to the individual member.

The case for assigning non-distributive collective responsibility is convincing. The profession has clear standards of acceptable practice that are within its responsibility to uphold. Individual practitioners have voluntarily assumed to fulfill, in Curtin's words, the promises of the profession. And yet there exists in nursing a "way of life" that permits and perpetuates operation at substandard levels, especially, for example, overwork and understaffing.

Muyskens believes that collective responsibility is a two-edged sword that exonerates the individual *qua* individual, but blames the nurse *qua* nurse. It can and should be used as a tool to educate the nurse to responsibilities beyond individual responsibilities and to upgrade the profession by mechanisms in place that handle reports of "incompetent, unethical or illegal practice" without fear of reprisal.

The article "Engineers as Moral Heroes" reports on an argument by philosopher Ken Alpern that has application to this issue.[3] The argument is that, contrary to Muyskens, nurses who risk their jobs to practice at professional levels are not acting as heroes. Rather, such nurses are exhibiting moral courage in fulfilling a duty of *ordinary* morality. Nurses are under this ordinary obligation because of their knowledge and position. According to Alpern's argument, nurses are in a position to avert harm and they cannot avoid this responsibility by appeals to job loss, the fact that other nurses have long condoned the unethical, incompetent, or illegal practice, or the lack of support from other nurses who may fear reprisals themselves.

The reading by Hayes, Hayes, and Kelly is an excerpt from a Catholic ethics text, *Moral Principles of Nursing*.[4] The reason for its inclusion in this debate is that it articulates excusing conditions for nurses participating in actions they feel are wrong. Although their discussion focuses on cooperating in immoral operations, the principles have broader application. The main point is that condoning an operation, system, or policy thought to be morally wrong may be permissible in some cases. What is required here is that the nurse have a sufficient reason. Greater evil and greater involvement require a correspondingly graver reason. A reason that will cover nearly all situations is "the threat of being dismissed immediately, combined with the knowledge that a new position will be almost impossible to obtain in the foreseeable future."

Thus, Hayes, Hayes, and Kelly can be construed as morally exonerating nurses for condoning practices about which they feel morally uncomfortable. And, as is also clear, this sort of exonerating defense has not been invented just for this occasion—the moral tradition here is very old.

SUMMARY

We have thus far considered the nature of professional obligations and how far a nurse must go in fulfilling such obligations. An additional consideration would be whether there are any legal inducements to carry out obligations concerning patients at risk. The literature has pointed to several court decisions that indicate a trend to hold hospitals liable for failure to monitor the competence of its staff or to assure that informed consent to treatment has been given.[5] To the extent that hospitals may be independently held to an independent standard of care, this may give prudent hospital administrations reason to give serious consideration to the patient-related concerns of nursing.

Crucial to the fulfillment of the promises of nursing is the commitment of nurses to those promises. What is not so clear is why the fulfilling of these promises remains difficult, who is to blame for that, and what can be done about it. The readings have variously suggested collective action, blame on individual practitioners, and greater fidelity to the promises of the profession.

NOTES

1. A similar argument can be found in American Nurses' Association, *Nursing: A Social Policy Statement* (Kansas City, Mo.: American Nurses' Association, 1980).
2. See James L. Muyskens, *The Moral Problems of Nursing: A Philosophical Investigation* (Totowa, N. J.: Rowan & Littlefield, 1982).
3. A version of this paper was later published. See Kenneth D. Alpern, "Moral Responsibility for Engineers," *Business & Professional Ethics Journal* 2(Winter 1983): 39–48.
4. Edward J. Hayes, Paul J. Hayes, and Dorothy Ellen Kelly, *Moral Principles of Nursing* (New York: Macmillan, 1964). The authors are two priests and a nurse.
5. Some noteworthy articles in this regard are: William J. Gargaro, "Hospital Liability for Failure to Monitor Competence of Its Staff—Part I," *Cancer Nursing* 6(October

1983): 387–388; Ibid., "Hospital Liability for Failure to Monitor Competence of Its Staff—Part II," *Cancer Nursing* 6(October 1983): 463–464; and Jane Greenlaw, "Should Hospitals be Responsible for Informed Consent?" *Law, Medicine and Health Care* 11(September 1983): 173–176, 187. Gargaro's article is on the implications of a California case, *Elam v. College Park Hospital* (1982) App., 183 Cal. Rptr. 156. Greenlaw is commenting on *Magana v. Elie* (1982) Ill. App., 439 N.E. 2d 1319. The rationale for the extension of liability to hospitals was influentially expressed in *Daring v. Charleston Community Memorial Hospital* (1965), 33 Ill. 2d 326, 211 N.E. 2d 253.

The Commitment of Nursing

Leah Curtin

*"It has given my heart a change of mood
And saved some part of the day I rued."*

Adapted from Robert Frost's *Dust of Snow*

The claim that nursing is a moral art emphasizes nurses' commitment to care for as well as to give care to other human beings. It involves a particularly intense form of the general moral imperative to care for one another. Understanding the content of this commitment is important because it constitutes the scope and depth of ethical concern in nursing and lays a foundation for an approach to any one ethical quandary. Moreover, an understanding of nursing as a moral art challenges the notion that considerations of ethics in nursing are limited to or even solely focused on the discrete ethical quandaries faced by nurses.

THE CONTENT OF COMMITMENT

Commitment in the profession of nursing raises at least two questions: What does being a professional nurse involve? Even more puzzling, what does it mean to be a practitioner of a moral art? Such questions entail an explication of the role, character, and behavior of individual practitioners.

The question of how the nurse is committed to the patient or client necessarily involves what it means to be a professional. The word profession has as its root the Latin word, *profitere*, which literally means "to declare publicly." It was applied to certain occupations because the practitioners of those occupations declared publicly, that is, promised publicly that they would meet certain standards and dedicate themselves to serve people through the fulfillment of certain needs.

The philosopher J. L. Austin developed the now famous distinction between two different kinds of statements: descriptive and performative.[1] Descriptive statements transmit a given fact in the world. For example, "The tree outside my window is 40 feet high." or "You have cancer of the lung." or "Your child was born with a condition called meningomyelocele." However, performative statements alter a reality in the world by introducing a new ingredient—something that would not be there *apart from the declaration*. For example, "I, Leah, take thee, Peter, to be my wedded spouse. . ." or "I will help you." or "I will not abandon you."

Because a promise is a link between what is and what will be, to make or to break a promise is a very serious thing to do. If we want to understand the nature of nurses' commitment to patients or clients, we must examine the performative declarations of the nursing profession. To what have nurses committed themselves? What promises are entailed in the practice of this profession? Briefly, nurses have promised to help those who are ill to regain their health, those who are healthy to maintain their health, those who cannot be cured to maximize their potentials and those who are dying to live as fully as possible until their deaths. The making of such promises entails an honest commitment to their fulfillment because their fulfillment significantly affects people's lives.

By and large, the question of honesty of health professionals has been limited to discussion of whether to tell the patient the truth (or part of it) or, more saliently, who should tell the patient the truth. To be sure, truth-telling in the context of health care is quite important because it involves the imparting of highly significant and risk-laden knowledge.[2] The squabble about who should impart such knowledge to patients is an interdisciplinary conflict that involves the qualifications and roles of various practitioners. However, the performative declarations of a professional expand the demands of honesty in a professional's life. The moral question for the professional (in this case, the nurse) is not simply a matter of telling the truth, but also of *being true* to the promises of the profession.[3] That is, honesty among professionals not only entails truthfulness, but also fidelity.

For professionals to practice effectively, they must have the public's trust. There is no such thing as an automatic right to be trusted; it is a privilege that one earns. To trust a professional, a patient or client must believe that this individual has the knowledge necessary to help him, and that this person will act in his best interests. The first involves knowledge: What special expertise does the professional have that enables her to address a specific problem? The second involves commitment: the promises the profession and the professional both make and imply—and whether the promises are kept.

Because the degree of trust granted by the public to a profession rests squarely on the shoulders of individual practitioners, the consequences of the presence or absence of fidelity in individual nurses are enormous. The total situation for patients includes not only the disease or disability they have, but also whether someone will care for them or abandon them through the course of the disease or through their dying. Taken as a whole, the performative declarations of the nursing profession commit nurses to work to improve the quality of living of those who seek or who receive their services.

While the fidelity of the nurse to these promises may not eliminate disease or prevent dying, it will affect the context in which the patient lives, that is, his or her quality of life. This is precisely why nurses are so concerned about preventing disease, promoting health, engaging in patient teaching and health counseling, maintaining health, and caring for the dying. If they are to fulfill the promises of the profession, they must become equally concerned with developing innovative ways of caring for persons who are chronically ill, handicapped, retarded, or aged. For nursing to be valued fully by the public, nurses must take the lead in developing innovative approaches to elevating the quality of life for those who cannot be cured.

The patient, specifically the institutionalized patient, is surrounded by nursing personnel twenty-four hours a day. Nurses create the atmosphere in which patients live or die. While it is true that some facts cannot be changed (the fact that a person is irreversibly dying; the fact that a child is born with a severely handicapping condition; the fact that a person is quadriplegic as a result of trauma or disease), the conditions under which people live out these facts can be changed. It is nursing's responsibility to create the opportunities and the atmosphere in which patients or clients can actualize their potentials and live their lives as fully as possible. Nursing assessments revolve around identification of an individual's quality of life to enable nurses to improve that quality of life. This is the moral imperative of nursing practice. Indeed, it describes how the nurse is committed to the patient. To the degree to which nurses are faithful to this commitment, they will alter the reality of the lives of patients or clients and their families.

PROFESSIONAL STANDARDS

Unfortunately, professions develop unevenly because the professionals who comprise them are in diverse states of awareness, intellectual attainment, and commitment. Practitioners' perceptions of their roles and their character traits affect the problems they see, the personal presence they bring to them, the manner in which they address them, and the reservoir of personal resources they can call upon to serve another day. At the same time, their moral commitments (or lack of them), as repeated in thousands of their colleagues, will create or destroy the profession.

The license to practice does not include a permission to practice poorly; it presupposes an obligation to practice well. The power to license that society grants to the professions exists prior to the granting of licenses to practice. If the license to practice entails an obligation to practice well, the power to license must include the obligation to judge and to monitor well the practice of individual practitioners.[4] As individual members of a profession, we share the obligation of assuring that established standards of practice are followed by all members of the profession. Practicing a profession involves internalizing a philosophy, perceiving what is congruent with reality and developing a discretion that enables one to recognize what is "fitting" or appropriate within this role. Among other things, it raises the questions of professional standards, self-regulation and self-discipline. The problem of maintaining professional standards goes to the heart of a profession's obligations to society. Professionals tend to avoid this problem because it involves questions of the virtue, style and character of the individual practitioner.

THE IMPLICATIONS OF NURSING'S COMMITMENT

In general, reflections on ethics in the nursing context have focused on the discrete quandaries faced by individual practitioners. The most obvious reason for this is that nurses naturally desire help in resolving the moral problems they face in every day practice. A less obvious reason may be that quandary ethics tends to ignore problems of professional discipline because it concentrates on particular problems of usually anonymous practitioners. As a result, professional ethics tend to concentrate only on exploring the moral principles that are applicable to concrete cases—what one might call abstract ethics for decision makers. In other words, analytic faculties are focused on how to reach a particular decision and generally fail to address how the decision should or can be implemented. Such an approach tends to obscure the fundamental philosophy that defines the profession and the degree of commitment the individual professional has to this philosophy.

Moreover, while professionals concentrate comfortably on procedural questions of appropriate decision making, larger questions about the social and economic structures within which the profession operates are left to others—political scientists, social engineers, health planners, economists, and administrators. For example, this proclivity tends to obscure nurses' obligations not just to share information with patients, but actually to teach patients and other lay persons about disease and health and to involve them actively in maintaining their own health. In the process of teaching, one does not just give words to people; one helps to interpret what is happening and why it is happening. Teaching has a therapeutic value that extends beyond the explanation of a disease; it can and should enable a person to understand his problem or potential problem, to ask critical questions about it, and to help make whole (or to heal) the individual and thus place him in a position of control over what happens to him. Health professionals really have committed relatively few of their professional resources to developing innovative systems for delivering preventive care and health knowledge to the public.

Concentration on only specific, individual problems may lead to neglect of the demands of social justice. Because the practice of a profession requires knowledge and skill that are essential to the public welfare, the principles of distributive justice require the delivery of such essential services to the whole community. In return, society accords the profession certain powers, status and privileges to the extent that its members help meet the needs of the public.

Clearly, no one professional or profession at large can meet all the needs of the public. In fact, a profession cannot even fulfill its own circumscribed mission without widespread communal support and assistance. However, professionals do have at least four obligations under the principles of distributive justice: (1) to do what they reasonably can do to meet the need for their services; (2) to do what they know how to do competently, whether or not the patient can pay for their services; (3) to help design methods for dealing with the health as well as the illness needs of the populace; and (4) to testify to the community about a social system that fails to meet the fundamental health needs of its citizenry. These obligations obtain not only because of one's role as a professional but also because a professional is in a position to know the injustices that result from the inequitable distribution of health resources. With this knowledge comes both the power and the responsibility to effect change.

In addition, health professionals have been lax in developing adequately systems for the care of long-term, chronic, and disabled individuals. While society has fostered elaborate specialization to handle problems in acute medicine, it has devoted a woefully small amount of its resources to the nursing care needs of large segments of the population. Thus, although medicine has been remarkably successful at prolonging life, nursing has yet to tackle effectively the problem of improving the quality of the lives so prolonged.

These problems of professional ethics require systematic, structural, and institutional reform. They do not fit easily (if they fit at all) into the conventional pattern of case-oriented ethics. The commitment of nursing demands that nurses develop an approach to ethics that is proactive rather than reactive; that nurses concentrate on the deeper aspects of preventive, chronic, and maintenance care rather than on the dramatic problems of acute care; and that nurses direct attention to the milieu in which they must make decisions, that is, environmental and personal factors that inhibit or advance the ability of individual providers to implement decisions.

For example, case-oriented ethics may lead nurses to the decision that it is not ethically defensible to kill an infant who is retarded, but they no longer can afford to ignore what this decision entails: it must address *how* the child shall live. That is, it logically entails a commitment to do what is possible to improve the quality of the child's life. To ignore this logical entailment is to abrogate the commitment of our profession: the commitment to improve the quality of living.

It has been said that knowledge and skill are the foundations of professionalism; this is not the case. Although knowledge and skill are integral to the practice of a profession, the foundation of a profession consists of the performative declarations professed by its practitioners and the fidelity of the practitioner to these promises. The fidelity of the practitioner is at the very root of the relationship between the individual and the professional and between society and the profession. Without fidelity there is no trust, and without trust the nurse cannot practice.

NOTES

1. May, William F. "Normative Inquiry and Medical Ethics in Our Colleges and Universities," in David Smith and Linda M. Bernstein, eds. *No Rush to Judgment: Essays on Medical Ethics* (The Indiana University Foundation, Bloomington, Indiana, 1978) p. 356.
2. Fletcher, John. "The Parent-Child Bond," *Theological Studies* 33 (September 1972) p. 458.
3. May, *op. cit.*, p. 357.
4. May, *op. cit.*, p. 360.

BIBLIOGRAPHY

Bandman, Bertram, "The Human Rights of Patients, Nurses and Other Health Professionals," in Elsie Bandman and Bertram Bandman (eds.). *Bioethics and Human Rights*. Little, Brown, Boston, 1978, pp. 321–330.

Bandman, Elsie L., "The Rights of Nurses and Patients: A Case for Advocacy," in Elsie Bandman and Bertram Bandman (eds.). *Bioethics and Human Rights*. Little, Brown, Boston, 1978, pp. 332–337.

Bok, Sissela. *Lying*. Pantheon Books, New York, 1978, pp. 220–248.

Fried, Charles. *An Anatomy of Values: Problems of Personal and Social Choice*. Harvard University Press, Cambridge, Massachusetts, 1970, p. 217.

Fried, Charles, "Rights and Health Care—Beyond Equity and Efficiency," *The New England Journal of Medicine*, Vol. 293, No. 5, July 13, 1975, pp. 241–245.

Fuchs, Victor. *Who Shall Live? Health Economics and Social Choice*. Basic Books, New York, 1974, pp. 52–58.

Gadow, Sally, "Nursing and the Humanities: An Approach to Humanistic Issues in Health Care," in Elsie Bandman and Bertram Bandman (eds.). *Bioethics and Human Rights*. Little, Brown, Boston, 1978, pp. 305–312.

Hiatt, Howard, "Protecting the Medical Commons: Who is Responsible?" *The New England Journal of Medicine*, Vol. 293, No. 5, July 31, 1975, pp. 235–241.

Kass, Leon, "Regarding the End of Medicine and the Pursuit of Health," *The Public Interest*, No. 40, Summer 1975, p. 39.

Murphy, Catherine P., "The Moral Situation in Nursing," in Elsie Bandman and Bertram Bandman (eds.). *Bioethics and Human Rights*. Little, Brown, Boston, 1978, pp. 313–319.

Pincoffs, Edmund, "Quandary Ethics," *Mind*, Vol. 80, 1971, p. 552.

Ramsey, Paul. *The Patient as Person*. Yale University Press, New Haven, 1970, pp. 252–275.

Urmson, J. O., "Saints and Heros," in A. I. Milden (ed.). *Essays in Moral Philosophy*. University of Washington Press, Seattle, 1958, p. 198.

The Nurse as a Member of a Profession

James L. Muyskens

Members of the nursing profession for a variety of reasons, including the nature of the profession but also economic exploitation and sexism (see Ashley, 1977), have been "caught in the middle." On the one hand, for example, the nurse is hired to carry out the directives of the physician and to support the policy of the hospital administration. The system cannot function as presently constituted without such cooperation and support to carrying out the decisions and policies of those higher up in the hierarchy. Yet, on the other hand, the nurse is legally and morally accountable for her or his judgments exercised and actions taken. "Neither physician's prescriptions nor the employing agency's policies relieve the nurse of ethical or legal accountability for actions taken and judgments made" (ANA, 1976, p. 10).

A common predicament of nurses is expressed in the April issue of *Nursing '78* by a nurse at a West Coast university hospital. She says:

> Our biggest problem right now is that our nursing leadership at the administrative level is completely impotent. They have no voting rights on any committee that has direct control over the hospital and/or nursing. Worse, the acting director and her associate have no idea of taking any power into their own hands, where it rightfully belongs. They ask permission to improve staffing ratios, by increasing or closing beds, and when they're turned down, say to us "Sorry girls! Work doubles" [Godfrey, 1978, pp. 101–2].

The overwork and understaffing not only make working conditions less than desirable for the nurse, they clearly endanger clients. When, for example, one registered nurse and an aide must try to care for 30 to 36 clients who have just undergone surgery, the situation is very dangerous and health care cannot be delivered in accordance with acceptable standards.

We can all sympathize with the nurse who wrote the following:

> I am supposed to be responsible for the control and safety of techniques used in the operating theatre. I have spent many hours teaching the technicians and the aides the routines necessary for maintaining aseptic conditions during surgery. They have learned to prepare materials and to maintain an adequate supply for all needs. They have learned to handle supplies with good technique.
>
> I find it is extremely difficult to have these appropriate routines carried out constantly by employees with little theoretical background or understanding. The surgeons are frequently breaking techniques and respond in a belligerent manner when breaks in technique are brought to their attention. I find a reminder of techniques often brings a determined response to ignore the remainder and proceed with surgery. For a male surgeon to be questioned by a female nurse is a serious breach of respect to them.
>
> One day a surgeon wore the same gown for two successive operations even though there were other gowns available. I quietly called this to his attention, but I had no authority which really allowed me to control his behavior for the good of the patient. In this situation even the hospital administrator was of no help to me [Tate, 1977, pp. 47–48].

This nurse is responsible for the control and safety of techniques used in the operating rooms. The conditions over which she is responsible have fallen below acceptable standards. Although she has done her best, the assigned task has not been accomplished. The clients who have a right to expect, and have paid for, a safe and aseptic operating room have been let down.

Nursing is the largest group of health care professionals within the vast health care delivery system—a system that, despite some dramatic achievements, is increasingly under attack as dehumanizing, exploitative, and cost-ineffective. Despite the seeming powerlessness of an individual nurse, taken collectively nursing, more than any other health care profession, is a necessary component in the delivery of health care. The present system could not have developed without nursing. If all nurses were to walk out tomorrow, the system would collapse. This cannot be said for any other group of health care professionals, including physicians. Hence, if the delivery of health care is substandard (as I believe it is), the nurse is not merely a victim of the system (along with the rest of us), but she or he is also an accomplice. As an accomplice she or he shares responsibility for the system's deficiencies. The nurse's plight is by no means unique. The paradoxical plight of the nurse who is both powerless and powerful, responsible yet not responsible, is a plight in which we almost all find ourselves in some aspects of our lives.

One way to try to make sense of these paradoxical situations—to be explored in this chapter—is to introduce the notion of collective responsibility. Two dramatic and widely discussed illustrations are the prosecution's case against certain middle-level Nazis after World War II and the defense's case for First Lieutenant William Calley, charged with murder at MyLai in southeast Asia.

In the prosecution case, blame for the actions of certain individual members of the collective is ascribed to all members. Karl Jaspers expressed this view when he said: "Every German is made to share the blame for the crimes committed in the name of the Reich . . . inasmuch as we let such a regime arise among us" (Quoted in Cooper, 1972, p. 86). In condemning every German, Jaspers is not merely blaming each German for his active or passive tolerance of the Nazis; he is saying that "the world of German ideas," "German thought," and "national tradition" are to blame. Collective responsibility is used as a net from which no member of the collective can escape.

In the defense case, the individual whose behavior has fallen below the acceptable standard is shielded from the full weight of blame, because the weight is shifted to the collective. It is the collective, the system, that must bear the brunt of the burden, rather than the individual. In the Calley case it was claimed that Americans as a group failed to perform as they could have been expected to.

In a recent survey of nurses' attitudes (Godfrey, 1978, Part II, p. 110), this defense strategy was tacitly used. It was reported that, although nurses saw themselves as performing well given the work conditions, they "felt they ought somehow to deliver even when the system won't let them." The writers of the report indicate that this blame is misplaced ("not deserved"). Although performing below the acceptable standard, the nurses were not to be blamed because as individuals each was doing the best possible for him or her in the situation. The system itself was to be blamed.

If the blame appropriately ascribed in a situation is no greater than the sum of all the ascriptions of blame to the individuals, we do not have a case of collective responsibility except in a weak (distributive) sense. By collective responsibility in the strong (nondistributive) sense, as the term is to be used here, we mean that the responsibility of the group is not equivalent to that of the individuals; that is, the whole is not equal to the sum of its parts.

It is incontrovertible that we do ascribe responsibility to collectives in this strong sense. To use an example of D. E. Cooper's, if we say that the local tennis club is responsible for its closure, we do not necessarily or usually mean that the officers of the club or any particular members are responsible for its closure. The blame cannot be attributed to any particular individual or to the officers of the club, since no person failed to do what was expected of him. Yet something was missing. "It was just a bad club as a whole." From the claim that the local tennis club is responsible for its closure, no statements about particular individuals follow. "This is so," as Cooper says, "because the existence of a collective is compatible with a varying membership. No determinate set of individuals is necessary for the existence of a collective" (Cooper, 1968, pp. 260–62).

As R. S. Downie has argued, "To provide an adequate description of the actions, purposes, and responsibilities of a certain range of collectives, such governments, armies, colleges, incorporated business firms, etc., we must make use of concepts which logically cannot be analyzed in individualistic terms" (Downie, 1972, p. 69).

The question to ask then is what set of conditions must obtain in order properly to ascribe nondistributive collective blame or responsibility. The conditions advanced by Cooper in his article "Responsibility and the 'System'" (1972, pp. 90–91) are sufficiently accurate and refined for purposes of this book. These conditions are:

1. Members of a group perform undesirable acts.

2. Their performing these acts is partly explained by their acting in accordance with the "way of life" of the group (i.e. the rules, mores, customs, etc. of the group).

3. These characteristics of the group's "way of life" are below the standards we might reasonably expect the group to meet.

4. It is not necessarily the case that members of the group, in performing the acts, are falling below standards we can reasonably expect individuals to meet.

A few comments about these conditions are in order. Clearly, we do not *hold* an individual or a group responsible—that is, following its etymology: having liability to answer to a *charge*—if undesirable acts have not been performed. When no undesirable acts occur, the question of blame or responsibility in the sense of liability does not arise. Hence the need for condition 1.

The second condition is not strictly necessary. It does seem, as Virginia Held has argued (1970), that when special conditions obtain even a random collection of individuals can be held responsible (a claim denied by condition 2). Nonetheless, for present purposes—consideration of collective responsibility of members of a profession—this stronger claim need not be defended. The most-plausible cases for ascribing collective responsibility are those cases in which the group has distinctive characteristics, has a sense of solidarity and cohesion (for example, feels "vicarious pride and shame" [Feinberg, 1968, p. 677]) and members identify themselves as members of the group (for example, "Who are you?" "I am a nurse"), and some of these group feelings or characteristics are appealed to in explaining the acts in question. An illustration: If the citizens of Syldavia can be characterized as being rather hostile and distrustful of foreigners, and their customs, laws, and policies reflect this, then when some border guards —overzealously carrying out the Syldavian policy— kill some visiting dignitaries, we blame not only the border guards but the Syldavians. In contrast, if these border guards steal from the visiting dignitaries, in accounting for this behavior we would not be inclined to appeal to any larger group feelings or characteristics, and we definitely would not wish to ascribe collective blame.

We have seen in the variety of cases discussed above that it is when a collective fails to live up to what can reasonably be expected of it—i.e., it falls below an acceptable standard—that it can incur collective blame. Hence the need for condition 3.

Condition 4 is necessary because the standards applied to groups may be different from those applied to individuals. For example, we may feel that the nurse (in the case cited above) who was charged with responsibility for the control and safety of techniques used in the operating rooms adequately met her obligations. She did not fall below standards we can reasonably expect an individual to meet. After all, as Joel Feinberg has argued, "No individual person can be blamed for not being a hero or a saint." Yet, as Feinberg goes on to say, "A whole people can be blamed for not producing a hero when the times require it, especially when the failure can be charged to some discernible element in the group's 'way of life' that militates against heroism" (Feinberg, 1968, p. 687). Although Feinberg was not referring to this case or to the collective responsibility of the nursing profession (he was talking about a Jesse James train robbery case), his remarks are especially apt for this case and in many other situations within the nursing profession.

One can readily see that conditions outlined for properly ascribing nondistributive collective responsibility obtain in many situations with professions. Professions more than most other collectives are bound together by common aspirations, values, methodologies, and training. In too many cases, they also have similar socio-economic backgrounds and are of the same sex and ethnic group. As we have seen, the more cohesive the group, the less problematic the ascription of collective responsibility. The fact that professions such as nursing promulgate codes of ethics or standards of behavior, toward which they expect members to strive, provides a clear criterion for judging whether the actual practices of the profession fall below standards to which we can reasonably hold the group.

In addition to meeting these formal criteria for ascribing collective responsibility, there are several other reasons unique to the professions for ascribing collective responsibility in certain situations.

A. There are several ways by which one becomes responsible. One can be *saddled* with it by circumstances, one can have responsibility *assigned* to one, or one can deliberately *assume* responsibility (Baier, 1972, p. 52). Typically a profession is chosen. In choosing the profession, one *assumes* the responsibility concomitant with being a professional. One chooses to adopt the values, methodology, and "way of life" of the profession. Such choice is much less prominent with most other basic group affiliations. One does not choose family membership, region of birth, usually not citizenship, and often not military service. Once in the profession, of course, as one goes about his or her job he or she will also sometimes be saddled with responsibility by circumstances and be assigned responsibility. But these assignments are all within the context of choice: to assume professional responsibility provides the backdrop for all his or her professional activities. Hence, as a professional, more than most other group affiliations, one sees oneself as a member of the group and has—with eyes open—chosen the identification.

B. Nurses (as is, of course, also the case in several other professions) have been vested by the state with the power to regulate and control nursing practice. This collective power or right—given exclusively to the profession—has a concomitant collective responsibility to see to it that acceptable standards are maintained. Since it is possible that each individual nurse, including officers of the American Nursing Association, is meeting acceptable standards in her or his own assignments and yet the group's "way of life" must be characterized as below an acceptable standard, appeal to collective responsibility is one of the tools the public has at its disposal to try to ensure adequate nursing and general health care. Obviously in these cases (when no individual has failed to meet her or his legal obligation), the public does not have recourse to law suits against individuals.

C. Supposedly as a means to protect the public, the licensing statutes of the states allow only those who have passed certain state requirements to practice nursing. One result of this is that the profession, which is by law also self-regulatory, becomes a protected monopoly. If a person is going to receive nursing care, this care must be provided by a member of the profession. If nursing care is to be upgraded, it must be from within with, at most, prodding from without. Quite clearly, one of the most-effective tools for such prodding is that of demonstrating collective responsibility, a responsibility that goes beyond the sum of each individual's responsibility.

From the discussion thus far, it is evident that the appeal to collective responsibility when some substandard behavior or undesirable act has occurred is a two-edged sword. It can be used to show that, despite undesirable performances or actions or conditions within a collective, a particular member of the collective is not individually responsible.

But it can also be used to show that, despite the fact that the behavior of individuals does not fall below standards we can reasonably require individuals to meet (given that we cannot *demand* that an individual be a hero), the group's conduct is below the standards we can reasonably expect the group to meet. One of the reasons the weapon of collective responsibility looks suspect in the widely discussed World War II prosecution of Vietnam conflict defense cases is that only one edge of the sword is used, while the other edge is conveniently ignored.

If conditions for properly ascribing collective responsibility are satisfied, to the extent that the individual is exonerated, the group is indicted. To the degree the individual *qua* individual is indicted, the group is exonerated. Either way the individual group member bears responsibility. For any member of a collective but especially (for reasons cited above) for a professional, it is not enough to know that one has done all that could be expected of him or her as an individual. The arm of responsibility for a professional has a longer reach than that of the individual.

Specific situations within the nursing profession illustrate the two edges of the sword of collective responsibility. These situations should be seen within the context of the rapid evolution of the nursing profession. In recent years there has been considerable effort both within and outside the profession (e.g., the medical profession) to upgrade the requirements for licensure. These efforts have borne results. The scope of the professional nurse has expanded greatly, as exemplified by medical assistant programs and their use by medical doctors in certain areas. The history of the struggle first to adopt a code of ethics for American nurses and then to revise it reflects this evolution. Tentative codes were presented in the 1920s, 1930s, and 1940s. These efforts were met by opposition from those who feared the professionalization of nursing. A striking instance of this is the advice given by a physician to one of the earliest advocates of a code of ethics for American nurses: "Be good women but do not have a code of ethics" (Dock, 1912, p. 129). Not until 1950 was a code of ethics adopted.

The code has been changed several times since then, the most recent being in 1985. Two of the most-interesting changes from our vantage point have been the following: early versions of the code stated that the nurse had an obligation to carry out the physician's orders. As we saw in Chapter 1, the 1968 and 1976 versions of the code instead stress the nurse's obligation to the client. The physician just mentioned who advised against having a code may have foreseen this development! Whereas earlier versions of the code pointed to an obligation to sustain confidence in associates, in the revised codes the nurse's obligation is to protect the client from incompetent, unethical, or illegal practice from any quarter. (See Sward, 1978, for a discussion of these and other changes in the versions of the code.)

With this background, it is apparent why nursing is an especially interesting example of collective responsibility in the professions. The fundamental issue in the ongoing struggle to upgrade the profession—reflected in the code changes—has been that of accountability, the willingness to make decisions and to accept responsibility for these decisions. The crucial question in the attempt to upgrade the profession is that of the interface of individual and collective responsibility.

The author of an article in the *Quarterly Record of the Massachusetts General Hospital Nurses Alumnae Association* wrote about "blame avoidance" behavior in nurses. As explained, blame avoidance behavior is exhibited when the nurse says such things as "I did this because the supervisor told me to do it," or "the doctor ordered it," or "the hospital rules demanded it." The author maintains that accountability requires that the nurse can say, "I did this because in my best judgment it is what the patient needed" (quoted in Durand, 1978, p. 19). Setting aside the many good qualities common to nurses, blame avoidance behavior does seem to be one of the more-prevalent, endemic faults of the nursing profession. As we have seen, a concerted effort by many within the profession has made inroads on this "way of life" of the profession.

These efforts have been made without explicit appeal to the concept of collective responsibility. As a result, judgment in cases of blame avoidance and other unacceptable or undesirable behavior has tended to be either too lenient or too harsh. That is, either (a) one judges that the individual nurse caught in the middle and in difficult circumstances has done all one can reasonably expect her or him to do. After all, we cannot expect or demand that she or he be a hero or a saint. Hence, the nurse is exonerated, but the unacceptable practice or condition continues unabated. Or (b) one focuses on professional responsibility and the fact that, if some individuals do not stand up against substandard practices—no matter what the odds of thereby improving the situation and no matter at what price to the individual— these practices likely will not be stopped. If the nurse does not take the action that would probably

cost her her position, but that would ensure the best care possible for clients in her care, the nurse is judged to be a moral coward.

For example, in the case of the nurse charged with responsibility for maintaining a safe and aseptic operating room, without appeal to the concept of collective responsibility we are likely to say one of the following: (1) She has done all we can require of her (she has asked the surgeon to comply; she does not have the authority or status to demand compliance to proper procedures; the lack of compliance quite properly was followed by a report to the hospital administration). Or (2) she has not done all we can require of her (she cannot allow dangerous violations of operating room aseptic standards to take place; in doing so, she is failing to carry out her assignment and is allowing the client's life to be placed in jeopardy; she should not be cowed by the surgeon's arrogance and sexism; even at the risk of losing her job, she cannot allow the operation to take place in these conditions).

The problem is that (1) is too lenient a judgment and (2) is too harsh. We cannot require the nurse *qua* individual to do more than she has done. But the nurse *qua* nurse shares blame with her colleagues in such cases, despite the much greater blame that must be placed on the surgeon who violates reasonable requirements. The lack of aggressive advocacy for the client's welfare and the willingness to be dominated by the (usually male) physician or surgeon (unfortunate if understandable "ways of life" of the nursing profession), which partially explain this nurse's behavior, are below the standard we can rightfully expect the group authorized to provide nursing services to meet. Appeal to collective responsibility yields a judgment neither too harsh nor too lenient.

This judgment conforms to the moral intuitions of the nurses surveyed who were mentioned earlier. Despite a feeling that as individuals they were doing all that could reasonably be required of them in their circumstances, they still felt dissatisfied with their performance. As nurses they felt blame for falling short of the mark set for the profession.

This dissatisfaction, when seen in the light of collective responsibility, can be turned to positive use. The nurse who has done all that is required of him or her as an individual need not suffer debilitating guilt. Guilt, in such cases, is misplaced; her or his individual actions do not warrant guilt. And, in contrast to nondistributive collective responsibility, there is no nondistributive collective guilt. "Guilt," as Feinberg has said, "consists in the intentional transgression of a prohibition . . . There can be no such thing as vicarious guilt" (Feinberg, 1968, p. 676). Nevertheless, although rightfully free of guilt, she or he cannot be complacent. She or he is a member of a group that stands judged (i.e., is liable) and must, with her or his colleagues, take appropriate steps to alleviate the undesirable conditions. It is not enough for a professional to do all that is required of her or him as an individual. Having freely accepted the privileges and benefits of the profession, one's responsibility in the areas of professional competence is greater than would be that of an equally skilled and knowledgeable individual who was not a member of the profession.

In order to meet this larger responsibility, as the American Nursing Association has recognized, "there should be an established mechanism for the reporting and handling of incompetent, unethical, or illegal practice within the employment setting so that such reporting can go through official channels and be done without fear of reprisal. The nurse should be knowledgeable about the mechanism and be prepared to utilize it if necessary" (Sward, 1978, p. 8).

Paradoxically, if such machinery which collective responsibility requires were put in place, individual accountability would increase and the need to appeal to collective responsibility would decrease. If reporting incompetent, unethical, or illegal conduct could be done effectively through official channels and without fear of reprisal, such reporting—which under more-dangerous and less-effective circumstances is not required—would be morally required of the individual. Hence, it may be that a profession should strive to organize itself and regulate itself to such a degree that the conditions for proper ascription of collective responsibility do not arise. But this is not the situation within the nursing profession at the present. Therefore, the notion of collective responsibility is a timely weapon of considerable force for those who are working toward upgrading the nursing profession and the delivery of health care.

REFERENCES

American Nurses' Association (ANA). 1976. *Code for Nurses with Interpretive Statements.* American Nurses' Association, Kansas City, Mo.

Baier, K. 1972. "Guilt and Responsibility." In *Individual and Collective Responsibility,* edited by P. A. French, pages 37–61. Cambridge, Mass.: Schenkman Publishing Co.

Cooper, D. E. 1968. "Collective Responsibility." *Philosophy* 43, no. 165 (July):258–68.

———. 1972. "Responsibility and the 'System.'" In *Individual and Collective Responsibility,* edited by P. A. French, pages 81–100. Cambridge Mass.: Schenkman Publishing Co.

Dock, L. L. 1912. *A History of Nursing,* vol. 3. New York: Putnam's Sons.

Downie, R. S. 1972. "Responsibility and Social Roles." In *Individual and Collective Responsibility,* edited by P. A. French, pages 65–80. Cambridge, Mass.: Schenkman Publishing Co.

Durand, B. 1978. "A Nursing Practice Perspective." In *Perspectives on the Code for Nurses.* Kansas City, Mo.: American Nurses' Association.

Feinberg, J. 1968. "Collective Responsibility," *The Journal of Philosophy* 65, no., 21 (November 7):674–88.

Godfrey, M. A. 1978. "Job Satisfaction—Or Should That Be Dissatisfaction? How Nurses Feel About Nursing." Part 1: *Nursing '78,* April 1978. Part 2: *Nursing '78,* May 1978.

Held, V. 1970. "Can a Random Collection of Individuals Be Morally Responsible?" *The Journal of Philosophy* 67, no. 14 (July 23): 471–81.

Sward, K. M. 1978. "An Historical Perspective." In *Perspectives on the Code for Nurses.* Kansas City, Mo.: American Nurses' Association.

Tate, B. L. 1977. *The Nurse's Dilemma.* Geneva, Switzerland: International Council of Nurses.

Engineers as Moral Heroes

Professor Ken Alpern advanced the seemingly paradoxical thesis that *"ordinary moral requirements"* frequently demand moral heroism of engineers. Alpern distinguished between two types of moral heroism. "The first type is supererogation or moral sainthood. It is to regularly do morally good things in excess of what is strictly required by morality. It is action above and beyond the call of duty. The second type of moral heroism is fortitude or moral courage. It does not involve exceeding ordinary moral requirements, but rather meeting ordinary requirements in the face of extraordinary obstacles, temptations, pressures and the like." Concerning the general requirements of morality, Alpern advanced the following principle as incontestable: "When one is in a position to contribute to greater harm or is in a position to play a more critical part in producing harm, one should exercise greater care to avoid doing so."

The foregoing principle, together with Alpern's specification of the second type of moral heroism, yielded the principal thesis of his paper: "Engineers in general exercise considerable control over technology—its design, quality, safety, use, and maintenance. They are thus in a position to affect the public's well being, for better or worse, to a greater extent than others. It is therefore appropriate to require of engineers greater care, including a willingness to make greater personal sacrifices in order to do what they ought in regard to the public welfare. This higher standard is not a matter of supererogation, but is merely the consequence of ordinary moral requirements applied in their situation. However, since there will often be significant pressures and disincentives to their meeting these ordinary moral requirements, engineers must exhibit moral courage in the course of their everyday work."

Alpern defended the above thesis against four objections which one might advance against it. First, he noted that individuals at times attempt to evade a difficult morally required action by complaining that doing so would cause them to lose their jobs. Second, one at times hears people disclaim moral responsibility by saying 'If I don't do it then someone else will.' Third, in some instances, a person insists that a given difficult but morally required action is not his job. Finally, the omnipresence of immoral practices on the part of employers is often cited as a reason for regarding them as unavoidable, that is, as practices one will have to engage in regardless of where one works.

Alpern presented a variety of grounds for categorically rejecting all four of the above kinds of arguments. He added, however, that engineers faced with situations that require moral heroism deserve sympathy. In addition, Alpern contended that society *owes* these engineers support because ". . . it is not neutral in the choice to become an engineer. To some extent society creates their problem by channeling students into a rigorous engineering curriculum which usually offers them little idea of what to expect on the job while extolling the virtues of the profession. Society thus 'owes' support, at least to the extent that it is responsible for the engineer's moral predicament."

Professor Lisa Newton of Fairfield University, who served as commentator for the first Friday morning session, warmly endorsed Alpern's conclusions. "As Alpern points out," she said, "no new rights and duties have to be derived to fit the case of engineers. The good old principle of due care will suffice, given the understanding long accepted in the law, that the duty bears with special force on the responsible professional. Only acceptance of this duty . . . will do the job we need done." "Government regulation," Newton declared, "is hopelessly ignorant, misguided, slipshod, and occasionally corrupt, not to mention expensive beyond belief. The responsible professional is guarantor ultimately of the moral conduct of the enterprise of engineering."

Engineers as moral heroes (1982, May-June). *Perspectives on the Professions*, 2, 3. Reprinted with permission of © Center for the Study of Ethics in Professions. All rights reserved.

The Morality of Cooperation

Edward J. Hayes, Paul J. Hayes, and Dorothy Ellen Kelly

The word "cooperation" comes from the Latin word *cum*, which means "with," and *operari*, which means "to work." This gives us an excellent definition of cooperation. *Cooperation is working with another in the performance of an action.* The action may be good or evil. However, moral problems arise only when the action is evil.

The principles we are enunciating in this section apply to assistance in any immoral action. However, for most practical purposes in the nursing profession, they pertain to assistance at operations.

Cooperation may be divided first of all into *formal* and *material* cooperation.

FORMAL COOPERATION

Formal cooperation is that in which the cooperator wills the evil, either by an explicit act of the will or by an actual sharing in the evil act itself. Those who share in an evil act sometimes say that they do so unwillingly. However, this is merely a way of saying that they are reluctant. If they were unwilling in the absolute sense of the word, they would not assist in the evil act at all. Since we are never allowed to will evil, formal cooperation in evil is always sinful. The assistant surgeon, who is actually performing some part of an immoral operation, formally cooperates in evil.

MATERIAL COOPERATION

Material cooperation is that in which the cooperator performs an act which in itself is not wrong, though it is used by the principal agent to help him commit sin. Under certain circumstances, such cooperation would be morally permissible. The ward nurse who prepares a patient for immoral surgery cooperates materially.

Here are examples of various types of cooperation: A gangster plans to murder a rival. He secures the cooperation of the local precinct police captain, who arranges that no squad car will be in the area while the crime is being committed. The captain's cooperation is formal because he wills the evil act. The criminal tells one of his henchmen to prepare the car by checking the gasoline and making sure that the motor is operating perfectly. This man cooperates materially but only remotely. Another member of the gang is assigned to drive the "get-away car." This man cooperates materially and proximately. A third man is assigned to hold the victim, while the leader of the gang kills him. This man cooperates formally by sharing the evil act.

MORAL NORMS

Formal Cooperation in Evil Never Allowed

The nurse, because of her training, is schooled in obedience. She carries out quickly and without question the orders of the doctor. However, we must never forget that the moral integrity of the nurse as an individual is superior by far to the commands of any doctor. Therefore, when the question of assistance at an immoral operation arises, it is entirely within the rights of the nurse to make a

Hayes, E. J., Hayes, P. J., & Kelly, E. D., (1964). The morality of cooperation. In *Moral principles of nursing* (pp. 79–83). New York: Macmillan. Reprinted with permission of © Macmillan. All rights reserved.

moral judgment and act in accordance with her conscience.

A nurse must never formally cooperate in immorality either by explicitly willing the evil or by directly sharing in the immoral act itself.

Material Cooperation in Evil Sometimes Allowed

Under what circumstances may a nurse materially cooperate by tolerating the evil?

Material cooperation consists in performing morally indifferent actions which make the operation possible. Those who cooperate materially do not perform immoral actions, but rather actions which are morally indifferent or good, and therefore allowable under certain circumstances. Such morally indifferent actions are performed by the anesthetist, scrub nurse, circulating nurse, and ward nurse.

A general rule which may be given regarding material cooperation is this: Material cooperation in

an immoral operation is morally permissible when a sufficient reason exists. No medical condition is a sufficient reason for the performance of an immoral operation. Certain circumstances may exist, however, which would constitute a sufficient reason for material cooperation; for example, the fact that refusal would probably result in dismissal.

Proportionate Reason Required for Cooperation in Evil

Just what constitutes a sufficient reason will vary according to the proximity to the immoral act itself. Material cooperation may be either proximate or remote. *Proximate cooperation* is that which is quite intimately connected with the immoral operation. An example of proximate cooperation would be that performed by the scrub nurse. Because of the very intimate connection of proximate cooperation with the evil act, a very grave reason is necessary in order that such cooperation be morally permissible. On the other hand, *remote*

Figure 1
The Morality of Cooperation.

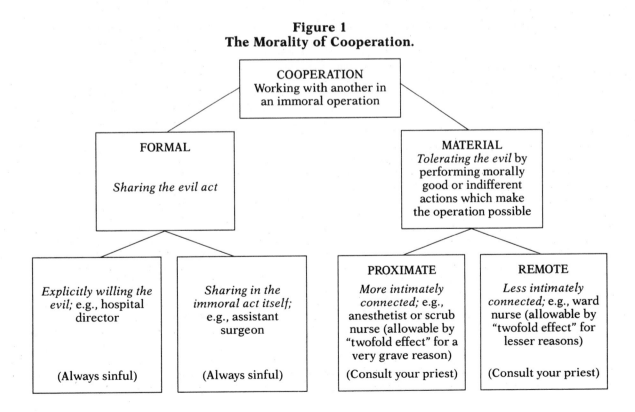

COOPERATION
Working with another in an immoral operation

FORMAL

Sharing the evil act

MATERIAL
Tolerating the evil by performing morally good or indifferent actions which make the operation possible

Explicitly willing the evil; e.g., hospital director

(Always sinful)

Sharing in the immoral act itself; e.g., assistant surgeon

(Always sinful)

PROXIMATE
More intimately connected; e.g., anesthetist or scrub nurse (allowable by "twofold effect" for a very grave reason)

(Consult your priest)

REMOTE
Less intimately connected; e.g., ward nurse (allowable by "twofold effect" for lesser reasons)

(Consult your priest)

cooperation, being less intimately connected with the evil act, is morally allowable for lesser reasons.

Exactly what reason is sufficient for cooperation in a particular case is a matter of accurate moral judgment. Some cases are very easy to judge. For example, the threat of being dismissed immediately, combined with the knowledge that a new position will be almost impossible to obtain in the foreseeable future, is a very grave situation and would constitute a sufficient reason for proximate cooperation in a particular case. On the other hand, the possibility of slightly hurt feelings on the part of fellow workers is obviously not a grave situation.

When material cooperation is habitual, a proportionately graver reason is required. An isolated instance of material cooperation in an immoral act is more easily justified than repeated acts of the same sort. The nurse who finds herself in a situation in which she is asked to cooperate in an immoral operation on rare occasions may more readily do so in good conscience than the nurse who constantly finds herself in this position. It is difficult, for instance, to justify continued employment in a hospital that is notorious for constant violations of the moral law, no matter how remote the cooperation.

The more necessary one's material cooperation is to the performance of the act, the graver must be the reason to justify it morally. If the withholding of one's cooperation would result in the principal agent's being unable to perform the action, a much graver reason would be required than if others could easily be obtained to cooperate.

Resolving Doubts
Regarding Cooperation

Between the obviously serious situations and those situations which are obviously not serious lies an entire field of situations which are difficult to judge. It is not possible to enter upon a detailed discussion of all the situations which arise in this regard. In practical cases concerning proximate and remote material cooperation in immoral operations, *a priest should be consulted* in order that a proper moral judgment may be passed. If it is impossible to consult a priest under the circumstances, the nurse will find it necessary to use her own judgment in accordance with her conscience. As soon as consultation is possible, a priest should be consulted, and a definite norm of conduct arrived at to govern future situations.

REFERENCES FOR FURTHER STUDY

Aikens, C. *Studies in Ethics for Nurses*, Philadelphia: W. B. Saunders Company, 1938.

Connell, F. *Morals in Politics and Professions*, Westminster, Md.: The Newman Press, 1951.

Finney, Patrick, and O'Brien, Patrick. *Moral Problems in Hospital Practice*, St. Louis: B. Herder Book Co., 1956.

McFadden, C. J. *Medical Ethics*, 5th ed., Philadelphia: F. A. Davis Company, 1961.

STUDY AND DISCUSSION QUESTIONS
PROFESSIONAL OBLIGATIONS OF NURSES

1. According to Curtin, a major source for the professional obligations of nurses are the promises of the profession. What has the profession promised to society? How well do you think nurses have kept their promises?

2. Do you agree with Curtin's judgment that health care professions have not addressed the needs for preventions of illness, chronic care, and maintenance?

3. Do you think nurses are equipped to deal with issues of social justice Curtin believes have been overlooked? Should they be?

4. Do you think you have obligations to the profession distinct from obligations owed individual clients? If so, what are they? If not, why not?

5. Consider the cases of nurses "caught in the middle" mentioned by Muyskens. What do you think is the appropriate judgment about their conduct?

6. Is being caught in the middle a frequent phenomenon in nursing?

7. Consider the conditions for ascribing collective responsibility to groups described by Muyskens. Do you think nursing as a profession meets these conditions?

8. Is "blame avoidance" a "way of life" in nursing?

9. Do you think the level of education of the nurse is related to the ability and willingness of nurses to challenge the system?

10. Muyskens believes that the concept of collective responsibility is "a timely weapon of considerable force for those who are working toward upgrading the nursing profession and the delivery of health care." Is it clear to you how this is so? Is Muyskens right?

11. Do you agree with philosopher Ken Alpern's thesis that implies that nurses have a duty (requiring great courage) to risk their jobs to protect their clients from harm or risk of harm?

12. Do you agree with Hayes et al. that the threat of job loss can provide a reason grave enough to go along with practices that may foster substandard care or create risks for clients?

13. As mentioned in the introduction to this chapter, do you think that hospitals should also be held liable for negligent acts of staff or the failure to assure that consents have been informed? Could the threat of this sort of legal liability be used to help persuade hospital administrators to listen to nursing complaints about quality care?

14. Just how far should a nurse pursue a complaint concerning substandard care? Is it beyond the call of duty to ask them to risk their employment? Or everthing but? What if refusing to take that risk allows substandard care to continue? Do you think that notions of collective responsibility or appeals to legal liability help?

9

The Nurse and the Institution

INTRODUCTION

The five articles in this chapter focus on the nurse–institution relationship. The articles by James L. Muyskens and Alice J. Baumgart discuss the moral permissibility of the use of the strike weapon and the use of collective bargaining within a profession. M. Josephine Flaherty presents a complex case study that illustrates, among other things, the conflicts that arise when hospital policies encroach on professional judgments. Finally, the articles by Roland R. Yarling and Beverly J. McElmurry point out the implications of greater professional autonomy in nursing. These articles focus on the issues of nurses writing do not resuscitate orders and examining the need for institutional reform, respectively.

THE CODE ON STRIKES AND WAGES

The attitude of the American Nurses' Association toward strikes and wages has shifted over the years. The 1926 suggested code stated, "No worker is welcome to the ranks of nursing who does not put the ideal of service above that of remuneration."[1] The 1940 suggested code declared that hospitals had "no claim for unremunerated service" but recognized the obligation of continuity of service to patients.[2] The first official code adopted by the ANA in 1950 said in Principle 9: "The nurse is entitled to just remuneration for services rendered and has a corresponding obligation to make a conscientious return in services."[3] The ANA Committee on Ethical Standards made this comment on Principle 9: "While the strike is considered an ethical means for many groups of workers, the danger to patients makes it undesirable and usually also unethical for nurses."[4] The code itself never carried such an explicit presumption against strikes in any of its revisions. By the 1968 revision, an explicit connection between the economic interests of the profession and public welfare were being asserted.

> The nurse must be concerned with the conditions of economic and general welfare within her profession because these conditions are important determinants in the recruitment and retention of well-qualified personnel and in the opportunity for each nurse to function to her fullest potential in the working situation. If the needs and demands of society for both quantity and quality of nursing care are to be met, the professional association and the individual nurse must share in the effort to establish conditions that will make it possible to meet these needs.[5]

This "recruitment and retention" argument for participation in efforts to establish and maintain conditions of employment conducive to high quality care did not survive the latest revision of the code in 1985, however. The argument emphasized in the current code notes, "Professional autonomy and self-regulation in the control of the conditions of practice are necessary for implementing nursing standards."[6]

In summary, the codes reveal a growing awareness of the economic interests of nurses individually and as a profession. The strike weapon is not explicitly mentioned in the code itself and when it is mentioned in commentary it is not absolutely forbidden, but there is an ethical presumption against its use. Control over working conditions is variously justified by more altruistic motives, including the recruitment and retention of nurses and the enforcement of nursing standards. These may seem to be for the good of the profession rather than the public, but it is argued that what is good for the profession is also good for the public, that being the availability and provision of quality nursing care.

James L. Muyskens, a philosopher, takes these arguments even further. In "The Nurse as an Employee," a chapter from his book *Moral Problems in Nursing: A Philosophical Investigation*,[7] he argues that under certain conditions not only is the use of the strike weapon permissible, it may be morally required. Admittedly, it is a weapon of last resort and care must be taken to provide emergency and life preserving services, but it ought to be used *if* it is the most effective means of securing quality nursing care.

Muyskens defends strikes against a series of objections. For instance, it may be felt that strikes for better pay and benefits are unethical and unprofessional since they place patients at risk. In addition, such "self-serving" goals are incompatible with the ideals of professional service. Muyskens counters that in many cases economic issues are not detachable from quality-of-care issues and that the latter *are* ethical obligations of the profession. He also counters the arguments that strikes are incompatible with client advocacy and that one must never allow future benefits to clients to outweigh duties to clients here and now. Finally, he appeals to conceptions of Rawlsian justice to justify the limited use of strikes.

MUYSKENS AND BAUMGART

Muyskens believes that binding arbitration is preferable to strikes in almost all cases for both parties. However, he concedes that employers may not be willing to accept the terms of arbitration unless a strike is likely to exact even greater concessions from them. Thus, Muyskens concludes that, "As client advocates, nurses should do all in their power to avoid strikes. But paradoxically, the best way to accomplish this is to be ready and able, in appropriate situations, to execute an effective strike."

Alice J. Baumgart, Dean of Queen's University School of Nursing, in "The Conflicting Demands of Professionalism and Unionism," examines the conditions in Canada that have led to a decline in nurse participation in professional organizations and a rise in union participation and nursing specialty groups. Many persons believe that greater socialization of medical services is inevitable for the United States and, therefore, the Canadian experience is of special interest. Baumgart's thesis is that unionism and professionalism are not necessarily conflicting. She surveys the various arguments for both incompatibility and compatibility and concludes that no hard lines should be drawn between unionism and professionalism. Many of the professional objections to unions—their self-investing nature, their concentration on short-term solutions, their substitution of seniority and security for merit, their use of the strike weapon and its adversarial nature—can be overcome. For example, unions can evolve and take into consideration issues of public welfare. Other professions have used collective bargaining without loss of status. Furthermore, she believes that the major argument against strikes—innocent people suffer harm—remains unproven. Thus, if unions can be flexible and adaptive, they can become an instrument for harmonizing professional and employee interests. Of course, the assumption of this argument is the continuing existence and flourishing of the professional organizations. The unions need healthy professional organizations for the articulation of public policy and nursing standards. "For example," Baumgart writes, "professional responsibility clauses are easier to negotiate when bargaining units can point to a code of ethics and competency requirements enforced by a self-regulatory association."

FLAHERTY

M. Josephine Flaherty, in "Insubordination—Patient Load," presents a case study describing a conflict between institutional policies and professional judgments. In this case, ICU nurses refused to take responsibility for a patient admitted from the Emergency Department on a ventilator because they were already understaffed. Ultimately, they were suspended for insubordination. Because the nurses were under a collective bargaining agreement, they were able to appeal their suspension to an arbitration board and have a judicial inquiry. The suspensions were upheld, however, because it was felt that their actions did not meet the conditions for exceptions to an "obey and grieve rule." There was not an exception for potential harm to clients, therefore the nurses could not sufficiently convince the board that their action was justified.

In this case, we have a situation of chronic understaffing, routine flouting of hospital policy, the overriding of nursing judgment by emergency room physicians, and the astonishing judgment of an arbitration board that would require nurses to risk the welfare of their clients in violation of their professional obligations.

On this latter and most important point, Flaherty argues that what nurses owe their employers is to act as professional nurses. Therefore, employee obligations can never subordinate professional obligations. Indeed, Flaherty believes that under the statutes of the locale where the nurses were practicing the hospital was requiring them to act unprofessionally and illegally. Or at least such a case could have been made.

YARLING AND McELMURRY

The final two articles by Roland Yarling and Beverly J. McElmurry, "Rethinking the Nurse's Role in 'Do Not Resuscitate' Orders: A Clinical Policy Proposal in Nursing Ethics" and "The Moral Foundation of Nursing," complement each other and in some ways recapitulate the themes of this anthology. In the first article, Yarling and McElmurry argue that nurses ought to be able to write do not resuscitate orders because such decisions are expressions of the client's values and are, therefore, moral rather than medical, legal, or nursing decisions. They believe that the patient is better served when nurses are able to write and document such orders. In addition, they believe that such a policy is compatible with the definition of nursing promulgated by the ANA; the nurse is usually best situated to have discussions with clients about do not resuscitate; nurses often initiate such discussions with physicians; and it is the nurses who usually carry out CPR or the do not resuscitate order.

Yarling and McElmurry anticipate some controversy over this simple policy that would improve patient care. The root of the difficulty is the domination of nursing practice by medical authoritarianism and repressive hospital policies that constrain nurses from honoring commitments made to the public. The authors believe that nurses are not free to be moral, that is, to practice at levels demanded by professional standards and excellence in nursing practice.

This last point is developed in the second essay, "The Moral Foundation of Nursing." Nurses are now taught to be patient advocates but in clinical practice they receive a different nonverbal message that places severe constraints on their commitment to the client's welfare. Nurses learn that open challenges to the system or powerful physicians within the system may mean putting "their jobs, their economic welfare, and their professional careers on the line, even if they are acting on behalf of the patient and have strong justification for doing so." Only by heroic action can nurses do the right thing. It is the pervasiveness of this coercive situation that constantly forces nurses to make choices between their integrity and their economic welfare, that leads Yarling and McElmurry to the conclusion that nurses are unfree to be moral, unfree to practice nursing.

As a result, Yarling and McElmurry call for a nursing ethic that aims at reform of the institution of the hospital as the culpable structure that has systematically created disincentives to responsible action. A greater professional autonomy is needed to free nursing from this "hospitalonian captivity."

Although Yarling and McElmurry offer reemphasis on the social reform tradition within nursing as one means of facilitating the necessary changes, their previous article placed the battle on a different venue. There they said that the war must be fought clinical issue by clinical issue. Do not resuscitate is but one illustration on which medical and institutional hegemony over nursing practice must be reexamined. Other areas are pain management, withholding or withdrawing life-sustaining treatment, informed consent procedures, and the use of placebos. These areas involve decisions that are moral rather than purely medical, legal, or nursing decisions.

There are two basic arguments for this sort of social reform ethic. The first is that if nursing does not reform the institution in which most of its practitioners practice and gain control over nursing practice, nursing will compromise the integrity of the nurse–patient relationship and betray its fiduciary relationship to the public. In effect, nursing will cease to be a profession. Second, public welfare will suffer having lost its most valuable ally within the health care system.

The ideal of professionally autonomous nurses armed with the appropriate mind set and capable of critical evaluation of the institutions that employ them is in the interest of a society concerned about quality care and individual self-determination.

SUMMARY

These articles have addressed the means of changing the institutions in which nurses work and the moral legitimacy of those means and goals. The authors have defended the strike weapon, warned against the dangers of myopic self-interest of unions unaffected by professional concerns and public welfare, and the need for professional autonomy to better serve the public interest.

NOTES

1. American Nurses' Association, Committee on Ethical Standards, "A Suggested Code," *American Journal of Nursing* 26(August 1926), p. 600.

2. American Nurses' Association, Committee on Ethical Standards, "A Tentative Code," *American Journal of Nursing* 40(September 1940):978.

3. American Nurses' Association, Committee on Ethical Standards, "A Code for Nurses," *American Journal of Nursing* 50(1950):196.

4. American Nurses' Association, Committee on Ethical Standards, "What's in Our Code?", *American Journal of Nursing* 53(September 1953):1099.

5. American Nurses' Association, "Code for Nurses," *American Journal of Nursing* 68(December 1968):2584.

6. American Nurses' Association, *Code for Nurses with Interpretive Statements* (Kansas City, Mo.: American Nurses' Association, 1985):14.

7. See James L. Muyskens, *Moral Problems in Nursing: A Philosophical Investigation* (Totowa, N.J.: Rowman & Littlefield, 1982).

The Nurse as an Employee

James L. Muyskens

Of all the moral issues facing the nurse as an employee, none is more difficult and divisive than deciding whether to go on strike, the issue we shall explore in this chapter. Its difficulty as a moral dilemma arises from the fact that compelling moral reasons can be given in support of both sides of the question.

A nurse is quoted in a recent article in the *New York Times* (March 25, 1980) as saying that when nurses strike, "they talk about better patient care, but the bottom line is 'How much are you going to give me?'" Since bill collectors are as persistent with nurses as with professors, plumbers, and police officers, it is hardly surprising if, for most individual nurses on strike, wages are of greater and more compelling concern than demands for improved client care. Yet it would be a mistake to conclude from this that the expressions of concern about quality client care are no more than smoke screens. Nurses as professionals have and take seriously the collective responsibility of maintaining and improving the quality of nursing care. The question to be discussed is whether (and if so, when) the strike is a morally acceptable weapon for nurses to use in attempting to maintain and improve the conditions necessary for proper nursing practice and their self-respect.

Too often, discussions of the moral duties of health professionals give the impression that the list of duties is exhausted when one has gone through those which pertain to the health professional as individual practitioner: the duty to respect a client's autonomy, the duty to obtain informed consent, the duty to maintain confidentiality, the duty to safeguard privacy. But health professionals do not work in a vacuum. Because of society's interests in their activity, their practice is regulated by the state.

Specifically, as mentioned in the previous chapter, the nursing profession is given the legal status of a protected monopoly (no one may practice nursing unless licensed by the profession) and the authority to control its own practice. In exchange, society asks the profession to deliver high-quality nursing services. By accepting the role of nurse, one—along with one's colleagues—assumes responsibility (1) for maintaining and improving standards of nursing, (2) for maintaining conditions of employment conducive to high-quality nursing care, (3) for contributing to the development and implementation of community and national health needs, and (4) for making the most-efficient and -effective use of nursing resources.

To exercise these duties, it is necessary for nurses to act in concert—for example, to work through professional associations or unions or to form independent groups within one's employment setting. If these collective efforts meet resistance or prove ineffectual, it may be difficult or impossible to fulfill these duties without taking further action, such as engaging in a strike or work slowdown. Yet such action may come into conflict with a variety of the nurses' other duties, including their collective duty to provide nursing care to all in need of it and their duties as practitioners to specific clients currently under their care. This potential for conflicts of duty is what makes the question of the nurses' right to strike a morally difficult and complex one.

The issue is compelling because many nurses find themselves in situations in which it is next to impossible to fulfill their collective responsibilities. Frequently (as we discussed in several previous chapters) nurses lack power relative to administrators and other health professionals, such as doctors. Their proper place is often seen as being "at the physician's side"—a position of low esteem. Nurse supervisors often have neither the ability nor the desire forcefully to defend members of their staff in disputes with other health professionals or administrators. Far too often nurses are assigned too many clients or ordered to do tasks that lie outside the range of their training or expertise. These and many other factors militate against high-quality nursing care.

We have already seen some of the causes of nurses' relative powerlessness and low esteem. Among the most important ones are the following:

1. The pervasive sexism of our culture. Sexist attitudes appear to have shaped society's expectations that nurses will perform the stereotypical female helping role. These same attitudes are reflected in (some) nurses' images of themselves as handmaidens of the physician or as surrogate mothers.

2. The class background of nurses. Whereas over the years most nurses have come from the lower half of the socio-economic spectrum, typically physicians have come from classes in the upper half.

3. Their relative lack of education. Many nurses lack a quality liberal arts education—a factor that sets them apart from most other professional groups. And their medical training is no match for that of doctors.

4. Their relatively low pay. This may be a consequence of the causes cited above, yet it in turn contributes to the low esteem accorded nurses. In our society esteem is, at least loosely, correlated with level of income. (The average nurse's salary in the United States is around $13,000–$14,000—considerably less than the pay of doctors and other professionals.)

High-quality nursing care is unlikely to be widely available if nurses' positions of relative powerlessness and low esteem persist. Only if the conditions just cited are ameliorated is there a possibility of change—change that is essential if nurses are to fulfill the collective duties outlined above. Of course, to change these conditions is no easy task. Yet there is a growing awareness that things can and should be different. Through sheer dint of numbers (there are more nurses than any other health professionals) and because of the importance of nursing services, the *potential* for power to make these changes is undeniable.

In a variety of ways, these offending conditions and attitudes are being challenged. Two examples

follow: New models of the nurse's role, such as the one discussed in Chapter 2, have stressed independent, professional judgment and action primarily on behalf of the client, as opposed to being primarily an extension of the physician. These models emphasize the distinctive contribution of nursing (e.g., *caring* for the sick as opposed to physicians' contributions of diagnosing disease and attempting cures). Discussion and adoption of these models help somewhat to overcome the negative effects of the traditional, weak model. A second example (also discussed in Chapter 2) is the American Nursing Association's diligent (and controversial) efforts to upgrade nursing education. The Association has been concerned that nurses' education be adequate to meet the challenges of high-quality nursing in today's world: care that requires skill in handling increasingly complex and sophisticated equipment, advanced training in nursing specialties and subspecialties, and the expertise to take on the lion's share of health education as our society places increasing emphasis on preventive care.

These are just two of any number of ways the nursing profession must work to satisfy its collective responsibility to provide quality nursing care. We turn now to the question of the appropriateness of a possible third way, collective action through strikes. Is the strike one of the paths nurses may follow in attempting to meet their collective responsibilities?

The strike is a technique usually used by labor organizations to exact economic concessions from management. It would be very unusual for a strike not to be premised in large part on demands for better pay and benefits. If such "self-serving" goals are incompatible with exercising professional responsibility, surely a strike by nurses could not be condoned. However, far from being incompatible with professional responsibility, the demand for better wages (we shall argue) is a requirement of professional responsibility.

An increase in compensation must go hand in hand with up-grading of the profession. Just as low pay is correlated with low esteem and low status, low status is linked to the lack of quality nursing care. Low status is a nearly insurmountable impediment to quality care. The economic issue is *not* detachable from the quality-of-care issue. The quest for higher wages as well as better working conditions is part and parcel of the struggle to fulfill the collective responsibilities of the profession.

It may be objected, however, that this line of reasoning blurs an important, traditional distinction between the professional and the laborer or worker.

The worker does his or her job for pay, in part because the required tasks lack intrinsic worth. A professional's motives, it has often been argued, should be different. A professional is committed to his or her profession for its own sake and for the sake of those who are its recipients and beneficiaries. Therefore, the argument continues, a professional must refrain from using the strike weapon.

Is this argument persuasive? Its persuasiveness depends on our being able to detach the economic issues from the quality-of-care issues. We have argued, to the contrary, that they are not detachable. Let us consider this issue further. It would appear to be an empirical fact that we are unlikely to get quality people to enter a profession with poor working conditions, low esteem, and low pay. Even if we were to succeed in attracting highly qualified and highly motivated people, it is unlikely that their enthusiasm and morale could be sustained over the years. High drop-out rates, cynicism, and discouragement—all of which presently obtain in nursing—would have to be expected. If all professionals were motivated solely by love of their art and service to humanity, as proponents of the view under challenge wistfully imagine, a strike would indeed be incompatible with professional standing. But since professionals are humans of complex motivation, the image of the professional on which the argument rests is unrealistic.

Since other professional groups (e.g., teachers, interns, and residents) now engage in strike action and appear not to have lost their professional standing, attempts to show that striking is incompatible with professionalism are unlikely to be effective. If we are to find that striking is incompatible with the professional duties of a *nurse*, the conflict will arise from specific nursing duties rather than from general professional obligations.

Before we turn to these specific duties of the nurse, it will be helpful to look more closely at one's activities when striking. To strike is to take collective action, including the refusal to work, with the aim of extracting concessions from one's employer. The refusal to work imposes inconvenience and possibly hardship on those in need of one's services. In the case of strikes by employees such as nurses, the detrimental effect of the strike on the public (those in need of nursing care) is often more immediate and more grave than on the employer. The public's inconvenience is the means by which pressure is put on the employer to come to a settlement agreeable to the striking employees. Were the public in no way inconvenienced, the strike would likely be ineffectual.

Consider the conflict that appears to arise for the striking nurse, given that the means for achieving admittedly worthy goals is the inconvenience and perhaps even the hardship of clients. The modern nurse who functions in accordance with the client advocate model developed in Chapter 2 is committed to working for the client, in that she or he has the special task of caring for the client as a person, of humanizing an otherwise impersonal and sometimes demeaning health care system. Of all health professionals, the nurse is uniquely situated so as to be the most-effective guardian of the client's interests and rights. Perhaps, then, it is this special role of the nurse that makes it wrong for nurses to strike. For a client advocate to be willing to sacrifice a particular client's interests, in order to achieve higher salaries for oneself and one's colleagues, or better care for future clients, at least appears to be contradictory and wrong.

One way out of this seeming impasse is to reject the special role of client advocate. But this is too heavy a price to pay. It would undermine the image and model of nursing that we have found is superior from the moral point of view and is one with which more and more responsible nurses are identifying themselves.

If—contrary to usual circumstances (as we have discussed)—a nurses' strike were *solely* for higher wages (if no quality-of-care issues were on the table and the situation happened to be such that the salary issue were unlikely to affect quality of care because the pay scale were already relatively high), we can see that a strike would be incompatible with the nurses' role as client advocate. Clients are being used as means for advancing nurses' interests. Clients' interests (which the nurse had pledged to advance) are being held hostage. What makes matters most difficult is that the especially stringent duty not to treat clients in this way is not counterbalanced by any other compelling moral duty. The moral duty of the nurse to her or his clients stands in conflict with self-interest—which, of course, does not provide one with a moral basis for failing to do one's moral duty.

On the other hand, if the strike were undertaken with an aim of advancing client care, the case would be quite different. We have the makings of a classic conflict-of-duty situation. The on-going, collective duty to maintain and improve the quality of nursing care appears to be in conflict with specific duties to one's current clients and the collective duty to provide nursing care to the public. When all of these duties cannot be fulfilled, one has to decide which duty ought to take priority over the others.

For those nurses who find themselves in work contexts in which wages, standards, and practice are deficient, our earlier discussion has made clear that concerted action to correct these conditions is obligatory. As is well known, the recent experience of many nursing groups within specific health care facilities is that the only effective way to affect the needed changes is strike action. If, as a matter of fact, a strike is the most-effective, or indeed the only effective, way in a particular situation to make the changes necessary for quality nursing care, the collective responsibilities of nurses require them to strike—*unless* there are other, more-stringent duties (to be considered below) which are binding on them and which would be violated were they to engage in a strike.

An initially appealing yet (as we shall see) unacceptable argument for giving priority to the duty to maintain and improve the quality of care (and, hence, to strike) is the following: the sacrifice of clients' interests resultant from a strike is for the improvement of future nursing care. That is, the sacrifice required of clients is for the good of clients. It would be short-sighted not to see that this is a reasonable price for clients to pay in order to have better care available in the future. Therefore, as in many other areas of our lives, it is reasonable to sacrifice the short-term interests for the long-term ones. Hence, clients cannot reasonably object to a strike under these conditions.

This argument would have some force if the *same* clients whose present interests and needs are sacrificed were the ones to benefit from the future gains. It is one thing to make X sacrifice now for X's (his or her own) later benefit. It is quite another to make X sacrifice now for Y's (another's) later benefit. But in most strikes, the sacrifice required now is for the benefit of others later. It is the yet-unknown client of the future, rather than the present client, whose welfare a strike can advance. The weakness of the argument is that it fails to consider the crucial question of justice (fair treatment of individuals to whom one already has obligations) and simply considers that of over-all consequences.

In an article discussing the morality of strikes by interns and residents, David Bleich asks:

> May a person on the way to a class on first-aid instruction ignore the plight of a dying man, on the plea that he must perfect skills which may enable him to rescue a greater number of persons at some future time? . . . No person may plead that an activity designed to advance future societal benefits is justification for ignoring an immediate

responsibility. . . . The "here and now" test is a general rule of thumb which may be applied to most situations requiring an ordering of priorities [Bleich and Veatch, 1975, p. 9].

No doubt we can all agree that the person failing to give aid on his way to first-aid instruction stands defenseless. Bleich suggests that this action violates a general principle to the effect that commitment to a course of action designed to increase future good is not a weighty enough reason to exempt one from immediate duties. Were we to apply this principle to the issue at hand in the manner Bleich proposes, we would conclude that a nurse going on strike even for the highest of motives, namely, to benefit future clients, is in the wrong, for she or he is violating immediate responsibilities to clients in need of nursing by inappropriately appealing to future benefits.

Such a conclusion need not be drawn even if we were to accept Bleich's argument. The sort of nurses' strike that would be analogous to his case of the man on his way to a first-aid class would be a case of nurses on strike to improve emergency nursing care and who refuse to respond to an emergency. In order to improve conditions so that more lives can be saved later, a life is lost here and now. Such a strike could not be morally justified—a fact that is generally recognized and honored by striking nurses, who see to it that nursing care in emergency rooms and intensive care units is not withdrawn. Bleich's example is useful in making it clear why withdrawal of services necessary for the maintenance of life cannot be justified.

The central moral question concerning nurses' strikes, however, is whether the withdrawal of non-emergency and nonlifesaving nursing services can be shown to be an acceptable means to the end of better nursing care for future clients. Bleich's general principle cited above (that one may not plead that one's attempt to advance future good exempts one from any immediate responsibility) prohibits withdrawal of these nursing services as well *if* doing so entails ignoring any immediate duties to clients.

Is Bleich's principle one we should accept? Whether or not we accept it will depend on how important we take considerations of consequences to be. We can imagine any number of cases in which greater overall good would be served if we were free to fail to meet an immediate conflicting responsibility. For example, suppose one were ready to proceed with a research project which, if successful, would probably provide us with the means to save numerous lives in the future. It has been determined that the only way the project can go forward is to select subjects from whom truly informed consent is not possible (for whatever reason). Most people would agree that, at least in general, one's immediate duty to his or her research subjects is to obtain genuine informed consent. Most would also agree that this is a very stringent requirement (as we have argued). Yet if the risk to the research subjects were truly minimal and the potential for gain for those benefiting from the research were immense, we may feel that it is appropriate at least to consider whether an appeal to future societal benefits is sufficient to outweigh this immediate and serious responsibility. If we feel such a consideration is appropriate, our position entails a rejection of Bleich's principle. On the other hand, we may feel consideration of consequences is illegitimate here.

In deciding for or against Bleich's principle, the crux of the matter is how weighty we consider the duty to work for future societal benefits to be. The ethical principles set forth in Chapter 1 allow for a middle position between that of the strict Kantian, who would see a consideration of consequences as illegitimate, and the utilitarian, who would see it as the only factor to be considered. We took the Kantian respect for persons principle and the principle of beneficence as basic. On this modified Kantian view, it is not wrong to consider consequences; however, in doing so one may not run roughshod over another's autonomy or fail to respect others as persons. The fundamental question that one must ask concerning this case is whether the proper balance has been struck between the duty to respect the research subjects as persons while carrying out one's duty of beneficence, which is the role of a research scientist.

We have established that nurses have a clear and compelling duty to see to it that future nursing care will be better than the substandard care available in certain facilities and locales. Contrary to Bleich, it is too stringent to declare *a priori* that all other immediate duties must take priority in conflict-of-duty situations. What must be determined is whether the duty to work toward better nursing care in the future should, in the particular situation at issue, take precedence over any other duty with which it conflicts.

In place of Bleich's principle, let us adopt the following procedural rule: all the various duties of nurses put forth in ethical codes, such as the *International Code of Nursing Ethics* and the ANA *Code for Nurses*, are binding on the nurse. The only time a nurse is excused from fulfilling any one of these duties is when doing so conflicts with fulfilling a more-stringent duty. As we have seen in the research example, how we determine which of several conflicting duties is the most stringent is a complicated issue that must be decided by an independent procedure (more on this later).

An obvious implication of following this procedural rule is that one must, in fact, be in a conflict-of-duty situation before one is relieved of any duties. If a strike could be conducted without violating any immediate responsibilities, such a course of action would be required. Certainly, in most situations ways can be found to minimize the failure to perform conflicting duties—for example, by directing non-emergency clients to other accessible facilities which provide nursing service and where nurses are not on strike, and by continuing to provide intensive care and emergency nursing services. A strike satisfying these conditions would not be morally objectionable. On the contrary, if a strike is the only means or clearly the most-effective way to change prevailing conditions that are incompatible with high-quality nursing care, then it is morally mandatory.

If other conditions obtain, it will be far more difficult to justify a strike. For example, if one were in a facility far from other facilities providing nursing care and a strike would leave many without the possibility of care, the duty to the public "here and now" might be the stronger duty. Or suppose a group of nurses has made a pledge to their employer not to strike or has signed a no-strike contract. Keeping that agreement is incompatible with strike action. Until 1968 the nursing profession (through the ANA) took a no-strike stance. The duty of fidelity (keeping agreements), which conflicts with striking in these situations, may also be one that cannot be outweighed by the duty to provide quality care to future clients. Fortunately, the ANA no longer adheres to a no-strike position, and most nurses are not working under no-strike contracts.

The moderate position defended here—condoning strikes in certain carefully circumscribed situations, claiming they are morally mandatory in others, yet not justified in still others—is a position that would be taken were nurses and the public to draw up an original contract. Consider the following hypothetical situation, following John Rawls, in which members of the public cannot know when or what nursing care they may need (they are under a veil of ignorance) (Rawls, 1971, 136–42) and nurses also do not know in what situation they will find themselves. Nurses as nurses would want to be able to provide the best care under the best conditions. They would seek sufficient power to be able to overcome any impediments to quality nursing care and self-respect. The public would be concerned to have available to them the best care possible within the limits of allocated resources. Under no conditions would they be willing to barter away a constant availability of emergency or lifesaving care. (They never know when such care may make the difference between life and death.) If it were determined that in some situations—due to factors outside the control of either nurses or the public—the only way quality care could be obtained would be by use of the strike weapon, nurses would insist on the right to use it, and the public would concur as long as emergency and lifesaving care could not be withdrawn. The public would agree to suffer the necessary inconveniences and hardship of a strike in the event that it were the only way to achieve high-quality nursing services.

The way to determine in a particular situation whether nurses' obligations to their clients and the public are weightier than the collective and future-oriented duty to take strike action is to appeal to the original contract. Would the public as party to the agreement be willing to make this required sacrifice in order to benefit from this sought-for goal? If so, the duties to one's clients or to the public that conflict with strike activity can justly be set aside in favor of the strike action. If not, they cannot.

Even if a strike can be morally justified, everyone would agree that it is an awkward and tortuous means of settling disputes. A better way would result from a three-party initial compact, a compact which also included the nurses' employers. Such an agreement would commit both nurses and employers to binding arbitration. That is, if a dispute between nurses and their employer could not be resolved by collective bargaining, it would be turned over to a mutually acceptable arbitrator. (The mechanics of this could be worked out in a variety of ways.) Strikes could be avoided while achieving the end of improved care. Clearly, such an agreement would be advantageous to the public; they would not have to pay the price for the failure of other parties to reach an agreement. Nurses would also find this to be in their best interest. They could avoid being forced into the extremely awkward position of causing hardship or at least inconvenience to those whose interests they have sworn to advocate. Employers in the original position would also see that they stand to gain. They could not count on nurses' inability or disinclination to vigorously press their demands. Faced with the prospect of having to concede just as much or more to striking nurses than in binding arbitration, they would prefer binding arbitration. Everyone would avoid the loss of income and goodwill that inevitably results from a strike.

Of course, in the present real-life situation the employer's lot is quite different. He or she has little to gain by accepting binding arbitration. Perhaps through moral suasion employers will come to see that they ought to accept it. More likely, however, binding arbitration will be accepted only when it is in a particular employer's interests to do so. This will be the case if nurses are able to exact as many concessions from their employers by striking as would be possible through binding arbitration. Only strong, united action on the part of nurses will achieve such a break-through.

As client advocates, nurses should do all in their power to avoid strikes. But paradoxically, the best way to accomplish this is to be ready and able, in appropriate situations, to execute an effective strike.

REFERENCES

Bleich, D., and Veatch, R. M. 1975. "Interns and Residents on Strike." *The Hastings Center Report* 5, no. 6 (December): 7–9.

Kant, I. 1949 reprint. *Fundamental Principles of the Metaphysic of Morals.* Translated by Thomas K. Abbott. The Liberal Arts Press, Inc. Indianapolis, Ind.: The Bobbs-Merrill Co.

Rawls, J. 1971. *A Theory of Justice.* Cambridge, Mass.: Harvard University Press, The Belknap Press.

The Conflicting Demands of Professionalism and Unionism

Alice J. Baumgart

INTRODUCTION

A recent letter to the editor of the *RN ABC News* (March 1983) stated in part:

I have just tried to phone toll-free, collect to the Association in order to use the library services. I was informed that there had been a change in policy and that members of the Association must pay for their own calls.

In light of the fact that the Association now occupies expensive new premises, has raised the fees 60 percent and has cut off loan assistance to members seeking higher education, could you please tell me what you are doing with my money that is of benefit to me?

I quite frankly am unable to see the Association as having my interests at heart. It seems to be an organization built upon a passive, disorganized mass with a very small elite at the top who are serving nobody's interests but their own.

The seeds of discontent. Such stirrings of discontent are not uncommon among Canadian nurses today. For many members of the nursing work force, provincial nursing associations are losing their relevance and their effectiveness. The erosion of their credibility may be traced, in part, to the establishment and growth of independent nurses' unions following the October 1973 Supreme Court of Canada decision that provincial professional associations were company-dominated. Thus, they could not be certified as nursing units for collective bargaining purposes (Rowsell, 1982).

Not too surprisingly, these events have confused and threatened provincial associations. Historically, these associations have enjoyed a pre-eminent position in representing and speaking for the interests of nurses. Now they face competition for resources and for political turf. For example, over three-quarters of Canadian nurses work in hospitals and nearly 80 percent of these nurses enjoy the protection of a collective agreement (Ponak, 1981). Unionism has provided them with a voice in determining their salaries and working conditions. It has also provided them with a sense of security and a feeling that there is a skilled organization to help them cope with the daily struggles of the workplace. Thus, many nurses are becoming increasingly reluctant to pay fees to both unions and professional associations. Heightening their allegiance to unionism is the work that nursing unions are doing to negotiate professional responsibility clauses and to lobby governments regarding financial cutbacks for health services. These developments have set the stage for a rapid escalation of mistrust and conflict between professional associations and unions.

Outline of presentation. In my presentation this morning, I would like to look at the conflict from three vantage points:

1) The changing sociopolitical and economic environment in which organized nursing groups function;

2) The price to be paid by the nursing profession if hard lines are drawn between professionalism and unionism;

3) The need for a political forum capable of generating large-scale compromise and achieving

Baumgart, A. J. (1983, September-October). The conflicting demands of professionalism and unionism. *International Nursing Review, 30,* 150–155. Reprinted with permission of © The International Council of Nurses. All rights reserved.

a broad-based consensus on nursing priorities for the 1980s and 1990s.

1. THE CHANGING ENVIRONMENT

In little over a decade, we have observed significant and, at times, dramatic changes in the environment affecting Canadian health care services.

The crisis of the welfare state: While public policies of cost containment and the corrosive effects of inflation have tended to capture most of our attention, we have, in fact, been dealing with fundamental shifts in the functioning of society. The classic aims of the welfare state since World War II—economic growth, full employment, the elimination of poverty, and the provision of a social security system (including government health insurance)—are no longer being reached.

Value shifts: The growing medicalization of society and bureaucratization of social institutions has also had a network of consequences. These include the assertion of various individual and collective rights to which Canadians now feel entitled. They are expressed in a host of code words such as the quality of life (including work life), the quality of death, self-care, health as a right, participative management, consumer rights, citizen's participation in decision-making, the regionalization of health services, and so on.

Structural changes: The demographic and disease patterns of society are evolving. The migration of the population from east to west, in combination with changes in the family structure, has enormous implications for shifting illness care from institutions to the community. Medico-legal decisions have been made which affect basic conceptions of life, death, the body, individuality, and humanity. Consideration of developments such as genetic engineering and life support systems together with concerns for social justice and the allocation of scarce resources has opened up far-reaching ethical issues.

The enlarging role of government: The advent of public financing of health services in Canada in 1968 has also meant that government has entered into the health sector in a more systematic and comprehensive way. In addition to increased control of economic resources, governments have tightened their control over the quality of services provided, the application of professional codes of ethics, the education of health care personnel, health research and the administration of health care institutions. A highly complex bureaucracy has emerged to maintain the new order and is having difficulties of its own.

This listing of environmental forces to which Canadian health services have been attempting to adapt is, obviously, incomplete. However, it is sufficient to suggest that the last decade has been a watershed era and has produced considerable instability and turbulence in many health care groups and institutions.

The mandate of professional associations: Certainly, some of the most crucial issues and conflicts confronting organized nursing interest groups stem from these trends. In drawing attention to them, it is useful to remind ourselves at the outset, of the three fold role of professional bodies:

1) to support individual practitioners;
2) to advance the interests of the profession through collective action; and
3) to serve society by providing a social mechanism for protecting the public and mediating between practitioners and social environment, of which the most important parts are the public, government, allied occupations, and educational institutions (Merton, 1958).

As Merton (1958) has noted, even in the best of times, professional interest groups face a difficult task in trying to reach and maintain an appropriate balance between these three functions. The balance can be lost at the expense of the individual or the profession as a whole, just as it can be lost at the expense of the public. The task is all the more difficult in the context of the dramatic social changes and the transformation of health services that we have witnessed in the past few years.

The evolving division of labour: Here, let me turn to the evolving division of labour between professional nursing associations and unions. In the early 1970s, several Canadian provinces commissioned reports to assemble and analyze data on health care needs and resources and to propose administrative and regulatory changes. The most comprehensive were the Castonguay-Nepveu Report in Quebec and the report of the Committee of the Healing Arts in Ontario. These enquiries identified at least two closely related issues which were central to the role of professional interest groups:

1) the self-regulatory powers of the health professions; and
2) the proper relationship between expert authority and democratic accountability in a publicly

funded and increasingly bureaucratized health care system.

A NEW REALITY

Among the important changes resulting from these reviews was a general agreement that professional associations could not simultaneously act to protect the public interest and also act exclusively in accordance with the profession's private economic interests. Thus, to retain self-regulatory powers, professional associations had to divest themselves of their functions pertaining to the economic return and the professional recognition of their members. New interest groups, namely unions, took on the latter role.

Other changes with which professional associations had to contend were the involvement of consumers in the governance of the profession and an increase of over 50 percent in the size of the nursing population between 1970 and 1975. To offer an attractive range of services to this growing and increasingly diverse membership was difficult. Additionally, there was a vast expansion in nursing interest groups representing particular spheres of activity such as critical care, nursing education and public health.

The era of the single, comprehensive association to serve a broad range of public and professional interests was over. Professional associations began to experience "the empty nest syndrome". Their decline began, ironically, just as government was beginning to accept the need for a broader range of interests to be represented in the formulation of health policy. This was intended to serve a dual purpose: to answer the democratic accountability critics and to serve as a countervailing force against the power of organized medicine.

Policy input and public accountability: For better or for worse, the health care system is dominated by the physicians. The politicization of the health care system has opened the door to other groups, including nurses, to participate in the policy process. Nursing's recent infatuation with politics reflects this new reality. However, in responding to it, professional associations have paid a price. Their relentless drive to master the art of politics and gain political leverage for issues of prominent concern for nurses has diverted attention away from the difficult task of maintaining membership support.

The growth of unionism: The problem of capturing the allegiance of individual nurses has been compounded by various factors which have favoured the growth of unionism. First, nurses are playing an ever-increasing role in the delivery of health services both absolutely and relative to doctors but they have reaped few rewards in terms of money, respect or status. At the same time, their increased numbers and concentration in large institutional settings makes mass organization against a common employer possible. Further, nurses are more career-oriented. They are staying in the work force longer, and so have a stronger commitment to changing the conditions of their work. Additionally, traditional cultural values respecting women, which have been useful to employers in setting one group of nurses against another, have been breaking down (Cannings & Lazonick, 1978, pp. 123–24). Thus, nurses have been brought together by their mutual identity as women as well as nurses.

Finally, as Badgley (1978, pp. 7–8) has noted, in few other institutions of society is social and economic inequality so marked and yet so generally unacknowledged as the health care system. Under government health insurance, workers at the top of the hierarchy have gained in income and social prestige while middle echelon workers such as nurses have suffered regressive consequences, resulting in a growing mood of dissatisfaction and militancy.

Nurses who have developed an identity of themselves as professionals serving the needs of patients, are outraged by their treatment as assembly-line workers giving their labour to employers to meet and diffuse corporate priorities.

These are ideal conditions for unionization. They are also provoking a new form of unionism in which the scope of collective bargaining is expanded to include issues reflecting distinctly professional concerns. Indeed, recent literature on the growth of unionization among professional employees suggests that they often attach more importance to professional concerns than the traditional union objectives of wages, hours and working conditions (Kleingartner, 1973; Ponak, 1981; Swan, 1978–79).

II. PROFESSIONALISM AND UNIONISM: A CONSTITUTIONAL STRUGGLE

What do these trends signify for the nursing profession and the means by which it takes collective action? Some experts see a future in which nurses must choose between professionalization and unionization (Hopping, 1976; Krause, 1977; Rotkovitch, 1980). For example, Rotkovitch, writing in *Supervisor Nurse,* asserts that unionization diminishes the nurses' self-image and public image and ultimately compromises standards of patient care. Others contend that the main difference between unionism and professionalism is simply that the former lacks respectability.

The case against unionism: The case that unionism is incompatible with professionalism tends to be built upon several familiar arguments. First, unions generally substitute seniority and security considerations for the principle of merit; thus, barriers are set up against rewarding nurses for clinical excellence or terminating incompetent employees. Also, in unionism, short-run solutions are favoured over long-term ones, often locking employing institutions into choices that discourage a search for better or innovative methods. The net effect is an undermining of the standards of nursing practice.

Probably the most troubling aspect of unionization for many nurses is the strike weapon and the conviction that its use is incompatible with the nurses' ethical code. Running a close second is the feeling that, since unionization is a conflict-based process, it involves significant threats to the service relationship between clients and professionals and the integrity of the nursing workforce. That is, nursing management and staff are social partners not adversaries.

The compatibility argument: The case in favour of professional unionism and the complementarity of the professional association and union roles is usually built around two propositions. A main argument is that as collective bargaining has spread to higher status, salaried professionals such as nurses, engineers or university faculty, it has taken on a new character.

Its adaptiveness and flexibility is much in evidence. Far from undermining professionalism, it has become an instrument for harmonizing professional and employee interests and obligations (Swan, 1978–79). As Beatty and Gunderson (1979), in their paper *The Employed Professional* have noted, collective bargaining is a bilateral exercise whereby the spheres of responsibility allocated to employers and employees are made clear and in a way that recognizes their civil liberties and public obligations. They conclude:

Collective bargaining, in short, insures that the occupational self-interest to monopolize and preserve the value of a property interest in an occupation is set against the equally compelling determination of the public to utilize resources and acquire services in the most efficient manner. Collective bargaining insures, then, that a check is provided against each of these powerful interests.

In other words, there is a more open and direct social responsibility, a change that is of benefit to the public as well as workers (Badgley, p. 10).

There is a second proposition in favour of professional unionism which centers on the strike issue. It argues, to quote Badgley (1978, p. 13) that:

if the rights and health of patients and the public are preserved, then strikes can serve as an important catalyst in converting a rigid and conservative health system into a more flexible democratic organization for all its workers. The argument against allowing strikes—i.e. that innocent people suffer harm—remains unproven. It is more often advanced to maintain a system's status quo and preserve an individual's stance in the name of ethics than to deal with the conditions causing workers dissatisfaction.

Proponents of this view point to the fact that doctors in Saskatchewan and Quebec went on strike in the name of their professional association. Further, where strikes by health workers were prohibited by law, penalties have been inversely imposed by the courts according to the status of the occupation. No sanctions were employed against striking doctors. In contrast, striking nurses or non-medical workers have been ordered back to work, fined, threatened with fires or firing, or given a prison sentence (Badgley, p. 11). There is an important lesson here for Alberta nurses.

My sympathies lie with the latter set of arguments. I believe that we need both professional associations and unions. To draw a hard line between professionalism and unionism is a costly bias. Unionism is a form of collective action to gain societal privileges that has proven to be a more potent formula for dealing with the immediate problems of the workplace than the professional association social consensus building models. In large part, this is the result of the special legal status unions enjoy in employment of settings. To argue that professionals should not use or, worse, do not need this means of advancing their interests is to seriously misjudge the power position of employers and employees in large bureaucratic organizations.

The constitutional struggle: How does this relate to the tensions now characterizing the relations between various provincial nursing associations and nursing unions? In my view, what we are seeing is a difficult and complex process of change and system learning. We are engaged in creating a new network of occupational support systems to advance the interests of nurses and to protect the public. The process may be likened to a constitutional struggle over how to achieve unity through diversity. Nursing is now a large, diverse and complex occupation, stratified both vertically and horizontally, and requires a multi-faceted approach to collective action.

III. THE RESTRUCTURING OF THE INSTRUMENTS OF COLLECTIVE ACTION

This brings one to the third aspect of the unionism-professionalism conflict I wish to address, namely, the need for a political forum capable of generating large-scale compromise and achieving a broad-based consensus on nursing priorities for the 1980s and 1990s.

There is virtually no process of change which does not impose losses. Professional associations have seen the range of matters over which they exercised jurisdiction narrowed considerably in the past 10 years. Their paranoia about unionism is understandable. Not only did the emergence of unions place their membership foundations in jeopardy, but they saw unions take on professional concerns which they felt were theirs to advance. Nevertheless, they could take comfort in the public and political credibility they still enjoyed and their broadened policy role.

Unions have also not been without a degree of myopic self-interests which perversely reinforced the conflict with associations. They have tended to have inexperienced direction and have been intimidated in their efforts by vested interest groups in the health care system.

Their analytic capacity has also been limited in terms of understanding the complexities of the political arena in which they were involved. The determining factors include their reluctance to form alliances with other unions, partly out of concern for compromising their professionalism, and their naive view of the power process in the health care system. In particular, they have tended to neglect a fact of enormous importance in political life—nurses are primarily women and the nurses struggle in the workplace is a women's issue. . .

Jenniece Larsen's address to this convention in 1981 eloquently addressed this point.

Permit me one final set of observations. If we need to restructure the instruments of collective action in nursing and work toward a complementarity of roles between unions and associations, what would the pattern look like? We can only speculate but some features are already visible. First, a variety of clinical and functional interest groups have been formed and are fulfilling the important role of knowledge diffusion and elaboration of standards for particular spheres of nursing activity. These groups also perform a role in creating a coherent moral order which can attach individuals to a group in a disciplined way. Professional associations have moved creatively into the policy input process in health care, and so are giving much greater visibility to the many contributions of nurses to Canadian health services.

Unions, for their part are beginning to recognize the limits of their political credibility. They are recognizing that bidding farewell to professional associations is foolish for it would deprive professionals in organizations of external leverage points in fighting internal battles. For example, professional responsibility clauses are easier to negotiate when bargaining units can point to a code of ethics and competency requirements enforced by a self-regulatory association (Swinton, 1979).

In this context, one of the most imaginative social experiments in creating a broad-based forum for reaching consensus on nursing priorities is the block or group membership concept endorsed by the R.N.A.O. As you know, by this provision members of O.N.A., the nursing union join R.N.A.O., the professional organization in the province on May 1, 1983. This provision also gives O.N.A. members greater access to a wide range of R.N.A.O.-affiliated interest groups.

CONCLUSION

Will new instruments of collective action follow which prevent the nursing profession from splitting apart into autonomous warring units? Recent developments such as the R.N.A.O.-O.N.A. initiative, and the proliferation of active and dynamic interest groups and unions offers considerable grounds for hope.

BIBLIOGRAPHY

Adams, G. W. Collective bargaining by salaried professionals. In P. Slayton and M. J. Trebilcock (eds). *The Professions and Public Policy*. Toronto: University of Toronto Press, 1979, 264–278.

Aiken, Linda H. The impact of federal health policy on nurses. In American Academy of Nursing. Linda H. Aiken (ed). *Nursing in the 1980s: crises, opportunities, challenges*. Philadelphia: J. B. Lippincott Company, 1982, 3–20.

Badgley, Robin F. Health worker strikes: Social and economic bases of conflict. In Samuel Wolfe (ed). *Organization of Health Workers and Labor Conflict*. Policy, Politics, Health and Medicine Series. Farmingdale, New York: Baywood Publishing Company, Inc., 1978, 7–16.

Baumgart, Alice J. Professional obligations, employment responsibilities and collective bargaining: a new agenda for the 1980s (Unpublished paper, presented at the R.N.A.B.C. Labour Relations Division, 4th Annual Convention, Vernon, B.C.), June 10, 1980.

Baumgart, Alice J. Nursing for a new century—a future framework. *Journal of Advanced Nursing*, 1982, 7, 19–23.

Beatty, David M. & Gunderson, Morley. *The Employed Professional*. Working Paper No. 14. Prepared for The Professional Organizations Committee, Ministry of the Attorney General. Toronto: Ontario Government, 1979.

Bellaby, Paul & Oribabor, Patrick. Determinants of the occupational strategies adopted by British hospital nurses. *International Journal of Health Services*, 1980, 10(2), 291–309. Baywood Publishing Company Inc., 1980.

Campbell, Marie. New directions for nurses. *Policy Options*, January–February, 1983, pp. 30–33.

Cannings, Kathleen & Lazonick, William. The development of the nursing labor force in the United States: a basic analysis. In Samuel Wolfe (ed). *Organization of Health Workers and Labor Conflict*. Policy, Politics, Health and Medicine Series. Farmingdale, New York: Baywood Publishing Company, Inc., 1978, 83–114.

Centre for Industrial Relations. Crispo, John H. G. (ed). *Collective Bargaining and the Professional Employee: conference proceedings, December 15–17, 1965*. Toronto: University of Toronto Press, 1966.

Cleland, V. S. Shared governance in a professional model of collective bargaining. *Journal of Nursing Administration*, May 1978, 39–43.

Cleland, Virginia. Nurses' economics and the control of nursing practice. In American Academy of Nursing. Linda H. Aiken (ed). *Nursing in the 1980s: crises, opportunities, challenges*. Philadelphia: J. B. Lippincott Company, 1982, 383–398.

Fraser, D. Bicameralism and the professional college. In P. Slayton and M. J. Trebilcock (eds). *The Professions and Public Policy*. Toronto: University of Toronto Press, 1978, 279–289.

Gaffin, J. (ed). *The nurse and the welfare state*. Aylesbury, England: HM & M Publishers, 1981.

Gilchrist, Joan M. Profession or union: who will call the shots? In School for Graduate Nurses, McGill University, *Nursing Papers*, November 1969, *1*(2), 4–10.

Goldenberg, Shirley B. Task Force on Labour Relations (under the Privy Council Office): Study No. 2. *Professional Workers and Collective Bargaining: An analysis of the problems which professional workers and their employers face when they adopt a collective bargaining relationship*. Ottawa: Queen's Printer for Canada, 1970.

Grescoe, Audrey. No more nurse nice-guys! *Homemaker's Magazine*, November 1982, pp. 92–104.

Hopping, Betty. Professionalism and unionism: Conflicting ideologies. *Nursing Forum*, 1976, *XV*(4), 372–383.

Kergin, Dorothy J. Nursing as a profession. In Mary Q. Innis (ed), *Nursing education in a changing society*. Toronto: University of Toronto Press, 1970, 46–63.

Kleingartner, Archie. Collective bargaining between salaried professionals and public sector management. *Public Administration Review*, 1973, 33, 165–173.

Krause, Elliot A. Power & Illness: *The Political Sociology of Health and Medical Care*. New York: Elsevier North-Holland, Inc., 1977.

Larsen, Jenniece. The effects of feminism of the nursing profession: And what is your excuse . . . (Unpublished paper, presented at the end of the 1981 Convention of the Alberta Association of Registered Nurses, Edmonton, Alberta), May 8, 1981.

Merton, Robert K. The functions of the professional association. In Bonnie Bullough & Vern Bullough (eds). *Issues in Nursing: Selected Readings*. New York: Springer Publishing Company, Inc., 1966.

Pepperdene, Barbara J. Professions, power and the state: Historical trends and their implications. (Paper presented at the annual meetings of the C.S.A.A., Session 78, Saskatoon, Saskatchewan), June, 1979.

Ponak, Allen M. Unionized professionals and the scope of bargaining: A study of nurses. *Industrial and Labor Relations Review*, April 1981, *34*(3), 396–407.

Rotkovitch, Rachel. Do labor union activities decrease professionalism? *Supervisor Nurse*, September 1980, pp. 16–18.

Rowsell, Glenna. Changing trends in labour relations: Effects on collective bargaining for nurses. *International Nursing Review*, 1982, *29*(5), 141–145.

Strauss, George. Professionalism and occupational associations. *Industrial Relations*, 1963, 2, 7–13.

Swan, K. P. Professional obligations, employment responsibilities and collective bargaining. *Interchange*, 1978-79, *9*(3), 98–110.

Swiercz, Paul W. & Skipper, James K., Jr. Labor law and physician's privileged position: An example of structural interest influence. *International Journal of Health Services*, 1982 *12*(2), 249–261.

Swinton, Katherine. *The Employed Professional.* Working Paper No. 13. Prepared for The Professional Organizations Committee, Ministry of the Attorney General. Toronto: Ontario Government, 1979.

Werther, William B. & Lockhart, Carol A. Collective action and Cooperation in the Health Professions. *Journal of Nursing Administration*, July-August 1977, pp. 13–19.

White, Julie. *Women and Unions.* Prepared for the Canadian Advisory Council on the Status of Women. Hull, Quebec: Minister of Supply and Services Canada, 1980.

Wolfe, Samuel. Worker Conflicts in the Health Field: An Overview. In Samuel Wolfe (ed). *Organization of Health Workers and Labor Conflict.* Policy, Politics, Health and Medicine Series. Farmingdale, New York: Baywood Publishing Company, Inc., 1978, 3–6.

Insubordination—Patient Load

M. Josephine Flaherty

BACKGROUND INFORMATION

About 2230h on February 26, Patient Mason was admitted with irregular breathing and an irregular heart rate to the Emergency Department of a large teaching hospital; various diagnostic tests were done. About 0200h on February 27, Mason went into respiratory arrest and was intubated and ventilated manually. Dr. Brown, physician in charge of the Emergency Department that night, deciding to admit the patient to the Intensive Care Unit, called the I.C.U. to advise the nursing staff of the admission. Nurse Ames, who took the call, said "John, we are very busy. We need more help. Do you want to call Nursing Supervisor Smith or do you want me to call?" Dr. Brown said that he was busy and asked that Nurse Ames call Supervisor Smith and let him know about her response. Dr. Brown called Dr. White, who was in charge of the I.C.U. to apprise him of the patient's condition and the decision to admit him; Dr. White concurred with this action.

Nurse Ames called Supervisor Smith, told her that there was a ventilator patient being admitted to I.C.U. and asked for more nursing staff. Smith said that she could not provide more help, told Ames to "do what you can do" and noted that she would ask the Emergency Department if the patient could be cared for there. She did so and Dr. Brown's response to this request was negative. Smith responded that if this were the case, the physician would have to be responsible for Patient Mason. Dr. Brown replied that he was unhappy with that remark, that he would report Supervisor Smith and that Mason was going to the I.C.U. Supervisor Smith accepted that decision.

Dr. Brown informed Dr. White by telephone that he was having difficulty having Mason admitted to I.C.U. and asked for Dr. White's assistance; White said that he would investigate the matter and call Dr. Brown.

Dr. White called I.C.U., spoke to another nurse, Miss Blank, and reprimanded her for "giving flak" to Dr. Brown. Nurse Blank said that no "flak" had been given and that Dr. Brown had been informed simply that the I.C.U. was at the saturation point in the work load of the nurses. When informed by Dr. White that nurses need only ask for additional help, Nurse Blank noted that Supervisor Smith had been informed and that no help was forthcoming. Neither Dr. White nor Nurse Blank disputed that Patient Mason appeared to need I.C.U. care, but Nurse Blank made it clear that the situation was such that there was no nurse available to care for the new patient. When questioned about this by Dr. White, she said, "No nurse feels capable of accepting the responsibility for another ventilator patient." Dr. White said that he would call Supervisor Smith. He testified later that he had noted to Nurse Blank that he would come in to help with the care of the patient if necessary and that this offer was motivated, not by recognition of the nurses' claim that they could not accept responsibility for more patients, but by recognition that, given the position taken by the nurses, he, as a responsible physician, had no alternative to coming in and providing care. Dr. White called Supervisor Smith and told her that the patient would go to the I.C.U. and that he and Respiratory Technologist Thomas would look after the ventilator so that the nurses could give nursing care. Supervisor Smith telephoned this information to Nurse Clark who replied that the nurses would not care for the patient; Smith told them to try anyway.

At 0520h, Patient Mason arrived in I.C.U. accompanied by Dr. Brown, Dr. Black (an intern), Nurse Evans (Emergency Department Nurse) and Technologist Thomas; they transferred Mason to a bed in an empty I.C.U. room. Nurse Evans attempted to give a report of the patient to Nurse Blank who told Evans that since no I.C.U. nurse would be caring for the patient, she should give the report to the doctors attending to him. Nurse Evans left the I.C.U. At this time, Drs. White and Gold (the intern in I.C.U.) arrived.

The room in which Patient Mason was placed had not been equipped for his care. Those attending him assembled the necessary equipment with the occasional assistance of I.C.U. Nurse Davis (although she was very busy with her own patient who was at least as ill as Patient Mason) and of Nurses Clark and Ames.

Subsequent to these events, Nurses Ames, Blank and Clark were suspended without pay for three days and were warned by the director of nursing that further similar behavior would "jeopardize" their relationships with the hospital as employees. The reason advanced for the suspension was "insubordination," as evidenced by their failure as registered nurses to carry out the following responsibilities:

—to appoint a team leader or nurse in charge (a policy of the hospital);

—to accept a report and a patient from the Emergency Department nurse;

—to offer to help in the admission of the patient to I.C.U. and in the care given by the medical staff during the remainder of the shift (approximately 3 hours); and

—to report fully the circumstances of the incident to the head nurse at morning report.

Supervisor Smith also was suspended without pay, for five days, because she was "not forceful enough in her supervision of the nurses in question." What are the ethical problems in this situation?

IDENTIFICATION AND CLARIFICATION OF ETHICAL COMPONENTS

This complex, real-life situation is not illustrative of one discrete ethical issue but involves a complexity of demands, needs, conflicting loyalties, and confusing lines of communication. This incident presents a picture of a health care situation in which the resources in the hospital do not appear to be adequate to the task of the provision of appropriate treatment for a seriously ill patient, a not unusual circumstance in large and small health care agencies today.

There are several types of rights and responsibilities involved:

1. The right of a patient to treatment
2. The rights and responsibilities of nurses as providers of the care
3. The rights and responsibilities of a health care agency to make decisions about who shall admit patients, who shall care for which patients and what the patient-nurse ratios shall be
4. The rights and responsibilities of physicians, as "guest practitioners" in the agency, to admit patients and to make decisions affecting the practice of other health practitioners over whom they have no authority.

Right of a Patient to Treatment

The hospital in question was a public hospital, defined in The Public Hospitals Act of the jurisdiction as "any institution, building or other premises or place established for the treatment of persons afflicted with or suffering from sickness, disease or injury, or for the treatment of convalescent of chronically ill persons that is approved under this Act as a public hospital." Under the same Act, a patient is a "person who is received and lodged in a hospital for the purpose of treatment"; and treatment means "the maintenance, observation, medical care and supervision and skilled nursing care of a patient. . . . " The jurisdiction concerned had a system of universal hospital care insurance by which Patient Mason was covered. Hence, since he was received and lodged in the hospital, Mason became a patient and had the right, by law and by the value system of the society in which he lived, to treatment, including skilled nursing care. A patient who is entitled to skilled nursing care should be able to assume that the nurses will practice competently, will consider the patient's needs paramount, will not harm the patient through acts of commission or omission, and will be faithful to both the patient and to the promises of the profession.

Rights and Responsibilities of Nurses as Providers of Health Care

As registered nurses, the staff members of the I.C.U. had statutory responsibilities to "exercise generally accepted standards of practice for the performance of nursing services." This includes making professional judgments about their ability to accept specific responsibility and the communication of their inability to accept such responsibility to their supervisors. When nurses are expected to practice according to the standards for registered nurses, they have the right to working conditions that make this possible. This includes work loads that are reasonable, including appropriate assistance and supervision. Registered nurses in the jurisdiction concerned are responsible and accountable, by statute, for the "effective supervision of . . . others who contribute to the provision of nursing care," for "the exercise of judgment in delegation of activities, . . . " for collaboration "with other members of the health team in the planning/ provision of care," for coordination of "nursing care with other aspects of health care" and for referring and reporting "pertinent information to other members of the health team." The Standards of Nursing Practice also include responsibilities for collaboration with other nurses and for seeking help and guidance when nurses are unable to perform competently. All of the nurses in this situation shared these responsibilities. One might ask how effectively they collaborated and communicated. Was the action of the supervisor appropriate? Should other nurses have been sent to the I.C.U.? Should the Emergency Department nurse have behaved differently? Do nurses have the right to "civil disobedience" in health care?

The Rights and Responsibilities of a Health Care Agency to Make Decisions About Who Shall Admit Patients and Who and How Many Persons Shall Provide Care

By admitting physicians to practice privileges in a hospital, either as full staff physicians or as resident or junior interns, does a hospital delegate *carte blanche* responsibility to these physicians to admit patients and to decide the wards or departments to which patients will be sent, in the absence of consideration of the occupancy and staff situations in the hospital? Does the hospital have the obligation to admit all patients needing care to its own wards or could Patient Mason have been sent to another public general hospital? In the city core area involved, there are several hospitals with a combined total of well over 3,000 beds, within a two-mile radius of the hospital to which Mason was admitted. Does a hospital have a right to permit extremely heavy patient loads in patient care areas?

The Rights and Responsibilities of Physicians as "Guest Practitioners"

Do physicians have the right to make decisions that affect directly the practice of members of another health discipline over which they have neither statutory nor organizational line authority in the work situation? Are physicians obliged to collaborate with institution managers and with other health professionals? Do physicians have the right and the qualifications to assess nursing care needs of patients as opposed to medical care needs?

ANALYSIS OF THE SPECIFIC SITUATION

Background Information

1. Mason was in need of intensive care including a ventilator. The ward of choice was the I.C.U.

2. The I.C.U. was staffed inadequately for its patient load. There were six nurses on duty, two of whom were relief nurses without experience in the I.C.U. and whose special care unit competence was limited. There were eight patients, five of whom were on ventilators or respirators and all of whom had monitoring equipment and/or indwelling tubes, drains, and so forth. One patient was on isolation technique for infection.

3. The nurses were on a twelve-hour shift that was supposed to include time for meals and coffee breaks. None of the nurses had a meal break; some had a cup of coffee in the Unit.

4. The nursing supervisor had a nondirective style of supervision and rarely gave direct orders.

5. No team leader had been appointed although the appointment of one was required by hospital policy. Since the supervisor had received reports from each of the nurses on the unit, she was aware of this breach of policy. The supervisor made no attempt to redistribute patient assignments.

6. The Emergency Department nurse who accompanied the patient to the I.C.U. returned to the Emergency Department without giving a report on her patient to the I.C.U. nurses.

7. The I.C.U. nurses requested additional help; they were refused help and were told to "do the best you can."

8. Hospital policy states that ventilated patients cannot be left unobserved or unattended.

9. No direct order or directive was given to all or any of the six nurses in the I.C.U. to care for Patient Mason.

10. Although the director of nursing had authority to hire more nurses, she noted during an arbitration hearing related to this incident that she had not done so because she had a budget to follow.

INDIVIDUALS INVOLVED IN DECISION MAKING

1. Physicians

A physician in the Emergency Department decided to admit the patient. The physician in charge of the Intensive Care Unit concurred. The Emergency Department physician notified the I.C.U. that the patient was coming and was informed that the nurses could not handle another patient. He asked an I.C.U. nurse to telephone the nursing supervisor about this. He informed the I.C.U. physician that he anticipated difficulties with the admission of his patient.

Although the Emergency Department physician had admitting authority, he also had responsibility to ensure that the area to which his patient would be admitted was appropriate. One would question how appropriate the I.C.U. was on this occasion when it was clear that there was a shortage of nurses. The I.C.U. physician telephoned the I.C.U. nurses and reprimanded them for "giving flak" to the Emergency Department physician. He said that he would talk with the nursing supervisor but the outcome of that conversation, if it did take place, is not known.

He did volunteer to come in to look after the patient if necessary but noted that this decision was motivated only by his responsibility as a physician and not by his recognition that the nurses needed help.

That four physicians and one respiratory technologist attended the patient in the Intensive Care Unit is indicative that they were aware of the complexity of the care demanded and of the fact that the nurses were unable to deal with this situation. In view of the fact that five persons were caring for one patient, one wonders why the physicians felt qualified to assert that the I.C.U. nurses should have been willing and able to care for this patient in addition to the other patients in the Unit. Since the two senior physicians involved were cognizant of the number and nature of patients in the Unit and the extent of the nursing staff on duty, one would question why they did not take action to ensure that additional nursing help was made available. Dr. White had noted that nurses who needed extra help need only ask for this. He was aware that such a request had been refused and yet he insisted that the patient be admitted to the I.C.U. and he believed that the nurses had been incorrect in their refusal to assume responsibility for this additional patient.

Why did physicians in this situation have the power to affect so directly the conditions of work for nurses—members of another health discipline over which they had neither statutory nor organizational responsibility? What was the quality of the communication between the physicians and the nurses in this agency, where a nursing supervisor was told that she would be reported for telling the physician that if he admitted the patient to the I.C.U. he would have to assume responsibility for the patient and where the same physician reprimanded a nurse in the I.C.U. for what he alleged was "flak" given to another physician by another nurse?

As health professionals, did the physicians have the responsibility to reassess the admission of the particular patient to their hospital in view of staffing problems that were apparent? Were the physicians exercising their responsibility to provide treatment, which by definition includes skilled nursing care, when they knew that this was not possible in that Unit?

2. The Nursing Supervisor

The nursing supervisor knew the conditions in the Intensive Care Unit on that shift as she had received reports on all patients at approximately

2200h in the evening. She was aware that no team leader had been chosen and she made no attempt to deal with this obvious breach of hospital policy. Although she had visited the Unit at 2200h, apparently she made no attempt to return to the Unit later to give nursing assistance to the staff and to see the new patient who had been admitted. In a conversation with the I.C.U. physician, she had told him that if he admitted the patient to the Unit, he would have to be responsible for the patient. When she was told that he would admit the patient anyway and report her for her comment, she accepted that decision.

When she was asked for nursing assistance by the I.C.U. nurses, she instructed them simply to "cope" and "do the best you can." At no time did she give a direct order to all or any of the nurses to care for the new patient. She noted later that her style of supervision recognized the fact that registered nurses are professional people with the responsibility to make professional judgments. However, there is no clear indication that she supported nurses in their resolution to refuse to accept responsibility for the new patient. There is no indication of the extent to which the supervisor communicated with the Emergency Department nurse. The fact that subsequent to these events, the nursing supervisor was suspended by the hospital for five days indicates that the hospital believed that the supervisor did not fulfill the responsibilities of her job on that occasion. It should be noted that the supervisor must also have been aware of the fact that although it was hospital policy that no ventilated patient be left unobserved or unattended, there were more ventilator patients in the Unit than there were nurses qualified to care for them. One would wonder also why the supervisor did not spend more time in the Unit that night when she was aware of the fact that carrying heavy patient loads were two relief nurses, neither of whom was an experienced or qualified I.C.U. nurse.

3. Nurses in the I.C.U.

There is no evidence to indicate that the nurses had asked for additional nursing help before the question of the admission of a new patient arose, even though they were understaffed for the patient population in the Unit. The nurses did explain to the physician who notified them about the new patient that no nurse was capable of assuming responsibility for the new patient. The nurses did contact the supervisor and ask for help. When the new patient was brought to the I.C.U., the nurses made clear that they would not accept the new patient and assume responsibility for him. Their reasons were related to the patient load they already were carrying. Although they claimed later that they were concerned about their responsibility for the provision of safe care for patients already under their care, apparently they did not make an issue of the safety factor on the evening concerned. While they might be faulted by some observers for this, it would seem reasonable to assume that they were extremely busy trying to do what needed to be done without becoming philosophical and providing detailed rationales for the stand they were taking.

The nurses were faulted by the hospital for failing to appoint a team leader according to the policy of the hospital. However, it was noted later (and this was not challenged) that the practice of failing to appoint a team leader had been going on for some time. The supervisor was aware of this and apparently did nothing to correct the situation.

The nurses acknowledged later that they gave limited help to the physicians involved in the care of Patient Mason. A physician noted that the nurses had "taken time to have a cup of coffee and yet they did not have time to care for the new patient." The nurses noted that one or two of them had drunk a cup of coffee at the nursing station while they were charting or speaking on the telephone. The nurses were faulted for not reporting details of the incident in the morning report when they went off duty. Their response was that they believed the situation had been handled and that their supervisor was aware of it and hence that a further report was not necessary. One would question their judgment on this issue in view of their professional responsibility to communicate appropriately with other members of the team.

It seems obvious that these nurses were aware of their professional responsibility to make judgments, to take action, and to be accountable for that action. Apparently they believed they were acting appropriately. It should be noted that they did not make a point of their legal responsibilities related to the abandoning of patients during the night in question. However, it cannot be assumed that this matter was not in their minds.

4. Emergency Room Nurse

In accordance with hospital policy, emergency room Nurse Evans accompanied Patient Mason to the Intensive Care Unit and attempted to give a report on him to one of the nurses present. When that nurse refused to take the report, because she was refusing to assume responsibility for the patient, apparently Nurse Evans left the Unit without giving a report. One would question why this nurse did not fulfill this responsibility and/or notify the supervisor that a report had not been given. It is not known how many other nurses were in the Emergency Department that night or how many other patients were there. However, there is little evidence that the Emergency Department nurse did anything in the Intensive Care Unit except assist the four doctors and one respiratory technologist to transfer the patient to an I.C.U. bed. Apparently she did not assemble equipment for the I.C.U. patient room. It may be that she was pressed to return to the Emergency Department immediately or that she was not aware of where some equipment was kept. One would wonder how much attempt she made to assist with the settling of the patient in the I.C.U. One cannot assume that she did not make attempts to do this. In view of the fact that the Emergency Department nurse failed to carry out her reporting responsibility and apparently failed to discuss this with her supervisor, one would wonder why the hospital did not discipline her for failure to carry out her responsibilities.

5. Hospital Authorities

This large general hospital was experiencing, no doubt, the same fiscal restraints that confront all health care institutions in these times. During a later arbitration hearing, the director of nursing acknowledged that she had been aware of the state of staffing in the hospital and in the Unit in question. One would wonder why she had permitted the Intensive Care Unit to be staffed as this one was. In view of hospital policy in relation to responsibilities of nurses in special care units, why were two of the six nurses totally inexperienced in intensive care unit work? By that policy, they were limited in their practice in that situation, because relief nurses who are not certified for specific procedures may not administer intravenous drugs and perform certain other activities related to hemodynamic monitoring. Why was a supervisor not available to monitor the work of these inexperienced nurses?

Although the director of nursing admitted later that she did have authority to hire additional nurses, she said she did not do so because she had a budget to follow. One would question the professional responsibility of a nurse manager who knowingly allows conditions to exist that threaten or make impossible the provision of skilled nursing care and the fulfillment of the standards of nursing practice in the agency. It is acknowledged that emergency situations in staffing can arise and this may well have been one. However, it must have been known for a great many hours before the new patient was admitted that there were too few nurses who were qualified to care for ventilator patients in that Unit. One would wonder why additional nurses could not have been found between the hours of roughly 1930h when the shift began and 0520h the next morning when the new patient was admitted to the I.C.U. One would question whether this situation had occurred before, whether it was one of long standing and whether it would continue. It is known that shortly after the occurrence of the incidents described in this situation, additional nurses were hired for the hospital and for the I.C.U. This and the disciplining of the nursing supervisor suggest strongly that the hospital was aware of its inadequacy. One would wonder, then, why the hospital felt justified in the disciplining of the I.C.U. nurses who took action that they believed was appropriate for professional nurses.

6. The Collective Bargaining Agreement

In this hospital, the nurses were covered by a collective bargaining agreement that was developed under the labor relations laws of the jurisdiction. It is recognized that the management level of an organization, including a hospital, has the right to decide what shall be done by whom in that organization and to regulate the distribution of resources, physical and human, within the institution. Hence, management has the right to assign responsibilities to members of the staff and this can lead to problems. For example, when members of the staff, such as nurses, are professionals who are accountable to the statutory body for the quality and scope of their practice, to the employer for carrying out the responsibilities of the job, to the patients who receive care, and to themselves for the character of their practice, which is carried out according to standards of nursing practice, statutory regulations, and the code of ethics of the profession, there may be conflicts between the nurses' loyalty to the employer and their loyalty to the profession and to the recipients of care.

It has been said for some time in the nursing profession that it is nurses who should make judgments regarding nursing practice and the nursing needs of patients. In this situation, it appears that physicians assumed the responsibility for making such judgments and this is not unusual in health care today. Nurses of the eighties believe they are qualified to make decisions about the nature and extent of nursing responsibilities that they can assume and, indeed, in the jurisdiction in which the situation under question occurred, the taking of responsibility for professional actions by nurses and their being accountable for their actions both are required by statute. One would wonder whether nurses have a right to "civil disobedience" in health care. Labor relations laws, largely in the industrial setting, allow for an *obey and grieve rule*, the rationale behind which is to give disaffected employees an opportunity to challenge a particular management decision in a way that recognizes both the interests of the employer in having work assignments carried out and the interests of the employee in obtaining a just disposition of his or her complaint. To allow employees to practice insubordination in light of their disagreement with a work directive could threaten the right of an employer to manage the organization. In the collective agreement at the hospital in question, there is a section that defines very clearly that the management of the hospital and the direction of working forces are fixed exclusively in the hospital and shall remain solely with the hospital, except as specifically limited by particular provisions of the agreement. The assignment of responsibilities to employees such as nurses rests with the hospital. Disaffected employees are expected to *obey* at the time and *grieve* later.

However, under the labor relations laws of the jurisdiction involved, there are several exceptions to the *obey and grieve* rule. These include the right of employees to disobey if they are asked to carry out a task that is unsafe or reasonably believed to be unsafe or if they are asked to do something illegal. It is noteworthy that under that law, although an employer cannot expect workers to do something that is unsafe for them, there is no provision for employees to refuse to do something that is unsafe for the recipient of their care. Hence, because of the failure of the law to deal specifically with the third set of interests, those of the patient, in a health care situation in the jurisdiction involved, it seems that the threat to safety of a patient is not sufficient to allow health care employees to disobey. It is partly for this weakness in the law that

the charge of insubordination of these nurses was upheld by an arbitration board and later by judicial inquiry.

If the nurses in this situation consciously had believed and had stated that by obeying the apparent directive to care for Patient Mason, they could be found guilty of abandoning other patients and hence of professional misconduct, or that they could be found to be incompetent because they had displayed in their professional care of patients a lack of judgment or a disregard for the welfare of patients, they would have pointed to their explicit responsibilities as professional nurses under the statutes that govern registered nurses in their region of the country. In this situation, they could have claimed that assuming responsibility for the new patient would have constituted an illegal act for them and their insubordination could have been upheld under the *obey and grieve* rule. It should be noted, however, that not all nursing statutes are as strong and as explicit as the ones in the jurisdiction in which these incidents took place.

It is important to distinguish between two dimensions of nurses' behavior: their professional responsibility and their obligation to their employer. Since nurses' main obligation to the employer is to behave as competent professional nurses if that employer has hired them to work as professional nurses, it is difficult to separate the two dimensions because nurses' obligation to the employer and their professional responsibility are one and the same. It could be suggested, then, that in refusing to take on the additional patient and thus acting as responsible professionals, these nurses in fact were fulfilling their responsibility or obligation to their employer to behave as competent professionals.

ETHICAL IMPLICATIONS

It appears that in this situation, there were several options or possible courses of action that might have been chosen by the persons who played parts in the decision making. Apparently, each of these decision makers acted the way he or she believed was right. One could wonder, however, if those people really did believe that their actions were right or whether some, pragmatically, were "going by the book" or were evading honest confrontation with reality. Although the actions taken may appear to be simply decisions based on facts, clearly they involve an ethical problem because the solution does not rest solely within science, it is perplexing to some or all of the people involved, and it has implications that touch many areas of human concern. That there are several types of rights and responsibilities involved has been acknowledged. It is questionable whether each of the actors in the situation projected fully the consequences of each possible course of action and identified fully the good and/or harm that could result.

It seems obvious that none of the possible options—refusal to admit Patient Mason and referral of him to another hospital, retention of him in the Emergency Department for care, the transfer of him from there to a unit other than the I.C.U., the assignment of nurses from another unit to either the Emergency Department or the I.C.U. to care for him, the co-opting of the nursing supervisor to care for him, the "calling in" of additional nurses to the hospital, *et al.*—was acceptable to all of the decision makers involved. However, there is little evidence that genuine attempts were made by any or all of them to explore the possible options in cooperation with the others. All persons and groups involved seemed to be determined to follow their own decisions for action, even though the issue had been reported to both a senior physician and a senior nurse. Some decisions (those of the physicians) seemed to be based on recognition of Patient Mason's human need for care without full enough consideration of the needs of other patients in the I.C.U. Other decisions (the nurses') did not deny Patient Mason's need for care, but appeared to be based on their recognition of other patient's needs, of their duties and obligations to provide care for them, and of their inability to fulfill those duties in addition to the new ones that would be imposed by the extra patient. Other decisions (the nursing supervisor's) appeared to be derived from the recognition that since she had spoken with the admitting physician and received no satisfaction, she should instruct the I.C.U. nurses simply to do their best, on their own, without her formal assistance. Her lack of action, and the hospital administration's, in the face of their knowledge about the level of staffing in the I.C.U. on the night in question, that clearly was in contravention of hospital policy with regard to number and qualifications of nurses assigned to the I.C.U., and their awareness of the failure of the nurses (on more than this one occasion) to appoint a team leader suggests evasion of honest confrontation with reality.

This particular situation required shared decision-making activity. There seems to be little evidence of sharing of deliberations and discussion of options. There is no clear evidence of recognition, by all persons involved, of the locus of authority for the decision making. The result was a series of incompatible decisions, with little indication that there was understanding of why dissenters were not in agreement with the decisions of other people. In this situation, there was confusion within and among the social expectations, held by some members of the hospital, for nurses to obey and conform, for physicians to make decisions that affect other disciplines over which they do not have line authority and responsibility and for the nursing supervisor to manage. There was confusion also in relation to the legal or statutory responsibilities of physicians as professionals and "guest practitioners" in the hospital, of nurses as professionals and employees, of the nursing supervisor as a professional nurse and an administrator, and of the hospital as a provider of treatment that included skilled nursing care.

The situation was a puzzling one but not a rare one. Each decision that was made had an element of right action that was perceived by the decision maker, and an element of wrong action that was demonstrated in the consequences. The situation provides an example of failure on the part of a number of health care professionals, all of whom perceived themselves to be competent and ethical, to behave in a collegial manner in the effort to find a solution for a practical and ethical problem. Mutual respect and cooperation and responsible leadership by both of the professions involved would have led to a more satisfactory solution. Nurses and physicians would do well to reflect on how they would or could have responded in this or a similar circumstance, on whether situations like this one will be repeated, and on what can be done to prevent them.

COMMENTARY BY LEAH CURTIN: INSUBORDINATION—PATIENT LOAD

The most important point Flaherty makes in her analysis of this case study is ". . . nurses' main obligation to the employer is to behave as competent professional nurses . . . [thus] nurses' obligations to the [hospital] and their professional responsibility are one. . . . " This simple and powerful statement provides a sound framework for nurse-employer relationships. The hospital has the authority to hire and to fire nurses, but it does not have the authority to coerce nurses to act contrary to their professional judgments. To attempt to do so is not a legitimate use of institutional power and is an unjustifiable interference with professional practice. The hospital has the authority and responsibility to articulate administrative policies and to insist on the maintenance by nurses of approved standards of practice and of professional behavior. Hence, it cannot reprimand or discipline nurses whose conduct in fact is in keeping with institutional policies and established standards of practice. That is, an institution cannot give lip service to its own policies and standards while insisting that its employees act contrary to these policies and standards. In this situation, the hospital disciplined the nurses for behavior that was in keeping with standards of practice and statutory obligations in the jurisdiction.

In addition, the hospital, as an employer of professionals, has an obligation to permit and to facilitate professional practice. Among other things, this obligation includes the provision of space for the making of discretionary professional judgments As Flaherty points out, administrative authorities were aware of the short staffing in the Intensive Care Unit. Six nurses were on duty, two of whom were relief nurses who had no previous I.C.U. experience, and there were eight patients, five of whom were on respirators or ventilators and all of whom had monitoring equipment and/or indwelling tubes, drains and so forth. One of the patients required isolation technique for infection. In the nurses' professional judgment, they were not sure that they could care adequately for the patients already in the I.C.U. and they certainly could not care adequately for another seriously ill patient.

Although the nurses clearly communicated this judgment to their supervisor and to the physicians involved in the case, they apparently were not as clear about the rationale for their decision. Communication probably would have been enhanced considerably if they had followed hospital administrative policies and designated one nurse to act as team leader or charge nurse. That they did not do

so, as Flaherty notes, weakened their position in this conflict.

The physician did communicate clearly both his decision to admit Patient Mason to the Intensive Care Unit and his rationale for the decision (the patient was critically ill). However, he failed to take into account the nurses' assertion that the care the patient needed could not be provided in the I.C.U. at this time. Apparently, the physician thought that he was competent to make decisions about the nursing care needs of patients and the amount of time a nurse would have to devote to this patient to care for him adequately—an interesting but invalid assumption.

Evidence is presented in the case study that it took four physicians and one respiratory therapist to care for Patient Mason; therefore, it reasonably could be assumed that one nurse who already was caring for other seriously ill patients could not safely assume the responsibility of caring for this incoming patient. Of course, one can question the competence of the physicians to practice nursing. Physicians are not prepared educationally or experientially to practice nursing and this could account for the extraordinary number of physicians required to deliver nursing care to this one patient.

Apparently the physicians learned nothing from this experience. They did not demonstrate an appreciation for the complexity and demands of nursing care because they maintained in a subsequent investigation that the nurses could and should have accepted the patient in the I.C.U.

In summary, the I.C.U. nurses made a professional judgment and there is evidence to support the validity of that judgment. The hospital and nursing administration, by allowing an Intensive Care Unit to be staffed in that fashion, exhibit a lamentable disregard for institutional policies and standards of nursing practice. What is astounding is that the arbitration board upheld the hospital's decision to discipline the nurses for acting in a manner that, in their judgment, was consistent with their obligation to protect their patients.

Rethinking the Nurse's Role in "Do Not Resuscitate" Orders: A Clinical Policy Proposal in Nursing Ethics

Roland R. Yarling and Beverly J. McElmurry

The question of when to use and when not to use cardiopulmonary resuscitation (CPR) is a problem familiar to the practitioners of nursing and medicine. It characterizes the complex issues that have developed in health care as a result of the advance of medical technology and the emergence of patient autonomy. It is now technically possible to do many things that from a moral perspective sometimes should not be done.

In the last few years, it has been common for hospitals to establish institutional policy in regard to "do not resuscitate" (DNR) orders, although many still do not have such a policy. These policies address specific questions including

- the conditions under which a DNR decision may be made (the terminal status of the patient),
- who should make the decision when the patient is competent (the patient),
- who should make it when the patient is not competent (usually the health care team and the family),
- who should implement it (the physician), and
- how it should be implemented (in writing).

Frequently, it is the nursing staff in a hospital who requests that such policy be established because DNR orders have long been a source of conflict and frustration for nurses. The problem has been discussed repeatedly in the nursing literature from a nursing perspective.[1-8] These discussions usually focus on the problem of physicians who give only verbal orders, order "slow codes," will not honor a patient's desire not to be resuscitated, write an order for a competent patient without consulting the patient, and/or do not communicate with the nursing staff about the orders they write. It is in response to such problems that nurses have urged the adoption of a responsible institutional policy to regularize decisions and procedures pertaining to DNR orders.

Given the relatively widespread policy activity by hospitals on this matter in the late 1970s, it might have been concluded that the corner had been turned and that the problem was being resolved. Whatever illusions may have been entertained in that regard were effectively dispelled with Curtin's 1979 editorial.[9] More letters were received in response to that editorial than to any editorial in the history of the journal, according to the editor. Curtin said that CPR is often misused and that conflict over the matter frequently puts the nurse in a difficult position. The issue is still being hotly contested in hospitals. It takes only a 1-page editorial to unleash the frustration of nurses. Many hospitals, regardless of size, still have no DNR policy, and even in those that have a policy, problems continue largely because physicians frequently disregard it even when it has been approved by the medical board.

Furthermore, the issue has symbolic importance. The conflict between nursing and medicine around this issue is paradigmatic of the general nature of the relationship of nursing and medicine historically. Medical authoritarianism and unjustifiable institutional constraints have long served to impede the practice of nursing as defined by the profession and to render nurses less able to act responsible vis-à-vis the needs and rights of their patients. The conflict around DNR orders is a microcosm of the larger picture.

WHY ONLY THE PHYSICIAN

This suggests that a more fundamental reassessment of the situation is in order. What kind of a decision is a DNR decision? It is *not* a medical decision, although it usually follows from a medical judgment concerning the irreversible nature of the patient's disease. The DNR decision must be clearly distinguished from a medical judgment about the irreversibility of a disease. This medical judgment is a necessary, but not a sufficient, condition for the DNR decision. It is *not a nursing* decision, even though the nurse as well as the physician may need to assist the competent patient in reaching an authentic decision about what he or she chooses to have done. It is *not a legal* decision, but it has strong legal entailments. It is a *moral* decision; therefore, it properly belongs to the patient.

In the case of an incompetent patient, it is still a moral decision and should usually be made by the family in consultation with the health care team. If there is no family, the decision rests by default with the health care team, including the physician, nurse, and clergy. The important point to be made here, however, is that the majority of patients could make this decision for themselves if those working with the patient would initiate a discussion of the question before the patient deteriorates into incompetence. Because such discussions can be difficult, they are too often postponed until the patient becomes incompetent, and then the difficulties of making the decision for the patient must be faced.

To assert that DNR decisions are moral decisions rather than medical, nursing, or legal decisions does not mean that medical, nursing, and legal decisions do not have a moral dimension. The point is that a DNR decision should not be based on extraneous criteria but rather on the moral values of the patient—values concerning the meaning, sanctity, and quality of life.

The decision is a moral decision because the criteria for the decision are moral values. The nature of a decision is not determined by its consequences but by its criteria. For instance, a DNR decision

entails the withholding of medical treatment, and it will have consequences for the medical status of the patient, but that does not make it a medical decision. So also, a decision of Congress not to provide funding for a totally implantable artificial heart for everyone who might reasonably be judged to benefit significantly from it would have tremendous implications for the field of cardiology and for the medical status of cardiac patients. However, such a decision would not be a medical decision. It would be a political-moral decision based on political and moral criteria.

Thus, a DNR decision, which is rightly based on moral considerations such as the value of life itself, the quality of life under given conditions, and the acceptance or denial of the imminence of death by the patient, is a moral decision, not a medical decision. Such moral decisions involve questions of values that are not related to the special expertise of the physician, the nurse, or the attorney. The proper basis for their resolution is the patient's value system. Therefore, it is a decision that belongs to the patient.[10]

If a DNR decision is not a medical decision, a nursing decision, or a legal decision, but a moral decision to be made by the patient, what is the logic of the situation that dictates that the decision of the patient be implemented by a physician? Why should the physician alone be the person designated in DNR policies to write the DNR order?

The question pertains to whether the patient is competent or incompetent. Although the patient is referred to as the decision maker in DNR situations, the arguments that follow apply equally to situations in which the patient is incompetent and the DNR decision must be made by the family and/or the health care team.

The most obvious recourse in response to the question is the legal requirements. It may be argued that writing orders, DNR orders in this case, is, by law, a physician function. The law on this question varies from state to state, but the Illinois Nursing Act does not say that writing orders is not a nursing function. It says that nursing shall not "include those acts of medical diagnosis or prescription of therapeutic or corrective measures which are properly performed only by physicians . . .," (*The Illinois Nursing Act of 1975*, Ill Rev Stat tit 91, §35.32-35.57), but it does not designate which acts of medical diagnosis or prescription are properly performed only by physicians. There is clearly much room for discussion in Illinois.

Furthermore, regardless of the wording of specific nursing acts in various states, legal requirements are often nothing more than a recognition of the way things have usually been done. This is what has been referred to as making medical law on the basis of the "may I-do you?" syndrome. The physician goes to the court and says, "May I do thus and so?" The court says, "Do you, ie, the medical community, ordinarily do thus and so?" The physician says, "We do." The court says, "Then you may." According to this model, the law deals more with the issue of what is than what ought to be. Appeal is implicitly made to the principle of the existing community standard of care.

Mill and Mill cogently observed that "laws and systems of polity always begin by recognizing the relation they find already existing between individuals. They convert what was a mere physical fact into a legal right, and give it the sanction of society."[11(p130)] But in so doing, the law may well sanction unjust situations.

From a moral point of view, can any good reasons be given for the status quo? Can a law or policy that designates the physician as the only person who can write a DNR order be morally justified? It is commonly stated and widely held that the physician in charge of a patient is fully responsible for the patient's full treatment and care. But this is not the case either in fact or law.

The physician in charge is responsible only for the patient's *medical* diagnosis and treatment, much of which must be implemented by the nurse; the nurse, on the other hand, is responsible for the patient's *nursing* diagnosis and treatment (*Darling v. Charleston Community Memorial Hospital*, 50 [Ill App 2d 253; 200 NE 2nd 149; (1965) *aff'd* 33 Ill 2d 327; 211 NE 2d 253 [1964] *cert denied*; and *Utter v United Hospital Center, Inc, and Lawrence Mills*, 236 SE [2d] 213 [WVa] [1977]),[12] in addition to implementing the physician's orders (or more properly, the physicians prescriptions). And nursing diagnosis and treatment are based on independent nursing judgments. If responsibility for the patient's diagnosis, treatment, and care falls primarily into two domains—the physician's responsibility for *medical* diagnosis and treatment and the nurse's responsibility for *nursing* diagnosis and treatment—the logical question is, again, why should this decision of the patient be implemented by the physician?

One viewpoint is that this task rightly belongs to the physician because the patient's decision is based on the medical judgment of the physician about the irreversibility of the disease. To the contrary, however, this medical judgment is not the *basis* of the patient's decision but is a *precondition* of the decision, like the disease itself. The proper *basis* of the patient's decision is the value system of the patient.

Another viewpoint is that the physician should write the order because the physician is usually the person to discuss the question with the patient. However, this assumption is questionable both in terms of what does happen and in terms of what should happen. In fact, patients probably discuss this matter more often with the nursing staff than with the medical staff.

With reference to what should happen, the best person to discuss the matter with the patient may or may not be the responsible physician because the decision is a moral decision based on the patient's value system. Technical skill does not translate into moral wisdom, so the best person to talk with the patient may be the physician, the nurse, clergy, a family member, or any other person with the appropriate sensitivity and a trusting relationship with the patient.

WHY NOT THE NURSE ALSO?

Since there is no logical reason for confining this function to the physician, the responsibility for writing a DNR order and documenting the discussion with the patient in the progress notes should be, rather, a responsibility shared by the responsible physician and the responsible nurse, either the primary nurse or the head nurse, depending on the system of nursing care used. The writing of a DNR order should be regarded as an *overlapping function* of medicine and nursing, which may be performed by either the physician or the nurse depending on the situation. The idea that the nurse as well as the physician should be authorized to write DNR orders seems so eminently reasonable that one must wonder how the present arrangement endured so long.

In view of the roles of the nurse and the physician in relation to patients with terminal illnesses, and given the nonmedical nature of a DNR decision, it must be concluded that the function of writing a DNR order, once the decision is made by the patient or whoever makes the decision in the case of an incompetent patient, belongs at least as much to the role of the nurse as to the role of the physician.

The issue here is not professional interest in territoriality. It is how the patient will be best served. It is apparent from experience and from the literature that the long-standing problems that nursing has had in this regard have generally been rooted in the frequent failure of physicians to function responsibly in writing DNR orders. When this happens, the nurse is often put in a difficult position, and most importantly, the patient is not well served. *The interest of the patient will be best served if the responsible nurse, as well as the responsible physician, is authorized by the DNR policy of the hospital to write DNR orders.*

This argument is strengthened by the following considerations: First, it is often the nurse who initiates a discussion with the physician about the possibility of a DNR order because it is often the nurse, due to the frequent and ongoing interaction with the patient, to whom the patient will first make known the desire to have treatment cease and to be allowed to die. The nature of the nurse's role is such that these conversations often occur more naturally with the nurse than with the physician. In such situations, it makes good sense for the nurse, after consultation with the physician and other appropriate persons, to write the DNR order and its justification in the progress notes. The decision of the patient is more likely to be honored in this arrangement than if the nurse must communicate the patient's wish to the physician, who must then take up the matter with the patient and then write the order. Too frequently, physicians cannot be persuaded to discuss the question with the patient, and conversely, the patient has a notoriously difficult time discussing anything with the physician during the brief daily visit. This problem becomes more acute for the patient with terminal disease.

Second, regardless of who writes the DNR order, it is almost inevitably the nurse who carries it out by deliberate inaction. Because of the frequent failure of physicians to communicate with nurses about DNR orders that they write and to provide justification for the orders in the progress notes, nurses are sometimes confronted with DNR orders without any supporting information.

This dilemma is compounded because it is not unheard of for a physician to write a DNR order for a competent patient without discussing it with the patient. Thus, when there is a DNR order that has not been discussed with the nurse nor justified in the progress notes, the nurse can never be sure that the patient has consented to it. If the patient has cardiac arrest before the nurse has the opportunity to clarify the situation, what should be done? Should the order be honored in the hope that the patient has consented to it or should it be disregarded, running the risk of violating the patient's decision and incurring the physician's wrath? If nurses were authorized to write DNR orders, the incidence of such situations would be reduced and the probability that the patient's decision would be implemented without complication would be greatly increased.

Third, the authorization of the nurse to write DNR orders is consistent with the definition of nursing set forth by the American Nurses' Association (ANA) in its *social policy statement*, which defines nursing as "the diagnosis and treatment of human responses to actual or potential health problems."[13] Although this definition has its origin in the language of the 1972 Nurse Practice Act of New York State, its present widespread currency within the profession seems to be largely due to its incorporation in this official ANA document. The proposal that nurses as well as physicians be authorized to write DNR orders is consistent with the understanding of nursing embodied in this widely cited definition (C. Murphy, EdD, written communication, April 16, 1982).

The decision of the patient to refuse resuscitation efforts is a "human response" to terminal illness and the resultant, radically reduced quality of life. The "diagnosis" of that response as coherent and genuine and the "treatment" based on that diagnosis, ie, writing a DNR order and the corresponding documentation of the patient's decision in the progress notes, are clearly within the domain of nursing as defined by the ANA. Even so, how does the fact that this function falls within nursing's definition of itself support the argument that the patient is better served when the nurse is also authorized to write DNR orders? The broader argument is that patients will be better served if nurses are allowed to practice nursing within the scope of nursing without the constraints of medical authority.

The medical profession must be reassured by the enthusiastic support by the nursing profession of a definition of nursing that confines nursing's focus to the human response to disease and illness. But even this modest definition of nursing clearly encompasses the writing of DNR orders. Can the medical profession be anything but grateful for such a proposal, which promotes a definition of nursing that is so modest in its relation to medicine and proposes to relieve the profession of sole responsibility for such a burdensome task?

It can be suggested that only the physician is sufficiently responsible to carry the burden of such a grave act. It is the height of incongruity to suggest that the nurse, who must bear the life and death responsibility for initiating CPR when there is no DNR order, is somehow not sufficiently responsible to write a DNR order in the patient's chart once the patient has made the decision.

But perhaps nurses do not *want* this responsibility. This should not occasion any great surprise. Probably physicians have not wanted the responsibility either, which may be, in part, why they have carried it out so poorly. It is irrelevant whether nurses want the responsibility. What nurses want is not the basis of the argument. Patients would be better served if nurses shared the responsibility with physicians. In light of this and light of the frustrations that nurses have experienced with physicians in regard to DNR orders, nurses will willingly assume the responsibility even though they may not "want" it.[12]

NOT FREE TO BE MORAL

Why should there be such a controversy over what may appear to be such a small matter? The answer is that this is one of several areas in patient care in which there are vestiges of the historical devaluation of the work of the nurse and violation of the autonomy of the nurse by physicians and hospitals, generally to the detriment of the patient. Ashley has eloquently documented the history of the oppression, exploitation, and devaluation of nurses by physicians and hospitals.[14] (This book should be required reading for every nursing student and perhaps, more importantly, for every medical student. A 4th-year medical student told us recently that he did not understand why nurses are so angry at physicians. We told him that his perplexity as a neophyte is understandable and recommended reading Ashley as a sure cure.)

The most recent witness to this reality is contained in the public hearing testimony before the National Commission on Nursing. Four of the five nursing problems most frequently mentioned corroborate Ashley's perception:

- the "status and image of nursing,"
- the "effective management of the nursing resource (staffing, scheduling, and salary),"
- the "relationship among nursing [staff] medical staff, and hospital administration,"
- and the "maturing of nursing as a self-determining profession."[15]

In its initial report, the Commission commented on "the fundamental unresolved nursing issues. One of the most fundamental of these is lack of recognition for nurses' worth in patient care."[16] One manifestation of this problem is the assignment of nursing responsibility in patient care without the authority necessary to fulfill that responsibility. The nurse is given a task that cannot be done without the pro forma cooperation of the physician; then it is often impossible to obtain the necessary cooperation. An excellent example is in the management of pain. Pain management is de facto a nursing function, regardless of its de jure status, but it cannot be performed without the pro forma cooperation of the physician, who sometimes does not order adequate medication and sometimes cannot be contacted when the order needs to be changed. The necessary authority is inappropriately vested solely with the physician. Because these kinds of situations abound in nursing practice, nurses have been aptly characterized as "the responsible powerless."[17]

In many situations involving DNR orders, pain management, or other aspects of patient care, Curtin's words are true: "Nurses are not free to practice nursing."[18]

The nurse in these situations is often not free to be moral, that is, a nurse is often not free to honor the commitment to the patient, whether that commitment takes the form of responding to the patient's request for no further treatment, of keeping the patient free from unnecessary suffering, or of performing whatever functions maybe required by professional standards of nursing and by excellence in nursing practice.

The fundamental moral predicament of hospital nurses is that they often are not free to be moral because they often are not free to exercise their commitment to the patient through excellence in patient care. Legal and institutional constraints hinder the practice of nursing sometimes in minor matters and sometimes in major matters of life and death. For the sake of patient care, the nurse must be set free to practice nursing, ie, set free to be moral.

There appears to be a growing consensus on this point among those concerned with nursing ethics. This concern found its way into the literature in 1978, for the first time, when Davis and Aroskar[19] asked the bold and fateful question, "Can the nurse be ethical?" The language is different from that of Curtin[18] in 1980, which was cited previously, but the point is the same. Most recently, in 1981, Mitchell argued that "nurses are unable to maintain their integrity."[8(p7)]

This analysis has implicit assumptions that need to be expressed. On the first level, the argument is that the interest of the patient is best served when the responsible nurse, as well as the responsible physician, is authorized to write DNR orders. The assumption here is that the interest of the patient lies in the preservation and actualization of patient autonomy. The policy objective is to serve the autonomy of the patient. Patient autonomy is honored when patients are effectively given final decision-making authority over their own care. Because the conditions of autonomy are often compromised by illness, special care must be taken to preserve patient autonomy. This is morally necessary because autonomy is the first principle of morality,[20] and it is psychologically important because patients, in the alien environment of the hospital, often experience a traumatic sense of loss of control and thereby a loss of social well-being as well as physical well-being.

Patients retain ultimate control over their own care insofar as those charged with that care involve them in significant decisions regarding their own care, provide them with all relevant information as a basis for decision making, enable them to reach decisions consistent with their considered and settled values, and then implement those decisions responsibly. The authorization of the responsible nurse, as well as the responsible physician, to write DNR orders will serve to promote the patient's autonomy in these ways. *If this argument holds, then the hospital is morally obligated to authorize the responsible nurse to write DNR orders.* If the preservation of the patient's autonomy is morally obligatory, then so is the best available means to that end. One cannot be obligated to the end without also being obligated to the best available means.

On the second level, the argument is that because of the historic domination of nursing by medical authoritarianism and repressive institutional policy, the nurse is often not free to be moral in the sense that she is often not free to exercise her professional commitment to the patient. The assumption here is that the patient will be best served if the nurse is empowered to actualize professional commitment to the patient. This assumption is not based on the further assumption that nurses are more virtuous than physicians or more committed to the well-being of the patient but rather on the assumption that the patient will be best served by a *balance of power around the bedside.* This precludes any one professional group from the unrestrained pursuit of its own interest at the expense of the patient. The presumed necessity for this balance of power rests on the same dim but realistic view of human nature that gave rise to the division and balance of power in government

in democratic to protect the citizen against the tyranny of the state.

SOCIAL ETHICS AND INSTITUTIONAL REFORM

The business of setting the nurse free to practice nursing, ie, free to be moral, must proceed on various fronts. It is partly a matter of nurses achieving internal or psychological freedom after generations of socialization into a subordinate role both as nurses and women;[21] it is partly a matter of nurses acquiring the appropriate paradigm to understand the nature of health care and their role in it,[22] and it is partly a matter of institutional reform. It is the latter that is the concern of these reflections. The reform of the hospital as the major institutional context of and constraint on the practice of nursing is a matter of the utmost urgency from a moral perspective. Historically, nursing ethics has taken the form of individual ethics with a focus on the individual practitioner and the nurse-patient relationship. The time has come when an adequate nursing ethic must address the problem of the structures and policies of the institutions that constitute the context of nursing practice. A nursing ethic that addresses these kinds of concerns is a social ethic, ie, an ethic concerned with the moral obligations of institutions rather than with the moral obligations of individuals.

As the institutional context of practice more and more determines the nature and quality of the nurse-patient relationship and the quality of nursing care that is possible to provide, nursing ethics must become, in part, social ethics, addressing those institutional constraints that keep nurses from practicing nursing in accord with professional standards and the interest of the patient. This theme of the importance of social or institutional ethics has recently been quite pronounced in the medical ethics literature. Since the bureaucratization of medical care has become an acknowledged fact,[23] there is growing attention to the necessity for hospitals and institutions to assume appropriate responsibility for the moral dilemmas current in the practice of medicine. Hospitals are being challenged to consider themselves as moral agents with significant moral responsibilities.[24-26]

Various institutional reforms would contribute to setting nurses free from the constraints of medical authority and institutional policies. One reform that is often suggested is upgrading the status of nursing administration within the power structure of the hospital. This may be accomplished, at least in part, by moving the director of nursing service to a vice presidential level and adjusting the salary to a level commensurate with the salary of the chiefs of staff of the various medical services. These are important strategies in setting nursing free from medical authority in the hospital, but no less important is the kind of reform that directly affects the clinical practitioners of nursing rather than nursing administrators.

It is essential to formulate specific policies that will invest the clinical nurse with the authority to perform, without constraint, those responsibilities that, by their nature, belong to the role of the nurse, such as requesting psychiatric or social work consultation,[27] writing DNR orders, and the writing of pain medication orders. (The federal law limiting the distribution of regulated substances to physicians is a legal constraint impeding the responsible practice of nursing in the management of patients with pain and will require reform to free nurses to be fully responsible to their patients [C. Duffy, personal communication, April 16, 1982].) This type of reform must proceed clinical issue by clinical issue as nurses claim the authority that is necessary in specific types of clinical situations to responsibly fulfill their commitments to patients.

The liberation of nurses and their enfranchisement as moral agents and autonomous providers in the patient care enterprise need to be accomplished at the clinical as well as at the administrative level. Situations requiring DNR decisions have long been a source of conflict and frustration for the nurse because the nurse has been "the responsible powerless." Policies and laws that legitimate this state of affairs are without justification and must be viewed as a hindrance to excellence in patient care. They are in need of reform.

One obvious place to begin is with hospital DNR policy. Hospitals that have yet to establish such a policy should consider authorizing the responsible nurse as well as the responsible physician to write DNR orders. Hospitals that have already established policy only to find that it is frequently not honored by physicians should consider the proposed reform as a way to help resolve these ongoing problems. Hospitals, as institutions that constitute the context of practice for both medicine and nursing, have a moral obligation to establish policies that require those procedures most likely to serve the interest of the patient.

The DNR policy is a clear instance of the type of moral issue in nursing in which the resolution is dependent on the assumption of moral responsibility by the hospital. Nursing ethics, as social ethics, calls for the moral maturation of the hospital as a responsible social institution. Clinical nurses who practice in hospitals and are embroiled in these issues must make themselves heard, and nursing administration must provide them with firm support. The 1965 ANA position paper on nursing education[28] set the terms for freeing nursing *education* from the domination of medical authoritarianism and the hospital. It now remains to free nursing *practice* from this same debilitating domination, through the reform of institutional policy that regulates the relation of medicine to nursing and impedes the responsible practice of nursing. If nursing fails to free itself from this historical bondage to medical authoritarianism, it will fail the patient as well as itself. As Ashley[14] has shown it is not only power that corrupts, it is also powerlessness.

REFERENCES

1. Alder DC: No code—The unwritten order. *Heart and Lung* 1977; 6(2): 213.
2. Aroskar M. et al: The nurse and orders not to resuscitate. *Hastings Cent Rep* 1977; 7(4): 27–28.
3. Berg DL: The right to die dilemma. *RN* 1977; 40(7): 1–7.
4. Cawley MA: Euthanasia: Should it be a choice? *Am J Nurs* 1977; 77: 859–861.
5. Johnson P: The long, hard dying of Joe Rodriques. *Am J Nurs* 1977; 77: 54–57.
6. Regan A: Nursing service problem: Verbal orders. *Regan Rep* 1977; 17(10): 4.
7. Steidl SN: Have you ever regretted doing the "right" thing? *RN* 1979; 42(8): 78D-78F.
8. Mitchell C: New directions in nursing ethics. *Massachusetts Nurse* 1981; 50(7): 7–10.
9. Curtin Ll.: The prostitution of CPR. *Supervisor Nurse* 1979; 10(8): 7.
10. Yarling RR: Ethical analysis of a nursing problem: The scope of nursing practice in disclosing the truth to terminal patients. *Supervisor Nurse* 1978; 9(5): 40–50 and 9(6): 28–34.
11. Mill JS, Mill IIT: *Essays on Sex Equality*, Rossi AS (ed). Chicago, University of Chicago, 1970, p 130.
12. Gewirth A: *Reason and Morality*. Chicago, University of Chicago, 1978. pp 49–52.

13. *Nursing—A Social Policy Statement.* Kansas City, Mo, American Nurses' Association, 1980, p 9.

14. Ashley JA: *Hospitals, Paternalism, and the Role of the Nurse.* New York. Teachers' College Press, Columbia University, 1976.

15. National Commission on Nursing: *Summary of Public Hearings.* Chicago. Hospital Research and Educational Trust. 1981, p 5.

16. National Commission on Nursing: *Initial Report and Preliminary Recommendations.* Chicago. Hospital Research and Educational Trust, 1981, p 10.

17. White AJ: Forum on DNR policy. University of Illinois College of Nursing, Mar, 1982.

18. Curtin L: Ethical issues in nursing practice and education, in *Ethical Issues in Nursing and Nursing Education.* New York, NLN, 1980, p 27.

19. Davis A, Aroskar M: *Ethical Dilemmas and Nursing Practice.* New York, Appleton-Century-Crofts, 1978, p 43.

20. Immanuel K: *Foundations of the Metaphysics of Morals,* Beck LW (trans). Indianapolis, Bobbs-Merrill, 1959, p 59.

21. Muff J (ed): *Socialization, Sexism, and Stereotyping: Women's Issues in Nursing.* St. Louis, CV Mosby, 1982.

22. Aroskar MA: Are nurses' mind sets compatible with ethical practice? *Top Clin Nurs.* 1982; 4(1): 22–32.

23. Mechanic D: *The Growth of Bureaucratic Medicine.* New York, Wiley-Interscience, 1976.

24. Pellegrino ED: Hospitals as moral agents, in *Humanism and the Physician.* Knoxville, Tenn, University of Tennessee, 1979.

25. Pellegrino ED: The hippocratic oath revisited, in *Humanism and the Physician.* Knoxville, Tenn, University of Tennessee, 1979.

26. DeGeorge RT: The moral responsibility of the hospital. *J Med Philos* 1982; 7(1): 87–100.

27. Donnelly G: Anatomy of a conflict. *Supervisor Nurse* 1975; 6(11): 28–38.

28. American Nurses' Association: ANA's first position on education for nursing. *Am J Nurs* 1965; 65(12): 106–111.

The Moral Foundation of Nursing

Roland R. Yarling and Beverly J. McElmurry

The moral foundation of nursing is crucial and determinative of the well-being of the profession. Professional ethics deals with matters that lie at the very core of a nurse's professional life.

Nursing ethics is discussed here in the context of nursing *practice*. The *conclusion* is presented first and is followed by supporting considerations. The conclusion, or proposition to be argued, is that *nurses are often not free to be moral*. A couple of qualifying statements are necessary to properly circumscribe this proposition. First, it is confined to those nurses who practice in hospitals. While it is true that important nursing activities take place in other settings,[1] the majority of all practicing nurses are found in hospitals. Second, the concept of freedom, as in "not free to be moral," is not a reference to transcendental freedom of the *will*, for freedom in this sense is a necessary condition of even being a moral agent and having moral problems. The reference is rather to freedom of *action* in the sense that acts are free from unforced choice.

The idea that nurses are not free to be moral was first raised by Davis and Aroskar in *Ethical Dilemmas and Nursing Practice*.[2] In a bold and pioneering chapter, entitled "Professional Ethics and Institutional Constraints in Nursing Practice," they identify several organizational and social constraints in hospitals that impede the ethical practice of nursing. These constraints include the role and social position of the physician and the nurse in the bureaucratic hospital's social system, the role and power of the nursing leadership in the system, sexism, and paternalism. The crucial question as to the nurse and ethical dilemmas is, given these factors, *can the nurse be ethical?*[1(pp42–43)]

The problem of nurses' freedom to be moral was also addressed by Curtin.[3] Clearly, she wrestled with the same problem when she stated that "ethical problems arise from the usurpation of the legitimate authority of the nurse over *nursing* decisions regarding care. The major ethical dilemma in nursing is that nurses are not free to practice nursing."[3(pp22–23,25)]

Further specifying the proposition, the moral situation of hospital nurses finds expression in a variety of clinical, patient care problems common to hospital nursing. Among these are care of patients in pain, cardiopulmonary resuscitation, withholding or withdrawing of life-sustaining treatment, informed consent procedures, refusal of consent to treatment, use of placebos, harmful care by another practitioner, and professional control of information. These problems are the locus of frequently recurring institutional conflicts involving nurses. The constitutive elements or preexisting conditions of these conflicts are

- established standards of nursing care as determined by the profession;
- consequent commitment of the nurse to the autonomy and well-being of the patient;
- responsibility of the hospital for all patients who receive care under its auspices;
- nurse's knowledge of actual or potential harm to the patient;
- divergence of the interest of the patient from the interest of the hospital or one of its power structures;
- employee status of the nurse in relation to the hospital;
- physician power structure in the hospital;
- nurse's subcollegial relation to the physician; and

Yarling, R. R., & McElmurry, B. J. (1986). The moral foundation of nursing. *Advances in Nursing Science, 8* (2), 63–73.

- vulnerability of the nurse to harmful action by the hospital as the employer.

These are the complex, preexisting conditions out of which conflicts arise around specific clinical issues. When these situations, with their potential for conflict, are translated into the perspective of nurses, they may be described in terms of the several obligations encompassed by the nursing role: to the patient, to the employer, to the physician, to the profession, to nursing administration, to the nurse as a moral being, etc.

The moral situation of nurses is most poignantly revealed when they perceive that the right to freedom and well-being of patients in their care and treatment is threatened or violated by a physician, another nurse, or some other health care provider for whom the hospital is responsible. In such instances, nurses experience conflict, with respect to their choice of action, between the prima facie right of the patient and the prima facie right of the hospital. The prima facie right of patients, as perceived by nurses, is to freedom and well-being with regard to treatment and care in the hospital; the prima facie right of the hospital, as perceived by the hospital in such situations, is usually the right to institutional maintenance, broadly construed, which is instrumental to its primary purpose of care for all its patients in general. This responsibility for and right to institutional maintenance for the sake of all patients served may be construed in such a way that it comes into conflict with the interest of particular patients or all patients in a particular way. This produces conflict for nurses because their role embodies obligations to both patients and the hospital.

At stake in this conflict, for nurses, is nothing less than the nurse-patient relationship. The nature of that relationship is fundamental to the nursing process and to the human quality of a patient's hospital experience. Furthermore, it is the necessary foundation for a nursing ethic. The conflict relative to this issue is acutely problematic for nurses because the hospital is usually able, as the employer, to force nurses to act in compliance with what it perceives to be in its interest. The threatened retaliation of a hospital against nurses, when they act or contemplate action on behalf of patients whose rights are in conflict with the interest of the hospital, generally causes a forced choice to refrain from such action.

Nurses then are not free to be moral in the sense of not being free from forced choice. They are not free to fulfill their moral obligation to the patient when the interest of the patient is in conflict with the interest of the hospital. They are not free to act apart from the risk of serious harm to their own well-being. They are forced to choose between patient interest and their own self-interest, between their commitment to the autonomy and well-being of the patient and the autonomy and well-being of their careers, between moral integrity and professional survival. The fundamental moral predicament of nurses is that they often are not free to be moral because they are deprived of the free exercise of moral agency.

The moral predicament of nurses arises from their commitment to patients, and that commitment is grounded in nurses' status as moral agents. Were nurses simply the instrument of those around them, as they are often assumed to be, then they would have no moral problem and no sense of not being free. An incident demonstrating this point occurred a couple of years ago when the first author, two nurses, and a physician formed a panel for a freshman medical school class in medical ethics. Under discussion was the role of the nurse in disclosing information to terminal patients. The question was, if the physician of a terminal patient has ordered that no information regarding the patient's prognosis be disclosed to the patient, and if the patient asks the nurse about the prognosis, what is the nurse's duty?

Every medical student who spoke in class that day held that the nurse had a moral duty to disclose and that the physician's order was unjustifiable. The physician on the panel, however, argued that the nurse had no such duty. One of the students asked, why not? The physician replied, "Because the nurse's relationship with the patient is different than the physician's. It does not require independent moral judgment by the nurse." That is to say, nurses have no duty to make autonomous moral judgments about what their relationships with patients require because their relationships with patients are different. They have no moral status. In this sample, the nurse-patient relationship—the moral foundation of nursing and of a nursing ethic—is negated and denied moral status.

HISTORICAL PERSPECTIVE

Having explicated this thesis, an examination of the historical perspective of the issue is in order. In its present form, the commitment of the nurse to the patient is a relatively recent phenomenon. This is not to say that there was ever a time when the nurse was not committed to the patient, but in earlier days that commitment was considerably diluted by the nurse's relationship to the hospital and to the physician. The following admonitions provide insight into how far removed current practicing nurses are from those pioneer nurses who established schools of nursing in the nineteenth century.

> Absolute and *unquestioning obedience* must be the foundation of the nurse's work, and to this end complete subordination of the individual to the work as a whole is as necessary for her as for the soldier.[4(pp96–97)] (Emphasis added.)

> Implicit, *unquestioning obedience* is one of the first lessons a probationer must learn, for this is a quality that will be expected from her in her professional capacity for all future use.[5(p57)] (Emphasis added.)

Even after the turn of the century, the theme continued.

> It is expected of all in training to do what they are told; no more, no less.[6(p452)]

> *Obedience* is the first law and the very cornerstone of good nursing. The first and most helpful criticism I ever received from a doctor was when he told me that I was supposed to be simply an intelligent machine for the purpose of carrying out his orders.[7(p394)] (Emphasis added.)

> Loyalty to the physician is one of the duties demanded of every nurse, not solely because the physician is her superior officer, but chiefly because the confidence of the patient in his physician is one of the important elements in the management of his illness.[8(p25)]

> She [a nurse] has a duty of charity as a faithful servant to a master to protect the good name and reputation of the physician under whom she is working.[9(p149)]

These quotations convey a sense of the difference in the professional identity of early twentieth century nurses and their contemporary counterparts. For nurses to be free to be moral, two necessary, but not sufficient, occurrences must take place: (1) the emergence of a strong sense of professional autonomy and (2) a shift in the locus of accountability from the physician to the patient. The evolution of a professional identity and commitment, which illustrates the above factors, began in nursing by the end

of World War II. Perhaps the most symbolic evidence of the changes that were afoot is the American Nurses' Association's *Code for Nurses*.[10] While this code, like most professional codes, has probably had minimal impact on practice, it is a reasonably accurate register of the changes that were taking place.

The first version of the code was adopted in 1950,[10] and the fourth and most recent one was adopted in 1976.[11–14] In that 25-year period, each version progressively reflected two emergent factors—professional autonomy and shift in accountability.

Present-day ideology of nursing, emphasizing nursing commitments to patients and autonomy in the exercise of that commitment, is a very recent development in the history of nursing. Nevertheless, it has had a pervasive and far-reaching effect. For example, few nurses graduating from basic nursing education programs in the past ten years think they owe physicians anything other than professional excellence in practice. Even the staunchest members of the old guard have been reindoctrinated with the new ideology.

So pervasive is this new ideology that it is surprising it is not being carried out in practice. The reality is that the ideological revolution in education has been a revolution in theory only; it has not pervaded the domain of practice. Nurses are not able to actualize their commitment to patients in the practice setting when the freedom and well-being of the patient is in conflict with the interest of the hospital. "Oh no," you say, "that can't be. Student nurses today are taught that nursing requires patient advocacy, that patient care comes first." Yes, that is what they are taught verbally and overtly; but in a thousand nonverbal and covert ways, they are taught by clinical example the limits of that advocacy. They learn quickly, by observing others, how to interpret the verbal message in terms of "what nurses do" and "what nurses do not do." They learn that their commitment to patients must be carefully contained.

Graduates from basic nursing education programs are psychologically part of the health care subculture, even though they verbalize patient-centered ideology. The nonverbal socialization process in the practice context is as powerful and thorough as the verbal and ideological socialization in the education context. In its construction of a new identity for the neophyte professional, it ultimately prevails. Professional nurses are conceived in moral contradiction and born in compromise. There is a profound moral dissonance between nursing education and nursing practice. This discord extends to the core of professional identity and leaves nurses essentially morally unintegrated professionals who are not self-determining, moral agents.

There is persuasive evidence, some systematic and some anecdotal, that this is the case. First, Swider et al[15] reported on a classroom exercise that examined the priorities reflected in the decisions reported by students when presented a case depicting the ethical dilemma in nursing. The exercise dealt with a primary nurse who was aware that the hospital was covering up the death of a patient as a result of a tenfold overprescription of a drug used in chemotherapy. The students were 175 seniors in baccalaureate nursing programs in 16 midwestern colleges and universities. Working in groups of five each, the students arrived at a course of action to deal with the dilemma. Categories for classifying responses were derived from the literature[16–18] in nursing ethics.

The categories used in content analysis of responses were (1) patient-centered responses, (2) physician-centered responses, and (3) bureaucratic-centered responses. The small groups of students made from 3 to 17 decisions trying to resolve the dilemma, with a mean number of 8 decisions per group. Of the 1,163 decisions, 9% were patient-centered, 19% were physician-centered, and 60% were bureaucratic centered. Selected characteristics of participants were examined for relationships to group responses. Group responses did not differ significantly according to education, clinical experience, previous experience with a similar dilemma, or RN status of group members. Students agreed on the first steps to take to resolve the dilemma, but failed to achieve a consensus on where the nurse's responsibility ended.

CASE STUDIES

Although the literature has oblique references to the conflict over the problem of nurse ethics, Stenberg says, "These cases are rarely documented in the nursing literature, due in part to a reluctance to confront or to publicize conflict within the profession or those between nursing and an agency.[19(p11)] One of the few specific cases in the literature is presented by Donnelly et al.[20] It concerns the firing of a director of nursing over conflicts concerning the right of nurses to practice nursing. Many nurses in the agency protested the firing on the basis that "Both medicine and administration had repeatedly interfered in the rights to practice professional nursing."[20(p28)]

In the final paragraph, they observe: "The price of speaking out can be a difficult one to pay. Some of those who resigned have been discredited in references. Others have been subjected to humiliating . . . job interviews. . . . the rewards for prudence are great."[20(p28)]

Donnelly, Mengel, and King resigned in protest, and later collaborated on this article, which explains why it was written and why many others like it are not.

Another case illustrating the "hospitalonian captivity" of nursing was discussed by McGuire.[21] She related a situation in which a patient, in her professional judgment, was being medically mismanaged and subsequently died. Her lament was that she did not insist on a consultation that might have saved the patient's life. She says, "Never again will I back down before a tradition-encrusted system or an ego-driven physician when a patient's well-being or dignity is at stake."[21(p56)]

A third case reported involved a physician who ordered a nurse not to disclose to a terminal patient her prognosis, even though the patient had asked the nurse direct questions.[22] The final lines in that case presentation indicate the conflict as the nurse followed the physician's order:

> She was very uncomfortable lying to a patient who had come to trust her. However . . . she was hesitant to act contrary to the wishes of the family, the physician, and the head nurse; and she was not sure what her legal rights were in the situation.[22(p28)]

It is difficult to imagine a more insidious violation of the fiduciary nature of the nurse-patient relationship than that in which this nurse found herself.

A fourth case, related by Curtin,[3] involved a young nurse having repeated confrontations with a resident over medication orders which the nurse repeatedly observed to be inappropriate and dangerous. Finally, a patient died from respiratory failure, apparently from an overdose of medication causing respiratory depression. The nurse's efforts to discover what had actually happened were systematically frustrated. The next day as she sat alone at a lunch table, she was joined by the chiefs of pharmacy, medicine, and staff; the director of nursing; and the hospital administrator. "To say the least, these were not the people with whom she ordinarily ate lunch. It seemed she was upset about something, they said. It seemed that the pressures of working on acute medicine were too much for her and that she needed to be transferred to a less demanding ward where she could recuperate from the rigors of acute medicine."[2(p21)] She was immediately transferred and subsequently harassed until she finally resigned. A hospital sometimes can be very persuasive.

There are also a couple of cases documented by Creighton[23] in the legal context of whistle-blowing. A staff nurse refused to carry out the following order: "Give the patient 200 mg of Demerol [meperidine hydrochloride] and 25 mg of reserpine, IV, and discharge her immediately." When the nursing supervisor and the director of nursing supported the staff nurse's refusal, the physician on the hospital board said he would have all three of them fired. Though not relating the denouement of that situation, Creighton, in commenting on it, referred to the significant legal case of *Rafferty vs. Philadelphia Psychiatric Center*. Mrs. Rafferty was a psychiatric nurse who was fired after her criticism of the medical and patient care at the center appeared in the newspaper. "During the time of her employment she had repeatedly tried to secure improvements by reports made through hospital channels. . . . While the nurse's comments did cause controversy, the court said: 'Mrs. Rafferty was engaging in precisely the sort of free and vigorous expression that the First Amendment was designed to protect.'"[23(p11)] And Creighton, commenting on the general situation, said, "The many, many tough situations in which the consciences of nurses ache and where nurses writhe in frustration over wrongs in patient care that they cannot at the moment change, set the stage for more whistle-blowing by nurses."[23(p57)]

In addition to these published cases, there are other kinds of anecdotal evidence. In teaching ethics to nursing students, nursing instructors have numerous conversations with them about such matters. Even older nurses volunteer stories about ethics from early in their careers about patients who suffered serious injury or harm, which they thought might have been prevented if they had acted more aggressively. They are stories in which the nurses felt helpless and painfully compromised. Why do nurses tell these stories? Because they represent the symbolic, socializing events through which their moral predicament was revealed to them in its full-blown dimensions. Although largely repressed, these are the experiences around which young nurses formulate their professional identity, however fractured that image may be.

In this same vein, the president of a state nursing association tells of receiving calls in the middle of the night, not just once or twice, but several times, from nurses who were too frightened to tell their names. They wanted to tell her a story about some experience that was wrenching their souls, but about which they felt either too powerless or too fearful to do anything. The pathos and tragedy of nurses whose moral instincts have been so repressed that they are divided within themselves is a concern that must eventually be addressed.

PRESENT-DAY REALITIES

Returning to the original proposition, how can it be said that nurses are not free to fulfill their moral obligation to patients? They can do whatever they choose to do. That is true in a sense. They are in some marginal capacity free, free at least to be heroic. And insofar as they are in some limited sense free, they are also in some limited sense culpable, for the risk attached to an action does not completely cancel the obligation to perform the action. If it did, nurses would have no moral problems, but unfortunately they do.

There is also a real sense in which nurses are not free. They are not free in the same sense that a victim is not free when a robber says, "Your money or your life." The victim can make a choice here, but one could not say the individual is free. The risks involved when nurses choose to act on behalf of patients whose rights are in conflict with the interest of the hospital are grave indeed. It is an indubitable fact for those who know the subculture of the health care professions and the power structures of hospitals that nurses who openly challenge established authority structures or powerful physicians in a hospital bureaucracy most often put their jobs, their economic welfare, and their professional careers on the line, even if they are acting on behalf of the patient and have strong justification for doing so.

In conflict over patient care situations, nurses often have the moral instinct founded on conscience, but will seldom act on their conscience when to do so is to act against the interests of a power structure that controls their professional and economic destiny. The average nurse is often expected to be a humble servant one moment and a heroic protagonist the next; it is not likely to happen. Nurses are confronted with situations that threaten to exact a price the average person is unwilling to pay. While nurses cannot be completely exonerated in this situation, their failure to make heroic sacrifices for patients is eminently understandable. While highly principled, heroic action is to be praised, it is also seldom to be found. The reason for this is not that nurses, as a group, lack principles. It is that they, like most ordinary mortals, are not capable of heroic action on a routine basis. When the institutional context of nursing practice is such that the commitment of nurses to patients embroils them in conflicts with powerful interests within the institution that employs them, it is unrealistic to expect that the commitment will be routinely honored. While it is common to offer praise for highly principled, heroic action in the face of great risk, it should not be expected as a routine attribute of institutional life. To do so is to fail to understand the institutional conditions necessary to foster consistently responsible moral action.

INSTITUTIONAL RESPONSIBILITY

It should be clear at this point in the analysis that the improbability of moral actions by the individual nurse under extremely adverse circumstances is not to be construed primarily as an indictment of the moral character of nurses (although their responsibility is inescapable). Rather, the principal indictment is intended for those institutional structures that systematically create formidable obstacles to responsible action. It must be clear to all that there is grave institutional culpability in a situation where the institutional disincentives to morally responsible action are so persuasive that the probability of moral action by the average person is rendered minimal. When social institutions are so construed that they systematically create overwhelming disincentives to responsible action, then they must be held responsible for the suppression of the moral impulse in everyday life. In a word, nurses are not free to be moral because they are deprived of moral agency by the repressive character of the hospitals in which they practice.

NURSING ETHIC AS A
SOCIAL ETHIC

The principal conclusion that can be drawn from the foregoing analysis is that a responsible nursing ethic must be a social ethic. That is, if the

fundamental moral problem of nursing is a consequence of the structure and policies of the social institution in which nursing is, for the most part, practiced, then any ethic that seeks to address this problem must seek reform of the policies and structures of that institution. An ethic that is concerned with structures and policies of social institutions is a social ethic. Hence, a nursing ethic must be first and foremost a social ethic. It must be one that seeks to free nursing *practice* from its "hospitalonian captivity," in the same way that the 1965 ANA resolution[24] on nursing education sought to free nursing *education* from that captivity. Ashley,[25] in making the same point, perceived the hospital as a demonic force in the history of nursing in this country. What is required from a moral perspective is a nursing ethic that will seek to free nursing from the hegemony of the hospital as a morally culpable social institution vis-à-vis its stance toward nursing.

GENERAL ALTERNATIVES

Precisely what policies and what structures are to be preferred in order to effect this liberation is not clear. It is a matter that will require extensive and ongoing deliberation in the councils of the profession. However, the general alternatives are clear. Either nursing must acquire sufficient power within the hospital, relative to medicine and administration, to create a balance of power in the control of the practice, or it must terminate its employee status with the hospital, move outside the hospital, and serve hospital patients from the vantage point of some new nursing-controlled organization. The most effective alternative will emerge in the years to come. The concern here is not so much the instruments and technologies of this liberation as the credibility of this general analysis of nursing's moral situation and the viability of a nursing ethic, which is primarily a social ethic.

The suggestion that a nursing ethic should be a special ethic interested in social reform, that is, the reform of one of our major social institutions—the hospital—is characterized by both discontinuity and continuity. Nursing ethics as reform ethics represents discontinuity in at least two respects. First, the bioethics tradition in general, including nursing ethics and medical ethics, has been staunchly nonreformist. In a word, medical ethicists have explicitly disclaimed any interest in reform. The second point of discontinuity derives from the traditionally apolitical posture of the nursing profession itself. The rank and file has always been more personal than political, more concerned with serving individuals than with reforming institutions. This propensity is natural to a caring profession, but it is inadequate as a professional style when social and political forces increasingly determine the context and conditions of practice. The beginnings of change in this regard appear to be emerging where nurses have formed political action groups and have established Washington, DC-based lobbies. However, the rank and file of the profession remains predominantly apolitical.

Despite these discontinuities, there is a significant precedent within the profession for viewing nursing ethics as reform ethics. This precedent resides in an obscure and neglected sector of the nursing tradition, the social reformers. Even though the nursing profession has historically been apolitical, there is a slender but distinct thread of social reform in the tradition. Such individuals would constitute an excellent resource for the reformation of nursing ethics. If nursing ethics is to become more than a footnote on medical ethics, and if the profession is to put into practice the values that it affirms in its professional ideology and code, then the social reform tradition and its major prophets must be enshrined in the memory of the profession, discussed in the classrooms of professional education, and honored in the convocations of the profession. Nursing has not always honored its prophets. The profession should draw upon the spirits of such reformers as Mary Adelaide Nutting, Lavinia Dock, and Annie Goodrich, not to mention Florence Nightingale, in order to translate its ethical commitments to patients into carefully designed strategies for institutional reform.

Unless nursing, through the reform of the institution in which the majority of its members practice, acquires a balance of controlling power in that institution or creates new structures for the organization of practice, it cannot effectively implement standards of care for its own practice. If it cannot realize reform it will compromise the integrity of the nurse-patient relationship, which is the moral foundation of nursing, and it will have lost its status as a profession. Furthermore, the public will have lost its most valuable ally within the health care system. The one action that would most improve the quality of health care in this society is simple and direct: Set the nurses free, set the nurses free.

REFERENCES

1. American Nurses' Association: *Facts about Nursing 82–83.* Kansas City, Mo: ANA, 1983.
2. Davis AJ. Aroskar MA: *Ethical Dilemmas and Nursing Practice,* ed. 1. New York, Appleton-Century-Crofts, 1978.
3. Curtin L: Ethical issues in nursing practice and nursing education, in *Ethical Issues in Nursing and Nursing Education.* New York, National League for Nursing, 1980, pp 22–23, 25.
4. Dock L: Nurses should be obedient, in Bullough B, Bullough V (eds): *Issues in Nursing,* New York, Springer, 1966, pp 96–97.
5. Robb III: *Nursing Ethics.* Cleveland, Koeckert, 1900.
6. Perry CM: Nursing ethics and etiquette. *Am J Nurs* 1906. 6:448–452, 513–514, 613–616, 861–863.
7. Dock S: The relation of the nurse to the doctor and the doctor to the nurse. *Am J Nurs* 1917; 17:394.
8. Aikens C: *Studies in Ethics for Nurses,* ed. 1. Philadelphia, WB Saunders, 1925.
9. Moore T: *Principles of Ethics,* ed 4. Philadelphia, Lippincott, 1943.
10. American Nurses' Association: Code for nurses. *Am J Nurs* 1950; 50: 196, 392.
11. American Nurses' Association: Revision proposed in code for professional nurses. *Am J Nurs* 1960; 60: 77–81.
12. American Nurses' Association: Code for nurses. *Am J Nurs* 1968; 68: 2582–2585.
13. American Nurses' Association: *Code for Nurses with Interpretive Statements.* Kansas City, Mo: ANA, 1976.
14. American Nurses' Association: *Code for Nurses with Interpretive Statements.* Kansas City, Mo: ANA, 1985.
15. Swider S, McElmurry BJ, Yarling RR: Professional decision making in a bureaucratic context. *Nurs Res* 1985; 34 (2): 108–112.
16. Aroskar M: Ethics of nurse-patient relationships. *Nurs Educator* 1980; 5: 18–20.
17. Gadow S: Existential advocacy: Philosophical foundation for nursing, in *Nursing: Images and Ideas.* New York, Springer, 1980, pp 79–101.
18. Murphy C: Models of the nurse-patient relationship, in *Ethical Problems in the Nurse-Patient Relationship.* Boston, Allyn Bacon, 1982, pp. 25–56.
19. Stenberg MJ: Search for a conceptual framework as a philosophic basis for nursing ethics. *Military Med* 1979; 144 (1): 9–22.

20. Donnelly G, Mengel A, King U: Anatomy of a conflict. *Superv Nurse* 1975; 6(November): 28–38.

21. McGuire M: Have you ever let a patient die by default? *RN* 1977; 8(November): 56–59.

22. Yarling RR: The scope of nursing practice in disclosing the truth to terminal patients. *Superv Nurse* 1978; 9(5,6): 28–34, 40–50.

23. Creighton H: The whistle blower. *Superv Nurse* 1975; 6(11): 11–12, 57.

24. American Nurses' Association: First position on education for nursing. *Am J Nurs* 1966; 66: 515–517.

25. Ashley J: *Hospitals, Paternalism, and the Role of the Nurse.* New York, Teachers College Press, 1976.

STUDY AND DISCUSSION QUESTIONS
THE NURSE AND THE INSTITUTION

1. Muyskens argues that some of the causes of the powerlessness and low esteem among nurses are pervasive sexism, the class background of nurses compared to physicians, nurses' relative lack of education, and nurses relatively low pay. Muyskens further believes that such conditions militate against quality care because few quality people are going to be attracted to a profession with poor working conditions, low esteem, and low pay. Is he right?

2. Muyskens asserts that the above conditions lead to high drop-out rates, cynicism, and discouragement and, therefore, nursing is unlikely to keep the well-qualified and motivated persons it attracts. What do you think of this argument that links the recruitment and retention of nurses to quality of care? Does higher wages and better working conditions for nurses benefit the public?

3. Should nurses strike? Do you agree with the limitations Muyskens puts on its use—emergency and lifesaving care must be provided and the strike must be the only or most effective means available?

4. Do you think the public would support strikes by nurses if they were aware of their purpose?

5. Muyskens does not mention the adversarial relationships and bad feelings strikes sometimes engender among nurses. Should he? How important is this factor?

6. Do you agree with the principle that it is always wrong to ignore here and now duties to clients in order to benefit future clients?

7. Do you know of any nurses that have gone on strike? How do they evaluate the strike weapon?

8. Baumgart says that professional nursing associations were losing their relevance and effectiveness in Canada. Do you think this is true in this country?

9. Do you think that unionism is incompatible with professionalism?

10. Do you agree with Baumgart that unions can be flexible enough to promote public welfare issues?

11. The ANA is a registered collective bargaining agent. Does this help address some of Baumgart's concerns or does it create other problems? Should the ANA be doing collective bargaining?

12. Why do you think unionization diminishes the public image of nursing?

13. Is the development of nursing specialty groups good for nursing?

14. Do you think the nurses in Flaherty's case study did the right thing in refusing to accept a patient they believed they could not adequately care for?

15. Should emergency room physicians dictate the appropriate patient load to ICU staff?

16. Was the suspension of the nursing supervisor justified?

17. How do you account for the fact that it took four physicians and one respiratory technologist to care for one patient on a ventilator and yet these same physicians later maintained that the ICU staff should have admitted the patient?

18. Is the director of nursing culpable in this incident because nothing was done about the chronic understaffing in the ICU?

19. Were the nurses in this hospital ICU free to practice nursing at the standards required by their profession?

20. Do you agree with Yarling and McElmurry's proposal to allow nurses to write do not resuscitate orders?

21. Is a refusal of treatment a medical or moral decision?

22. Do you agree that nursing authority to write do not resuscitate orders is in the best interests of patients?

23. Yarling and McElmurry argue that their proposed policy is consistent with the definition of nursing as "the diagnosis and treatment of human responses to actual or potential health problems." Do you agree?

24. Yarling and McElmurry dismiss the objection that nurses may not want this authority. Do nurses want this authority? Ought they to have it? Does it matter what nurses want on this issue?

25. Do you believe that Yarling and McElmurry are correct in their assessment that nurses are not free to be moral, not permitted to practice nursing as it ought to be practiced?

26. Yarling and McElmurry claim that there is a profound moral dissonance between what nurses are taught in school—patient advocacy—and the realities of nursing practice where open challenges to the system can cost a nurse economic security. Do you think this is true?

27. Does nursing need to be freed from the "hospitalonian captivity" described by Yarling and McElmurry?

28. What do you think of Yarling and McElmurry's suggestion that if nurses cannot gain power and control over their own profession within the hospital they should terminate their employee relationship and serve patients from some new nursing controlled organization?

29. What do you know about the social reform tradition in nursing? Do you know much about Mary Adeline Nutting, Lavinia Dock, or Annie Goodrich?

30. Would greater nursing autonomy serve the best interests of the public as Yarling and McElmurry claim?

31. What clinical issues, aside from do not resuscitate orders, do you think Yarling and McElmurry would claim as nursing functions?